VISUAL ATTENTION
IN CHILDREN
Theories and Activities

VISUAL ATTENTION
IN CHILDREN
Theories and Activities

Kenneth A. Lane, OD
Lane Learning Center
Lewisville, Texas

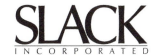
SLACK
INCORPORATED

MT

ISBN: 978-1-55642-956-9

Published by: SLACK Incorporated
                   6900 Grove Road
                   Thorofare, NJ 08086 USA
                   Telephone: 856-848-1000
                   Fax: 856-848-6091
                   www.slackbooks.com

Contact SLACK Incorporated for more information about other books in this field or about the availability of our books from distributors outside the United States.

Library of Congress Cataloging-in-Publication Data
Lane, Kenneth A.
 Visual attention in children : theories and activities / Kenneth A. Lane.
    p. ; cm.
 Includes bibliographical references and index.
  ISBN 978-1-55642-956-9 (alk. paper)
 I. Title.
 [DNLM: 1. Attention--physiology. 2. Eye Movements--physiology. 3. Child Development. 4. Learning Disorders--rehabilitation. 5. Occupational Therapy--methods. WW 105]

 618.92'85882--dc23
                        2011046554

Printed in the United States of America.

Last digit is print number: 10 9 8 7 6 5 4 3 2 1

10/9/13

DEDICATION

This book is dedicated to my wife and best friend, Janet.

CONTENTS

See the Color Atlas after page 174

ACKNOWLEDGMENTS

This book would not have been completed without the help of the following individuals:

- Brien Cummings of SLACK Incorporated, who had faith in this book.
- Vicki Neville, who spent hours trying to read my handwriting and doing a great job organizing this book.
- Randy Webb, who did all of the artwork and illustrations.
- Jo Beth Coyle, who helped with the organization of this book.
- Kim Solari, OT, and Jennifer Suggs, OT, at S.P.O.T.S. in Dallas.
- Gifted occupational therapists who helped with proofreading.
- The American Optometric Association library, which helped me obtain journal articles.
- My wife, Janet, who put up with my very cluttered office in our house for more than 2 years.

ABOUT THE AUTHOR

Kenneth A. Lane, OD is a doctor of optometry and a fellow with the College of Optometrists in Vision Development. Since his first book, *Reversal Errors: Theories and Therapy Procedures,* in 1988, Dr. Lane has published *Developing Your Child for Success, Developing Ocular Motor and Visual Perceptual Skills,* and a series of workbooks that deal with eye tracking and perception. He started the Lane Learning Center to help learning-disabled children in 1980. *Visual Attention in Children: Theories and Activities* is the result of 3 years of research. Dr. Lane lives with his wife, Janet, in north Texas and spends his leisure time in Ruidoso, New Mexico.

PREFACE

The idea for this book began with an observation and then a question. Over the years, I have noticed that at each re-evaluation of our vision therapy children, their visual motor skills almost always show dramatic improvement even though we do not specifically train visual motor skills. An example of this is shown in Figure A, which shows a 7-year-old child's drawing in the Developmental Test of Visual-Motor Integration.

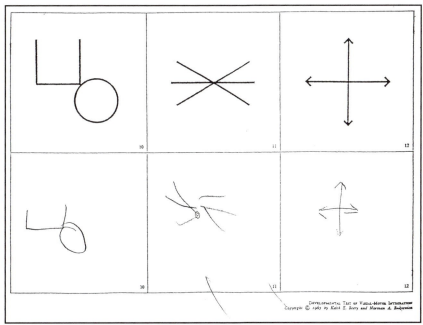

Figure A. Seven-year-old child's drawing. (*Beery-Buktenica Development Test of Visual-Motor Integration, Fifth Edition [The Beery VMI]*. Copyright © 1967, 1982, 1997, 1989, 1997, 2004 Keith E. Beery and Natasha A. Beery. Reproduced with permission of the publisher NCS Pearson, Inc. All rights reserved.)

Figure B shows the same child 6 months later.

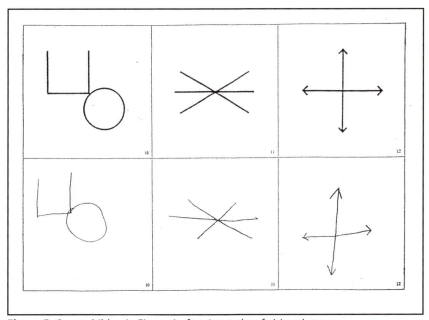

Figure B. Same child as in Figure A after 6 months of vision therapy.

Figure C shows a second-grade student and then 4 months later in Figure D.

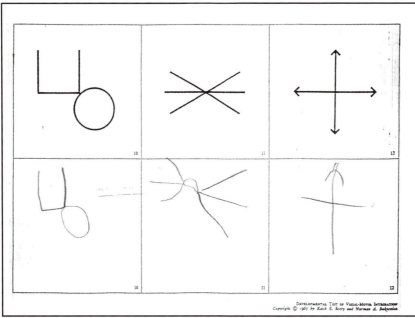

Figure C. Second-grade student's drawing. (*Beery-Buktenica Development Test of Visual-Motor Integration, Fifth Edition [The Beery VMI]*. Copyright © 1967, 1982, 1997, 1989, 1997, 2004 Keith E. Beery and Natasha A. Beery. Reproduced with permission of the publisher NCS Pearson, Inc. All rights reserved.)

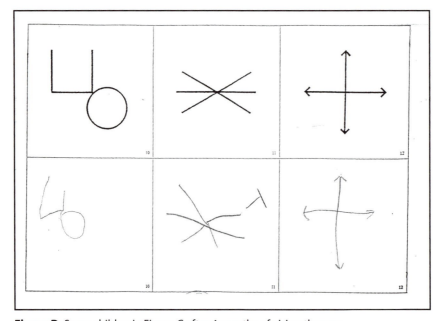

Figure D. Same child as in Figure C after 4 months of vision therapy.

Because of these observations, I decided to investigate what area of the brain dealt with visual spatial skills and also what other areas that brain region may control.

Copying geometric shapes is not only a fine motor task but is one of spatial analysis and motor planning. All of these require attention. The functions of spatial attention and motor planning are, by and large, controlled by the posterior parietal cortex (Steinman, Steinman, & Lehmkuhle, 1995). Other functions of the parietal cortex include shifting of visual attention, saccadic and pursuit eye movements (Mirsky, 1991), and hand projection movements (Robinson, Goldberg, &

Stanton, 1978). The parietal cortex is therefore involved with attention and spatial organizations and, along with the frontal cortex, executes eye-hand and eye movements.

What this information showed me was that many of the areas that are included in vision training (VT), such as smooth pursuit and saccadic fixations, are controlled by the parietal cortex, which also controls visual attention and motor planning. Therefore, is VT training attention?

The principles of VT are centered on the development of eye movement, spatial concepts, and integration of visual systems, such as oculomotor, convergence, and visual fixation. These are the very skills that, one way or the other, are mediated by the parietal cortex. If VT improves the skills mediated by the parietal cortex, this would explain why children's visual motor skills improve. Because VT stresses saccadic and smooth pursuit eye movements along with fixation training, it also improves visual attention and, along with it, motor planning and better visual motor performance.

One way to test this theory was to evaluate the visual attention of children who went through our vision therapy program and to compare their results to control children who did not go through our program.

The Test of Variables of Attention Continuous Performance (TOVA) is a test of visual attention. It was specifically designed to measure attention and impulse central processes in five areas: inattention (omissions), impulse control (commissions), response time, response time variability, and a cumulative measure of attention deficit/hyperactivity disorder (AD/HD). This test requires a child to perform a task on a computer for 23 minutes. During the test, one of the two stimuli is presented for 100 milliseconds every 2 seconds. The task is for the child to respond to the appropriate target as soon as possible. He or she is to push a microswitch when a target appears in the top half of the screen but not in the bottom half. By varying the target-nontarget ratio, the program allows the examination of the effects of differing response demands on inattention and impulsivity. Impulsivity is measured in the second half of the test by increasing the target presentation and forcing the child to inhibit responses. A previous study showed that 80% of AD/HD children were correctly identified using the TOVA when AD/HD was defined as being 1.5 standard deviations from age- and gender-adjusted means (Forbes, 1998).

The TOVA responses are then compared to other children within their age level. This test has been normed on children 6 to 19 years and can be given multiple times without affecting the reliability of the results. It is, therefore, useful in testing the effect of medication. However, the test is boring. The results of the TOVA, given after the initial test, are usually worse because the child knows it is going to be boring and the novelty factor has decreased.

Because difficulties in attention are linked to the posterior parietal cortex, it was hypothesized that visual therapy procedures aimed at the posterior parietal cortex, emphasizing oculomotor function, might improve attention.

To test this hypothesis, a pilot study was completed. Children of both genders aged 7 through 11 who were being enrolled in a VT program (experimental: N = 9) were administered the TOVA, along with a matched control group of children (control: N = 5) who did not undergo VT. At the completion of the VT program, or 6 months for the control group, all of the children were then retested with the TOVA. The experimental group was compared to the control group.

The two groups' TOVA scores were compared after approximately 6 months. Members of the experimental group had completed their prescribed VT program while members of the control group followed their normal routine. The experimental group was found to have statistically improved in every category except response time. The control group evaluation was not found to be statistically different from the first test.

This unpublished study showed that visual attention improved, and, in some cases, dramatically improved, in the children who received VT. While this was a small study, the results showed that VT improved the visual attention in the experimental group.

REFERENCES

Forbes, G. B. (1998). Clinical utility of the test of variables of attention (TOVA) in the diagnosis of attention deficit disorder/hyperactivity disorder. *Journal of Clinical Psychology, 54*(4), 461-476.

Mirsky, A. (1991). Analysis of the attention function upon the excitability of the light-sensitive neurons of the posterior parietal cortex. *The Journal of Neuroscience, 1*(11), 1218-1235.

Robinson, D. L., Goldberg, M. E., & Stanton, G. B. (1978). Parietal association cortex in the primate: sensory mechanisms and behavioral modulations. *Journal of Neurophysiology, 41*(4), 910-932.

Steinman, B. A., Steinman S. B., & Lehmkuhle S. (1995). Visual attention mechanisms show a center surround organization. *Vision Research, 35*(13), 1859-1869.

INTRODUCTION

Visual Attention in Children: Theories and Activities was written for occupational therapists, developmental optometrists, teachers, and others who work with children. This book is designed to show the connection between vision and attention. It is a not just a textbook but is a combination of textbook and workbook. All of the therapy activities in *Visual Attention in Children: Theories and Activities* are based on vision and attention theories.

The goal of this book is to give those who work with children the knowledge to develop activities that can be added to their existing programs to improve children's visual attention. These activities are not intended to replace, but to be added to, existing programs.

Attention is a critical component of a child's success in learning. Anyone who has worked with children knows the importance of attention. If a child's visual attention can be improved, his or her success in school and life can be improved.

This book is divided into nine chapters and attention activities:

- Chapter 1: Vision and Attention—This chapter discusses how the brain processes light and the concepts of vision and sight. Young children's vision is discussed, as well as tests that can detect a visual problem. Attention and vision are discussed in length along with color and vision. The chapter also discusses ambient vision, inertia, and change blindness, along with lazy eye. It ends with tips and training suggestions.

- Chapter 2: Attention—This chapter discusses theories on attention. Two theories (Premotor and Feature Integration) are discussed at length. Areas of attention are reviewed. These include focused, sustained, selective, divided, and shifting. Young children's attention is discussed along with perceptual areas of binding and conjunctions.

- Chapter 3: Memory—This chapter discusses attention and memory and stresses how they cannot be separated. Long- and short-term memory are explained and compared. Working memory and especially the executive function are discussed in detail. Chapter 3, like the other chapters, ends with tips on attention and training along with specific activities to help working memory.

- Chapter 4: Attention Deficit/Hyperactivity Disorder—This chapter reviews the history of attention disorders and shows the areas of the brain involved in attention. The etiology of AD/HD is discussed, including fetal alcohol syndrome, along with statistics. Chapter 4 also stresses the role of TV and attention in young children.

- Chapter 5: Autism—Chapter 5 evaluates the etiologies of autism and the diagnostic criteria needed to label a child as autistic. Asperger's syndrome is discussed along with attention and autism. The chapter ends with a discussion on yoked prisms.

- Chapter 6: Reading Disability—Chapter 6 begins with the case history of three children who had greatly improved their reading with visual training activities. The chapter discusses the definition of reading difficulties and the visual theory of dyslexia called the magnocellular theory of dyslexia.

- Chapter 7: Plasticity—This chapter discusses the adult and child brains and how they can be affected by experience. Attention is a critical part of plasticity, and TV can be very disruptive for the young brain.

- Chapter 8: Cerebrovascular Accident and Traumatic Brain Injury—Cerebrovascular accidents and traumatic brain injury are investigated along with acquired brain injury. Warning signs, along with brain areas, are discussed in detail.

- Chapter 9: The Training Program—This chapter discusses the training program and is followed by a section of activities to improve attention.

Vision and Attention

The human eye is remarkable. It is so remarkably sensitive that the mechanical energy of a pea falling from a height of one inch would (if translated into luminous energy) be sufficient to give a faint impression of light to every person who ever lived (Fischler, 1987). The following are some other facts concerning the eye:

- There are 120 million rod cells in each eye (in the peripheral retina for night vision).

- There are 6 million cone cells in each eye (for color and detailed vision).

- There are 1 million nerve fibers in the optic nerve exiting the eye and traveling to the brain.

- There are 250 million receptor cells in the two eyes versus 250,000 independent elements in a TV picture.

- Rod cells are on the order of 500 times more sensitive than cone cells.

- Object distance from the eye for depth perception: 10 inches to 1,500 feet (Fischler, 1987).

When light first comes into contact with the eye, it hits the cornea. This is the clear part of your eye and is responsible for most of the bending of the light waves (refraction) that hit your eye. The light then goes through your lens, which helps to focus the light on the back part of your eye, called the retina. If your cornea or lens has an uneven curvature, then you have astigmatism, as light from different directions will hit an uneven surface and will focus unevenly on the back part of your eye. If your eye is too long and the light focuses in front of the retina, you are myopic (nearsighted). If your eye is too short and light focuses behind the retina, you are hyperopic (farsighted).

At birth, the eyeball is relatively short, so that the rays of light are focused behind the retina, creating hyperopia. The eye grows 5 mm in the first 3 years of life and then about 1.5 mm up to age 14, when the adult size of 24 to 25 mm is reached (Trobe, 2001). If the light is focused on the fovea (Figure 1-1), it is called emmetropia, and you do not need glasses. Approximately 30% of adults are emmetropic, and the remaining 70% need glasses.

When light strikes the retina, the decomposition (bleaching) of pigments in the rods and cones results in electrical activity, which is integrated in the bipolar and ganglion cells comprising the sixth and eighth levels of the 10-layer system of the retina. As a result of this chemical transformation, bursts of neural energy begin a complicated and relatively long and slow journey from the back of the eye to the visual areas of the brain 6 inches away at the back of the head. The impulses from approximately 120 million light-sensitive cells in the retina (where the neural messages originate) will be thinned out over a hundredfold; when they get to the optic nerve, it consists of barely a million neural pathways (Smith, 1994). The actual nature of the impulses that pass to the back of the brain is much different from our conception of what the light stimulus is like. Every nerve in our body is limited to conveying only one type of signal. Either it fires, or it does not. It is the organization of this firing that gives us vision. The nerve impulses are also slow, not the speed of light that most of us think. They travel at about 200 miles an hour. They also go through a relay station called the lateral geniculate body (LGB) before they reach the back of the brain and the visual areas. What is critical for our understanding is that only a small number of the inputs to the LGB come from the

Lane, K. A. *Visual Attention in Children:*
Theories and Activities (pp. 1-28).
© 2012 SLACK Incorporated.

eyes. The rest come from other parts of the body, including the visual centers in the brain and lower brain areas that deal with primitive functions such as motor and balance. All of these have an influence on the signals sent to the brain. The LGB probably screens relevant from irrelevant visual information before it is sent to the visual cortex. The foveal region of the eye, which occupies less than 10% of the retinal surface, projects to 50% of the surface area in the LGB. This "magnification factor" reflects both the volume and importance of the foveal projections, but this magnification of the foveal region is perpetuated in the visual cortex, which occupies a much larger brain volume. The impulses now continue on to the primary visual cortex (V1), also called the striate cortex, and then are sent to the rest of the visual areas, V2 to V5. There are three principles of the transmissions from the retina to the visual areas in the brain.

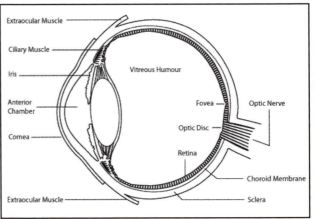

Figure 1-1. The fovea of the eye, which is 1.5 mm in diameter.

1. Retinotopic mapping: Each point in visual space is neurologically represented on a specific geographic region of the retina, a specific bundle of retinocortical axons, and a specific portion of V1, V2, and V3.

2. Parallel processing: Separate processing of form and/or color and spatial information begins at the retina and is carried out in distinct channels. Spatial channels may be selectively damaged in glaucoma, amblyopia, or dyslexia. This may explain why most dyslexics have very poor visual spatial skills (e.g., disorganized printing).

3. Hierarchical processing: Uncoding of visual information proceeds from a primitive to a more complex level. Retinal receptors encode an array of spots of different light intensities, retinal ganglion cells enhance edge contrasts and encode spectral information, and the primary visual cortex encodes orientation of line segments (Trobe, 2001).

What all of this means is that the eyes are not windows and the brain does not look through them. Not only what we see, but our conviction of seeing is a fabrication of the brain.

A small unit of time is the millisecond, usually abbreviated msec. One millisecond is a thousandth part of a second. Ten milliseconds are about the time the shutter of a camera is required to be open to get an image on the film. It is also the amount of time the brain takes to form a single perceptual experience. It takes more time for neural impulses to get from the eye to the brain than for the brain to make a perceptual decision. An exposure of 50 msec is more than adequate for all of the information the brain can memorize on any one occasion. This does not mean that 50 msec is adequate for identifying everything in a single glance. For example, you cannot inspect a page of print for less than 1 second and expect to have seen every word. But 50 msec is a sufficient exposure for all of the visual information that can be gained in a single fixation (Smith,

1994). This is why when you pause to read (a fixation) and that fixation lasts on the average 250 msec, the word is identified in the first 50 msec. The rest of the time (200 msec) is used to decide when and where to move your eyes for the next fixation. This means that your eyes pick up usable information for only a fraction of the time they are open. Therefore, the more familiar you are with what you are looking at, the more you can identify. It will make no difference if the source of the visual information is removed after 50 or 250 msec; nothing more will be seen. If you saw a random string of letters such as k, y, b, e, o, u, you might remember four or five letters. If, however, the letters were in word form, then two or three words might be identified in that time. If the words happen to be in a sentence, then maybe four or five words could be identified or up to 25 letters in the same 50-msec exposure (Smith, 1994). Because of this limitation on the amount of visual information the brain can process, the average person can only read about 250 words per minute (about four words per second).

Our eyes cannot see the entire visual field (everything in our view) with high acuity. The fovea, which is where the light from each eye has to focus for clear vision, is only 1.5 mm in diameter (see Figure 1-1).

This is the area of the retina that has all of the cones for good acuity. In order for the entire visual field to be in high acuity and focus on cones, the fovea would have to be 200 times larger in cross-section to accommodate the additional nerve fibers. Instead, what has developed is a small area of high-quality vision surrounded by a low acuity periphery. This narrow "searchlight" beam of high visual acuity is directed at and held on visual objects of interest by the muscles of the eye.

Occupational therapists (OTs) need to be aware of symptoms that may be visually related. Do not assume that because the child just had an eye examination that all visual functions have been evaluated. Most optometrists and ophthalmologists are mainly interested in the health of the eye and the refractive status (eyeglasses). They often do not have time or do not believe that some of these other areas are important enough to test. To give you an example of the different thinking by the medical community concerning vision and school achievement, the American Academy of Pediatrics considers 20/40 vision as acceptable for a 4-year-old or younger and will not refer in the absence of very severe problems. They consider 20/30 as acceptable for children 5 and older. I can tell you that children are very capable of squinting out two lines of letters, and when the pediatricians say 20/30, the child may be 20/50.

There are also problems with the school nurse's eye screening. For example, the Texas State Department of Health Bureau of Children's Health states that most children's visual problems can be detected with distance testing. This means that they almost totally ignore any visual skills at reading distance. This is worrisome because visual problems that affect reading occur at 16 inches, not 20 feet. If a child is farsighted, he or she would still pass the school's visual screening because he or she can see the distance letter chart. Also, there is not much, if any, testing of binocular skills and oculomotor skills (eye tracking). Both of these areas can greatly affect a child's school performance. Therefore, as OTs, be alert. The first thing to make note of is the child's symptoms. The following is a list of symptoms that are visually related and, in parentheses, the most likely cause.

1. Makes mistakes copying from the board or text (oculomotor or binocular skills)

2. Loses his or her place or has to use his or her finger as a marker to read (oculomotor)

3. Complains of words running together or moving during reading (binocular skills)

4. Sloppy or disorganized printing or handwriting (visual motor, oculomotor)

5. Excessive reversals of letters or words (visual motor, visual memory)

6. Complains of words blurring (accommodation)

7. Headaches after prolonged reading (binocular skills)

8. Blurred distance vision (needs glasses, refractive error)

9. Repeatedly omits words during reading (oculomotor, binocular skills)

10. Fails to recognize the same word in the next sentence or paragraph (working memory)

11. Blinks excessively when reading but not at other times (binocular skills, refractive error)

12. Comprehension declines as reading continues (refractive error, binocular skills, oculomotor)

13. Covers one eye when reading (binocular skills)

14. Has to move his or her head while reading (oculomotor)

15. Holds book very close (refractive error)

16. Reports seeing double (binocular skills)

17. Very slow reader (decoding problem, oculomotor)

Only four of the previous symptoms are usually remediated with glasses (8, 11, 12, 15). The rest are remediated through visual training (VT) by a developmental optometrist. OTs are also capable of remediating some of the symptoms (1, 2, 4, 5, 9, 10, 12, 14, 17). Many vision therapy symptoms are also occupational therapy symptoms. If you have a child with poor gross motor, balance, or visual motor symptoms, he or she is most likely to also have oculomotor problems.

The main problem that OTs face when they see a child who they know has visual problems is determining where to send him or her. If the child goes back to the last person who tested his or her vision, he or she is going to come back with, "There is nothing wrong." So what do you do? The patient should be referred to a developmental optometrist, also called a behavioral optometrist. This is an optometrist who has special interest in binocular vision and learning disabilities in children and adults. He or she has taken extra continuing education in these areas and usually offers vision therapy in the office. Unfortunately, just because he or she claims to be a developmental optometrist does not mean that he or she is qualified. Watch out for optometrists who just prescribe prism glasses or a home therapy program. Just as you cannot get as good results in sensory integration training with just home therapy, you cannot with vision therapy either. Also, there is no quick cure. A pair of glasses, whether it is tinted lenses or prism, is not going to replace a good therapy program. The ideal situation is to find an optometrist who has been tested on his or her knowledge by peers. This is the situation with optometrists who receive their fellowship through the College of Optometrists in Vision Development (COVD). In order to receive a fellowship, the optometrist must pass a written and oral test and show competency by submitting case reports for review. He or she must also take continuing education courses each year, in addition to the courses needed to keep his or her license. Not all optometrists in COVD have a fellowship. Anyone can join and be a COVD member. This does not mean that a regular optometrist or a nonfellow is not qualified to examine a child; however, you may get better results with a COVD fellow.

The area that OTs need to be concerned with is oculomotor. As I mentioned earlier, if the child has poor visual motor skills, he or she probably also has oculomotor problems. There are two very simple and quick tests that you can do to test a child's oculomotor system. The two areas you should be concerned with are smooth pursuit movement and saccadic functions. There will be a lot more on these later in the book; however, smooth pursuit movement is the ability to track a moving object. I feel that this ability is almost entirely related to visual attention. To evaluate this,

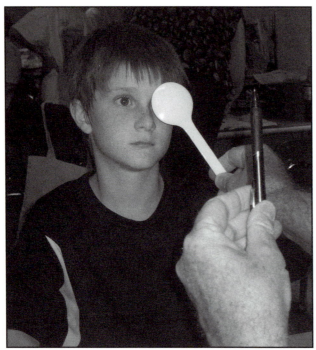

Figure 1-2. A child doing pursuit testing.

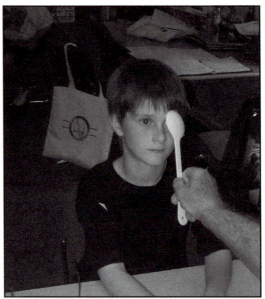

Figure 1-3A. Strabismus testing.

have the child in front of you and use something to cover one of his or her eyes. You need to test pursuits one eye at a time (Figure 1-2).

Slowly move a pencil in a left to right horizontal direction in front of the patient at about 16 inches. Watch the uncovered eye to see if he or she loses fixation. The child may also move his or her head or body, which indicates difficulty separating gross and fine motor skills. Also, watch to see if there is any midline tremor as you cross his or her midline. Poor eye movement or midline tremors are indications of poor oculomotor skills. The second area is saccadic fixation, which is the ability to move the eye accurately to a stationary object. This is what the child will do as he or she moves his or her eyes across a line of print to read. One way to test this is with the Developmental Eye Movement (DEM) Fixation Test, which can be given and graded in less than 10 minutes. It will list percentiles that you can use for re-evaluations to see if you are making any progress.

While I do not expect you to replace an optometrist, there is one other area with which you need to be familiar. This is in binocular vision and is called convergence insufficiency (CI). Most eye doctors agree that CI can interfere with school and reading. A CI means that when a child looks from far to near, his or her eyes have a tendency to drift "out" instead of "in." A normal convergence at reading distance is slightly "in" compared to the distance convergence. In CI, the near convergence is slightly "out" compared to the distance convergence. You can do a quick cover test and determine if a child has CI. Have the child seated in front of you (Figure 1-3A) just like you did for pursuit testing.

Slowly move the cover over one of his or her eyes while you are looking at the uncovered eye. The uncovered eye should not move. If it moves, it means that it was never straight in the first place and when the other eye is covered, it had to move to pick up fixation. This is strabismus and should be referred. Now, move the occluder to the other eye, and watch the eye that was just uncovered (Figure 1-3B).

In which direction did it move and how far? When the eye is covered, it will go to its position of rest, which should be slightly "out." Therefore, the eye should follow the direction of the occluder. If it moves in the opposite direction of the occluder, this is an overconvergence and could be helped with reading glasses. The idea is to do this test twice—once with the child looking across the room and once looking at your pencil 16 inches in front of him or her. If the eyes show a larger following movement when looking at 16 inches compared to 20 feet, this means that the child's eyes drift out when he or she looks at things up close, and this is CI. You will need to refer for this. You can also move a pencil slowly toward his or her nose (Figure 1-4) and see how close you move it before one of his or her eyes drifts "out."

A normal situation is about 6 inches in front of the child's nose before an eye drifts out. If his or her eye drifts out at more than 6 inches from his or her nose, this can also indicate a CI problem and should be referred.

Over the years, I have noticed a large percentage of children who are learning disabled and/or have attention deficit/hyperactivity disorder (AD/HD) and have CI. A study showed that 16% of AD/HD children have CI. This is more than three times what you would expect (ScienceDaily, 2000). CI has been said to occur in 1% of normal children and in 15% of adults; however, it can be as high as 7% in children (Ciuffreda, 2002; Cooper, 2000). My experience

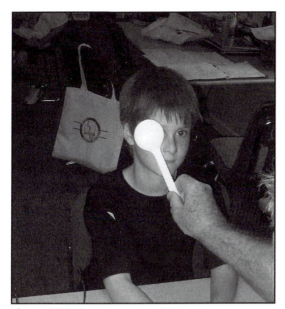

Figure 1-3B. Convergence testing.

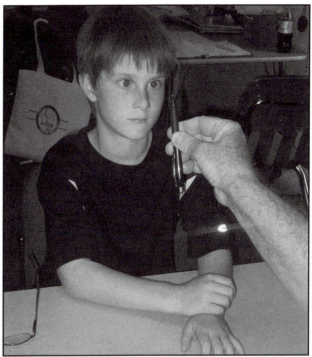

Figure 1-4. Convergence insufficiency testing as you slowly move the pencil toward the nose.

from examining learning disabled and AD/HD children puts it much higher than 16% and closer to 30% or higher. The question is, why the high number of CI cases? There has to be a correlation between an area in the brain that might deal with vergence movements and poor visual attention. The same can be said for oculomotor problems, AD/HD, and learning disabilities. I have seen an extremely high correlation between poor eye movements, attention, and reading disabilities. Is it possible that the areas of the brain that deal with visual spatial attention also deal with eye movements and by improving eye movements, including oculomotor and vergence, the spatial visual attention network is also improved? I feel the answer is perhaps; however, I know of no study that has proven the correlation. The area of the brain that would be responsible for both spatial attention and eye movements is the right parietal lobe, especially area 7 in primates. Area 7 in the inferior parietal cortex of primates has been suggested to be an important center for neural control of directed visual attention, of spatial perception, and of spatially oriented movements including pursuit eye movements and visual tracking (Dillon-Crunly, 1991). Area 7 also receives and processes neural signals transmitted via the retina-collicular system and its upward thalamocortical projections. These signals are thought to provide information about the spatial locations of objects. There is also considerable evidence to suggest that this area, together with the cortical and subcortical structures with which it is linked, plays a role in the direction of attention and the interested fixation of gaze. There are several classes of neurons in area 7 of the parietal lobe. These include the following:

- Unidentified cells (31%)
- Fixation and fixation-suppression cells
- Light-sensitive cells (10%)
- Refixation neurons
- Tracking neurons
- Vergence neurons (Motter & Mountcastle, 1981)
- Visual and eye position neurons
- Somatosensory and reach-related cells (Zipser & Andersen, 1988).

The parietal lobe is mentioned often in this book. It may be the main area that we need to target in our training programs to improve a child's visual attention.

There is an essential difference between light and sound. Reflected light from different surfaces (and emitted light from different sources) can converge at points in space essentially without interaction or interference. Sound waves from different sources, on the contrary, interact; they summate and form a complex wave form. Visual information is already spatially sorted out on the retina; in the ear, sound is not. Visual information processing is intrinsically spatial; spatial direction is merely one of the computable properties of auditory information. In hearing, the wanted information has to be undone from unwanted information coming from other sources. In vision, the potential objects of attention have well-defined locations and can be chosen by selecting this location. The main problem is a problem of choice among parallel events over the entire visual field. The choice of one event can leave the others undisturbed. This is the solution chosen by evolution for attentional selection in vision (Heijden, 1992).

Vision has intrigued people for centuries. The ancient Greeks thought that the eyes sent out rays to select objects to view (Cave & Bichot, 1999). When we think of vision today, most of us will think of seeing our surroundings, objects in our environment, or vision perception and reading. Vision is much more than conscious perception, a function that appears to be a relative newcomer on the evolutionary scene. Vision evolved in animals to help guide their movements. Indeed, the visual system of most animals, rather than being a general purpose network dedicated to reconstructing the rather limited world in which they live, consists instead of a set of relative independent input-output lines or visuomotor "modules," each of which is responsible for the visual control of a particular class of motor outputs. Although the need for more flexible control was one of the demands in the evolving brain, others were related to the need to identify the objects, to understand their significance and causal relations, to plan a course of action, and to communicate with other members of the species. In short, the emergence of cognitive systems and complex social behavior created a whole new set of demands on vision and the organization of the visual system. These cognitive systems involved memory, semantics, spatial reasoning, planning, and communication. Even though higher-order systems permit the formation of goals and the decision to engage in a specific act without reference to particular motor outputs, the actual execution of an action may nevertheless be mediated by dedicated visuo-motor modules. Vision in humans has two distinct but interactive functions: (1) the perception of objects and their relations, which provides a foundation for cognitive life, and (2) the control of actions directed at (or with respect to) those objects, in which specific sets of motor outputs are programmed and guided (Goodale & Humphrey, 1998).

The eye and the visual system were developed to control action. This amazing system started with a single strip of cells. It is now believed that during the Cambrian period, between 544 and 539 million years ago, a strip of light-sensing cells and associated neurons developed on the dorsal (back) surface of sea animals to improve their ability to properly orient and position themselves relative to the surface illumination (Fischler, 1987). This was the first primitive eye. By creasing and folding inward, this strip of nerve cells first formed a tubular nerve cord and eventually developed into the spinal cord that distinguishes the vertebrates (Fischler, 1987). The first fossils containing an eye were trilobites, which lived 543 million years ago. It was probably the development of eyes that started the Cambrian explosion from three animal phyla (same internal body plan) to the 38 phyla that exist today.

SIGHT VERSUS VISION

One of the most confusing issues with parents and professionals, such as teachers, is the issue of sight versus

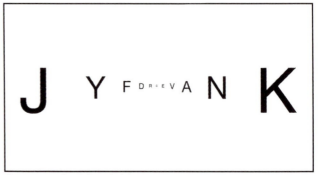

Figure 1-5. Peripheral vision.

vision. Most people equate vision with needing glasses and seeing the 20/20 line. They do not realize that seeing the 20/20 line is not vision but sight (acuity). This is only one small part of the whole package called vision. Vision is sight plus oculomotor, binocular vision, accommodation (focusing), and perception.

The way the eye has evolved indicates that, because the brain cannot process all of the visual information available to it all at once, it selects areas of the visual field to evaluate. It does this by putting most of the cones, which are used for color and detail analysis, in one small area called the fovea.

Retinal acuity is defined in terms of the minimal separation that the eye can resolve. As a measure, the reciprocal of the visual angle (in minutes of arc) subtended by a just resolvable stimulus is used (Heijden, 1992). You do not need to remember this definition. The thing you need to know is that 20/20 means average vision. It means that if you have 20/20 vision, you see at 20 feet what the average person sees at 20 feet. If your vision is 20/200, it means that you see at 20 feet what the average person sees at 200 feet. So, 20/20 is not perfect vision—it is average. There are many people who can see better than 20/20 and many who have never seen 20/20. The main function of the visual system is to make sure the light that enters the eye focuses on this small area in both eyes at the same time. Think of a degree of arc as four letters on a page of print. Your acuity is decreased to half its maximum value at an eccentricity between 0.5 and 1.5 degrees of arc (Figure 1-5).

Figure 1-5 was drawn so that each letter was made 10 times its threshold height. Each letter should be equally readable when the center of the figure is fixated. You can see how much your acuity drops off by looking at a letter on this page and seeing how far in your peripheral vision you can still identify letters. Acuity is sometimes best explained in terms of hardware (i.e., neurons and their connections). First, in the center of the fovea, the receptors of the daylight visual system—the cones—are packed very tightly together. Their numbers fall off very rapidly toward the periphery of the retina. Second, from the bundle of axons of retinal ganglion cells that leave the eye, most are devoted to the transmission of information from the foveal region that has the highest receptor density. Third, also in the striate

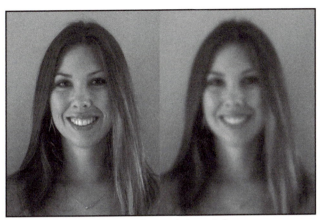

Figure 1-6. Blurred vision of a newly born infant.

cortex (V1), the amount of neural tissue representing each degree of visual field declines monotonically with eccentricity from the fovea (Heijden, 1992). All of the areas of the visual system are devoted to either getting light to focus clearly on the fovea in each eye or interpreting the visual information sent from the fovea in each eye. For the visual system to function properly, all of the components must work together. The first job of the visual system is to move the eyes to the object of interest. This is accomplished by rapid (saccadic) eye movements to objects that are detected in our peripheral vision. If the object moves, the eyes follow it through pursuit eye movements. It is important that both eyes are pointing to similar targets. This is accomplished by eye movements called vergence. We converge our eyes to look at closer targets and diverge to look at objects further away. This must be accomplished so that each eye fixates on the same object at the exact same time, regardless of head or body position. Once the target is fixated by both eyes (binocular vision), the object must be clearly focused on each fovea. This is accomplished by the accommodative system of the lens in the eye. The resultant clear, single image is then sent to the brain to be identified. Any problem in the visual system to keep the eyes from performing their functions correctly can cause eye strain or blurred or double vision.

A CHILD'S EARLY YEARS

"Rich experiences produce rich brains" (Eliot, 1999).

Unlike other senses, such as hearing, that are used before birth, when a child opens his or her eyes for the first time, it will be a completely new experience. What does your newborn see when he or she opens his or her eyes? The old thinking was that the newborn only saw a world of "blooming, buzzing confusion." New research now indicates that this is not the case. A baby opens his or her eyes to a two-dimensional, very blurred world of limited colors. His or her vision is so blurred that he or she can only see about 8 inches and only notices the boldest of patterns. Figure 1-6 shows what a face looks like to a newborn.

Several lines of evidence suggest that newborn infants come into the world with some innately specified representation of faces. Newborns who were only 9 minutes from birth and had never seen a human face turned their heads more to follow (i.e., track) a two-dimensional, schematic, face-like pattern than either of two patterns consisting of the same facial features in different arrangements. Not only are they attracted to faces but they prefer attractive faces. This was noted in infants 14 to 15 hours old. It was noted, however, that this may be the result of a preference to faces they have seen in their first few hours (Slater, 1998).

A newborn has some color vision but not the full spectrum. Reds and greens are seen, but not blues. An analogy would be looking through a frosted window (Eliot, 1999). A child comes into this world with some primitive perception because newborns can tell the difference between a cross and a triangle and can perceive an object as being whole rather than only separate elements. Newborns tend to move their eyes in jerky, horizontal steps known as saccades. This is because at birth, their eye movements are controlled by lower brain areas. It usually takes 2 months before the higher brain areas take over visual functioning and a child will be able to follow a moving object with smooth eye movements called pursuits. By 6 months, however, all of his or her visual abilities, such as color vision, depth perception, fine acuity, and controlled eye movements, will have developed (Eliot, 1999). There is some visual organization at birth. For example, an object may change its orientation, or slant, relative to the child but, despite these changes, the newborn sees the object as the same shape. This is known as object shape constancy. A newborn will perceive an object as being the same despite changes to its distance and, hence, changes to its retinal size. This is referred to as size constancy and is also present at birth. It is also known that 4-month-old infants are able to perceive angular relationships and, hence, have some degree of form perception (Slater, 1998).

Children who are 3 years old or older will habituate to repeated representations of simple stimuli. It is well-documented that infants older than 2 or 3 months prefer to look at novel stimuli rather than ones that have been made familiar. The nature of attentional preferences (other than faces) in infants younger than 3 months is not clear. With infants, it is a two-stage process. An initial attraction for the familiar is followed by a preference for novelty. It has been suggested that 8 weeks may mark the end of the phenomenon of "attention to the familiar." Starting at this time, an infant may have developed a basic change in cognitive functioning (about 10 to 11 weeks postnatal). A study showed that 8 week olds preferred familiar stimuli while 10 week olds preferred novelty (Wetherford, 1973). Dramatic changes occur in the distribution and quality of waking and sleeping across the first 3 months. There is a dramatic increase in the amount of time spent in alert states over the first 10 to 12 postnatal weeks (Colombo, 2001).

The first 4 months of life show infants' attention to be drawn most consistently to objects with greater light-dark contrast, those with a moderate amount of edges, and those that move. One ability that emerges in the first 6 months is the tracking of visual stimuli, particularly smooth pursuit eye movements (eye movement following a moving object). At birth and up to 1 month of age, tracking of visual stimuli is relatively poor, occurs only at relatively slow stimulus speeds, and generally involves saccadic eye movements rather than smooth pursuit eye movements (Richards & Holley, 1999). Saccadic eye movements are rapid eye movements to stationary objects and were the first eye movements to emerge during evolution. Between 8 and 24 weeks of age, smooth pursuit eye movements appear to rapidly develop but only at very slow target speeds. It does not reach adult-level speeds until near 6 months. From 6 weeks until 6 months of age, the speed at which targets are pursued with smooth pursuit eye movements gradually increases. The ratio of pursuit to saccadic movements also increases over this time period. It is hypothesized that the development of attention during this age range would be reflected in age-related changes in pursuit tracking involving sustained attention (Richards & Turner, 2001). When we have a child do a smooth pursuit test (follow our finger), we are really watching his or her ability for sustained attention. Pursuit training is a very powerful way to train attention and should be included in every therapy program. Interaction between child and adult may be crucial to the development of the ability to direct attention voluntarily. When an adult directs an infant's attention to stimuli of interest by alternating the stimulus characteristics in some way, the child's voluntary attention is developed. By about 4 years of age, children develop the ability to scan their environment actively, rather than being drawn by the novelty or salience of a stimulus. This internally driven attention is believed to be well established by 5 or 6 years of age (Lyon, 1996).

Fixation is another area of eye movement in infants we need to analyze. This is when the infant does not move his or her eyes but analyzes an object. It appears that fixation duration may give us a clue in the child's predicted IQ scores. Prolonged fixation at 4 months of age predicted poorer IQ scores at 8 years in a large preterm sample. If we accept duration of fixation as an index of cognitive processing, it appears reasonable to hypothesize that infants with shorter peak fixations may process stimuli faster or more efficiently than infants with larger peak fixations (Colombo, 1987, 1996, 2004; Saxon, Frick, & Colombo, 1997).

If an infant looks at an object for a long time, it may indicate that he or she is slow at processing information. A short fixation might indicate that the infant is processing the more holistic or configural properties of the stimulus. One study showed that long-looking infants appear to rely on local visual analysis. They showed no evidence of recognizing the similarity of degraded visual forms that did not share common local contours. Short-looking infants, however, appeared to abstract the complete form from the presentation of its partial contour, thus supporting the hypothesis that these infants (like adults) engage initially in a scan of the "global" components in the visual field. These results might be attributable to more specific mechanisms; short-looking infants may be better able to "fill in" missing contours, and/or long-looking infants may be confused by the similarity of the angular local features that comprise stimuli (Colombo, 2001). It has been reported that the developmental cause of visual scanning in infancy proceeds from a concentrated saccadic inspection of specific features in early infancy to a more widely distributed inspection of the "whole" stimulus after 2 months of age. This change has been theoretically linked to the maturation of the magnocellular visual pathway of the geniculostriate visual system in infancy (Colombo, 1996).

To think that an infant begins life with these primitive visual skills and that in 5 years he or she is expected to do the most difficult neurological processing a human can do—reading—is really amazing. Vision is learned. As I have explained, we come into this world with very few visual skills. Unlike other senses, such as hearing, which is quite advanced at birth, vision emerges late and matures quickly (Eliot, 1999). By birth, babies have had about 12 weeks of actual listening experiences compared to none for vision. The thing that is critical for a child's successful visual development is experience.

The first year of a baby's life is busy. During the first 2 months, the brain's higher centers explode with new nerve connections (synapses). Before 2 months, it is the brainstem (primitive brain area) that controls everything.

CRITICAL PERIODS

By the age of 2, a child's brain contains twice as many synapses and consumes twice as much energy as the brain of a normal adult (Nash, 1997). The number of synapses in one layer of the visual cortex rises from around 2,500 per neuron at birth to as many as 18,000 approximately 6 months later. It reaches its highest permanent densities (15,000 synapses per neuron) at around the age of 2 years and remains at that level until the age of 10 or 11. Because the number of synapses in the visual cortex explodes between 2 and 8 months of age, new visual skills emerge and improve until the end of the first year when a baby's vision is nearly as good as an adult's (Eliot, 1999). It is experience that influences vision after the first 2 months, and experience is the reason for the rapid growth of the brain's visual centers. Scientists now believe that experiences underlie the development of every circuit in the visual cortex.

A baby's brain at birth contains 100 billion neurons, the same as the number of stars in the Milky Way (Nash, 1997). While the brain contains all of the neurons it will ever need, the wiring between them has to be established. While the brain gives us what we need, it is early experiences that determine the correct connections. Early experiences are critical to shape a child's visual-perception, eye-hand coordination, and so on. The more a baby sees and experiences, the stronger and better the brain will be wired to do the complex visual skills needed for success in school. Also, higher levels of infant functioning have been linked to maternal encouragement of infant attention to objects at very early ages (Lawson, 1992). The brain will eliminate synapses that are seldom used. It is important to remember that the brain's greatest growth spurt draws to a close around the age of 10 when the balance between synapse creation and atrophy abruptly shifts (Nash, 1997). During the next few years, it will destroy its weakest synapses (the ones not used), and only the ones that have been transformed by experience will survive. Therefore, therapy activities designed to strengthen these circuits in the brain's wiring are extremely important in the early school years. With appropriate therapy, researchers say even serious disorders, such as dyslexia, may be treatable (Nash, 1997). Every time I hear a teacher say that a child does not need therapy because he or she will outgrow it, I cringe. There are critical time periods in a child's life to improve his or her developmental and visual skills, and we need to work with him or her during these periods, not wait until he or she "outgrows it."

Just as there are critical time periods for a child's perceptual and developmental skills, there are also critical time periods for his or her binocular skills and the development of his or her visual acuities. Unless it is exercised early on, the visual system will not develop. Binocular vision (and depth perception) must be developed by 3 years of age and visual acuity by 7 to 8 years. *Amblyopia* (lazy eye) is a term most of us have heard. It means that the child's vision cannot be corrected to 20/20 with glasses. It usually involves only one eye but can occur in both eyes. Amblyopia can only develop during the first 7 years of life (American Optometric Association, 1995). It is estimated that amblyopia affects 1% to 4% of preschool children and is the most common cause of unilateral (one eye) vision loss in patients under the age of 70 (Nelson, 2005). The criteria to be diagnosed as having amblyopia are as follows:

- Reduced visual acuity in one eye. This usually varies from 20/25 to 20/70; however, I often see 20/100 or worse.

- Difference in visual acuity of two or more lines on the eye chart between the two eyes.

In order to explain how amblyopia develops, we need to remember how the brain develops circuits of neurons, and if a certain group of neurons is not used, it will be eliminated later or replaced by another group. Because various aspects of the visual system undergo refinement at different times, the period during which they are sensitive to visual input also varies so that various aspects of vision—acuity, binocularity, and the like—are vulnerable to abnormal experiences at different times in a baby's life. Visual abilities are highly malleable until the age of 2 and then somewhat less until 8 or 9. The most critical time period for a child's visual acuity is from 4 months (when the higher brain areas take over), peaks between 9 and 11 months, and is largely over by 2 years of age. Even after this, however, binocularity and acuity can still remain vulnerable up to 8 years of age (Eliot, 1999).

What are the abnormal experiences that can affect a child's vision? The two most common are refractive error (needing glasses) and strabismus (eyes crossing or drifting out) (Eliot, 1999).

It is estimated that 5% to 7% of preschool children have refractive errors and need glasses (American Optometric Association, 1995). The problem arises when only one eye is affected. If this happens, that eye's neurons in the visual cortex do not develop because the other eye is used all the time and the weaker eye is not used at all. The brain has a simple solution to one eye with blurred vision. It subconsciously shuts it off. This is called suppression. What makes suppression serious for a child is that he or she does not know that only one eye is being used. Because the good eye is doing all the work, the child is not aware he or she is not using the bad eye. The first time the child is aware of this is usually when his or her eyes are examined and when he or she covers up the good eye, he or she cannot see out of the bad eye. Unfortunately, this is often missed at some vision screenings at the pediatrician's office. In fact, one recent study showed that trained vision screeners still missed up to 30% of children who had these visual disorders. I have seen many children who had amblyopia, and neither the child nor the parent had any idea anything was wrong. One experience sticks in my mind more than the others. A mother brought one of her children in for our vision therapy program twice a week for 9 months. She would sit in the reception area with the child's younger sister. When her son graduated from our program, she decided to have the sister's eyes examined. When I tested her eyes, her vision in one eye was only corrected to 20/100 because it was very farsighted. This was a child who sat in my reception area for 9 months, and neither she nor her mother thought she had a problem. The good news is that, if found early enough, we can patch one eye for several hours a day and force the other eye to develop the circuits in the brain that it needs for good vision. Treatment that is started by the time a child reaches 4 or 5 years is usually partially successful, and we can usually get the vision in the bad eye down to at least 20/30. Even older children (7 to 10 years old) who have been treated with occlusion (patching) have been improved (Nelson, 2005). The key for success is finding the problem early. Unfortunately, in the United States, only 21% of children receive a vision screening between the ages of 3 and 5 (Nelson, 2005).

To give you an example of how amblyopia can be helped if caught early enough, I will tell you about Randy. Randy is a 7 year old who was sent to us by another optometrist because of amblyopia. When I saw Randy, acuity in his left eye was 20/200. A pair of glasses improved his acuity to 20/100. We then put Randy through a combination of patching and vision therapy programs to strengthen his left eye. We started patching for 3 hours a day and did activities to improve his visual skills in his left eye. I retested Randy 2 months after the start of his program, and his vision had improved to 20/40 in his left eye. His vision was eventually improved to 20/25. This shows the importance of early diagnosis and treatment. The second factor that can cause amblyopia is strabismus. This means that one eye drifts "in" or "out" and the vision in that eye does not develop. Strabismus affects 2% of full-term babies and 10% to 20% of premature babies (Eliot, 1999). You would think it would be easy to see if a child's eyes drifted in or out, but many times, it is not. Often with young infants, one of the eyes may appear to turn in. In fact, convergence deviations in infants in the first month of life are common and normal. They reflect the early exercise of the vergence system and rarely prove to be true strabismus. This is because in the first month of life, good acuity, cortical binocularity, and active accommodation are not present yet. There is a condition called neonatal misalignments (NMs) that reflects the child's first exercise of his or her convergence system (Horwood, 2003). It makes one of the eyes drift "in" and is normal for an infant younger than 4 months. Often, parents will notice their baby's eyes occasionally turning in, and they become concerned. If you notice a child's eye turning in occasionally during the first 4 months, you need to know this is normal. If it continues past 4 months or if one eye consistently turns "in," it is not normal.

You need to be aware of the critical times for a child's development of a normal visual system. Remember, unless exercised, the visual system will not develop properly. Binocular vision must be developed by 3 years, and the time period that may cause amblyopia in a child is from birth to 7 or 8 years (Nelson, 2005). Give a child as many experiences as you can. One study showed that children who do not play much or who are rarely touched developed brains that were 20% to 30% smaller than normal for their age (Nash, 1997). Remember that rich experiences produce rich brains.

CAPACITY LIMITS

The human brain is extremely complex. Its hundred billion neurons and several hundred trillion synaptic connections can process and exchange large amounts of information over a distributed network of brain tissue in a matter of milliseconds. Such massive parallel processing capacity permits our brains to analyze complex images in one tenth of a second, allowing us to visually experience our world.

The brain also has a huge storage capacity that is almost infinite. During our lifetime, our brain will have stored more than 50,000 times the amount of text contained in the U.S. Library of Congress or more than five times the amount of the total printed material in the world (Marcois, 2005). Yet, with all the processing power, the average person can barely attend to or hold in his or her mind more than a few objects and can hardly perform more than one task at a time. The brain faces several limitations. The first concerns the time that it takes to consciously identify an object. We think we do this instantaneously when, in fact, this process can take more than half a second before our brain is free to identify a second object. The second limited capacity is the number of objects that can be simultaneously maintained in working memory. This is estimated to be about four objects. In fact, even a person with very good memory will have difficulty remembering more than seven digits that are shown to him or her. The last bottleneck arises when we must choose the proper course of action for an object or event. For example, when you are driving and are not sure of the exit, this will probably keep you from answering questions asked by someone riding with you. As we will see later in this book, you have a difficult time dividing your attention. A child with his or her mind on one thing would have difficulty following what you are saying. This very likely goes back to our primitive ancestors. It is possible that our brains did not need to be built to maintain a detailed representation of the visual world because why should we have to remember something when a new representation is just one look away? That piece of fruit on a tree is still going to be there. It is not going anywhere. It is unlikely during evolution of the brain that there was any strong pressure for our nervous system to fully identify visual objects or events in very rapid succession. Even under fight-or-flight situations, probably only one predator needs to be identified at a time. Sequential processing was not very important in our past; however, it is today with events such as reading. It is also unlikely that our ancestors had to make several split-second decisions at once. For example, reaching for a piece of fruit or escaping from a predator did not require more than one decision at a time. This has all changed now in our fast-paced world. This is why when you are presented with images very quickly in succession, say 10 a second, and are asked to determine if two particular objects were presented among eight other objects, you will be able to detect only the first of the two targets presented, but will fail to perceive the second one if it was presented within half a second of the first. Because of the severe limitations of the brain, our visual system was developed to work in a divide-and-conquer fashion. The visual information coming through the retina and transmitted to the cortex is processed by different regions of the visual cortex in the occipital lobe with each region being specialized in the processing of different attributes, such as color or motion. The first actions of the visual cortex appear to process simpler features of the visual scene, such as the contours of a face, whereas, later, deeper areas of the visual cortex may be more specialized, for instance, for identifying a particular face. Research has shown that the early stages of visual processing can quickly process a large amount of information in parallel (not serial). In contrast, later stages are more limited in their processing power—they can process only one item at a time. Therefore, the early stage of visual processing permits the rapid, initial categorization of the visual world (a quick look) while later attention-demanding, capacity-limited stages (detailed looks) are necessary for the conscious reporting of and action upon the stimuli (Schall, 1999).

Visual processing from the retina is processed first by a pair of small structures deep in the brain called the lateral geniculate nuclei (LGN). Individual neurons in the LGN can be activated by visual stimulation from either one eye or the other but not both. They respond to any change of brightness or color in a specific region within an area of view called the receptive field, which varies among neurons. From the LGN, visual information moves to the primary visual cortex known as V1, which is at the back of the head. Neurons in V1 behave differently than those in the LGN. They can usually be activated by either eye, but they are also sensitive to specific attributes, such as the orientation of a contour or the direction of motion of a stimulus placed within their receptive field. Visual information is transmitted from V1 to more than two dozen other distinct cortical regions, called the extrastriate visual areas. Information from V1 moves through areas known as V2 and V4 before winding up in regions known as the inferior temporal cortex (ITC). The ITC is important in perceiving form and recognizing objects. Neurons in V4 are known to respond selectively to aspects of visual stimuli critical to discerning shapes. In the ITC, some neurons behave like V4 cells, but others respond only when entire objects, such as faces, are placed within their large receptive fields. Other signals from V1 pass through regions V2, V3, and an area known as V5/MT (the medial temporal cortex) before reaching a part of the brain called the parietal lobe. Most neurons in V5/MT respond strongly to items moving with a specific velocity (speed and direction selective). Neurons in the other areas of the parietal lobe respond when an animal pays attention to a stimulus or intends to move toward it. The parietal lobe will be mentioned often in this book as it is a very critical area of the brain for attention, eye movements, and motor planning. These pathways are mentioned because, in order to understand visual attention, you have to have an idea of how the visual pathway progresses from the retina to the parietal lobe. Attention effects have generally been found to increase in magnitude as one processes from V1 up the visual pathway into the parietal and temporal lobes. We also have to keep in mind that the control of motor output is precisely why vision evolved in the first place and that attention directs motor actions.

TWO VISUAL PATHWAYS

We now know that the visual system has evolved for two different functions, and there are two visual pathways involved. One pathway involves directing motor movement such as eye or hand movement. This is also called several names, including M pathway, dorsal pathway, the "where" system, or magnocellular layers. It deals with spatial and motor skills and ambient vision. The other pathway directs object identification and is called the P pathway, the ventral stream, the "what" system, or parvocellular layers. The phylogenetically older pathway from the retina to the superior colliculus deals with movement. This is the ambient (peripheral) system used for guiding whole-body movements, such as locomotion and position, while the newer system is used for focal vision guiding fine motor acts such as manipulation and object identification. These two pathways were discovered in the late 1960s and indicate that there is not one pathway from the retina, but at least two independent channels from the retina to the brain (Milner, 2006). The M and P systems differ in at least four functional ways: color sensitivity, contrast sensitivity, temporal resolution (motion), and visual spatial resolution (acuity). The M system has poor color sensitivity and poor acuity; however, it is very sensitive to movement and low spatial frequency stimuli. Though the exact role of the M pathway (called dorsal after the LGN) is not fully understood, it is known that it carries information on movement, stereopsis (depth) spatial localization, figural grouping, illusory border, perception, and figural ground segregation (Patel, 2004). We have to remember that the brain is trying to deal with an incredible amount of information. To deal with this, the visual systems involve a surprising degree of division of labor by which a seemingly single function is carried out by multiple specialized systems that operate in parallel (Farah, 2000). In the visual systems, if many receptor cells are pooled, lower levels of light can be detected. But this gain in sensitivity comes at the cost of lower spatial resolution (detail). This is because once the outputs from different points on the retina are pooled, the information concerning which of those points were stimulated and which were not has been lost. Good resolution can be maintained by limiting the number of photoreceptor outputs that converge on later cells, but this results in poor sensitivity to low levels of light. Rather than choose one trade-off or the other, the visual system partitions the image into two: one that favors sensitivity and one that favors resolution. The duplex retina, therefore, has a system of rods, with greater individual sensitivity to give us a low-resolution image of the world that persists under conditions of low illumination (our peripheral vision) and also a system of cones (central vision) with their much more limited convergence to give us a high-resolution image of the world provided there is ample light (Farah, 2000). A consequence of color vision's reliance on cones is that we are effectively colorblind in low illumination.

It is apparent that vision and action systems evolved together to enable successful interaction with the environment. The ability to extract information to guide goal-directed behavior, such as pursuit of prey or avoidance of predators, is fundamental to an organism's survival. Hence, massive evolutionary pressure has ensured that the most exquisitely efficient systems have evolved (Gazzaniga, 2004).

As a result of evolution, perception and action cannot be considered separate and independent systems. It is motor and actions that train perception, not just looking at a computer screen. There is also increasing evidence that attention can interact with action-based representations; therefore, attention, action, and perception cannot be separated. You train one, you train all of them. Most early work studying links between attention and action have examined saccades (rapid eye movement to a stationary target). For example, the premotor theory is based on two complimentary ideas. The first is the notion that preparation of eye movements automatically involves shifts of attention. The second idea concerns the alternative relationship between attention and saccades. That is, orienting attention to a location automatically activates motor responses such as saccades to the location (even though no overt saccades need to be produced). A substantial amount of information now supports a link between attention and saccades (Gazzaniga, 2004). This is why I feel that vision training has been so effective in helping children in school. Vision training deals with eye movements, and eye movements involve attention. Also, there is abundant evidence that visual processes can flow automatically into actions, such that the latter can be evoked with little or no conscious intention to act (Gazzaniga, 2004). The following are three examples of automatic links between vision and actions involving the levels:

1. The first example is what is known as the Simon Effect. In this task, subjects might be asked to report the color of a stimulus with a key press; for example, they are asked to press the right key with the right hand if the color is red and to press the left key with the left hand if the color is green. When subjects are asked to report the red color with the right key press, reaction times are faster when the stimulus is on the right side of the screen than when it is on the left. An intuitively obvious explanation for this is that the right-sided stimulus is closer to the responding hand, and this reveals an automatic link between a stimulus and goal-directed reading actions.

2. The second example of automatic encoding of vision and action required subjects to report with right and left key presses whether an object was in its normal orientation or inverted. If a right key press was required, an object such as a frying pan with the handle oriented toward the right hand was classified faster than if the handle was oriented to the left hand.

3. The third example of automatic visuomotor processing demonstrates the important interactions between the ventral and dorsal visual streams. These streams both appear to receive inputs from the parvo (P) pathways and magno (M) pathways. Most of the input to the dorsal stream is magno in origin (Milner, 2006). It has been demonstrated that unconscious processing of information in the ventral stream (P pathway; central vision), such as analysis of color, can automatically prime motor responses encoded in the dorsal (peripheral vision) stream, such as painting. For example, when subjects were required to reach for a target of a particular color, a color prime briefly presented at the same location facilitates reaching if it is the same color as the target (Gazzaniga, 2004). What do these three examples tell you?

    a. If a child uses his or her right hand, he or she is faster at finding a target in the right side of a display.

    b. A child will more likely be faster at picking up an object with his or her right hand if the handle is facing to his or her right.

    c. A colored target will be identified faster if the target is an object of the same color. For example, reach the red cup. This will be faster if the red cup is on a red cloth rather than a green one or if the child had just finished playing with a red ball.

Research has shown that luminance contrast is an important determinant for evoking visual attention (brighter or darker than the background). We also know that visual attention favors stimuli that preferentially excite the M pathway (such as motion). In fact, the M pathway has priority in triggering visual attention. The simultaneous presentation of M- and P-biased clues would result in excitation of visual cortex by the M-biased cue first. Even if the P-biased cue precedes the M-biased cue by as much as 100 msec, the M-biased cue always dominates the attentional responses. The notion that the M pathway has a superior capacity to drive the neural processes responsible for visual attention is consistent with several features of the M pathway. The M pathway, which is prevalent in the peripheral retina, produces fast, transient responses to luminous changes. The rapid initial responses of the M ganglion cells in turn modulate subsequent processing of retinal information transmitted by the slower P pathway. Therefore, the quicker M pathway could serve to prime information about the retinal location of a new stimulus (Steinman, Steinman, & Lehmkuhle, 1997). The location of a new stimulus would alert the brain to prepare for a saccadic eye movement.

Priming and localization functions often associated with the M pathway have also been attributed to visual attention. It is not surprising that deficits in attention have been linked to deficits in posterior parietal cortex, the primary projection of the M processing stream. The M pathway is the oldest of the pathways and, therefore, is primary for attention. Saccadic eye movements are the oldest eye movements and evolved before pursuit movements. It is, therefore, not surprising that saccadic eye movements and attention go together. You cannot do one without the other, and if you are going to train attention, you have to train saccadic and peripheral eye movements. A peripheral target will dominate over a central target for attention.

Attention can be focused by either voluntary concentration on a particular location or as an involuntary response to the sudden onset of a stimulus. Sudden stimulus-induced attention is dominant and will always override voluntary attention. So, you can see how a child can lose attention when something comes into his or her peripheral vision. We also know that attention causes visual processing to be accelerated. The greatest acceleration is in the region closest to the stimulus cue and falls off with separation from the stimulus cue. At even greater separations from the stimulus, visual processing is actually decelerated.

SACCADIC EYE MOVEMENT

Vision is somewhat of an illusion. We regard our visual world as "just there," not as something that is only acquired after sequential sampling and reconstruction. It appears that vision occurs in parallel, yet our actual contact with the world is essentially serial (Nakayama, 1990).

Sequential sampling is coordinated by the use of saccadic eye movements. The term *saccade* is derived from the French word *squer*, to pull, which refers to the jerking of a horse's head by a tug on the reins or to the flicking of a sail in a gust of wind. The function of voluntary saccades in primates is directly linked to the presence of a fovea because images are best seen if located there. Saccadic velocities cannot be voluntarily controlled, although they may become lower with fatigue or inattention. Saccades are about 10% slower when made in complete darkness (Leigh, 1983). Saccades are the eye movements often termed *eye tracking* when reading and dyslexia are involved. Some patients with dyslexia do show unusual patterns of saccades during scanning of written materials, although the relationship between eye movement abnormalities and childhood dyslexia is not clear; however, patients with certain types of acquired ocular motor abnormalities do have significant reading difficulty (Leigh, 1983).

The average person makes three to four saccades every second of his or her life. Another interesting fact is that the brain shuts off visual information during the saccade. We have vision at the fixation and at the end of the saccade but not during the saccade. If the brain did not shut off vision during the saccade, our world would be a series of smeared images as our eyes move. The shutting off of vision during the saccade is called saccadic suppression. If you do not believe your brain shuts off the visual images during eye movement, try to see your eyes move when you look into a mirror and move your eyes.

Attention is critical for proper eye movement, especially during visual scanning and reading. When the eye fixates a word (or letter in a word), attention is initially allocated to the stimulus at the fixation point. Attention is then reallocated to some location in the periphery, and the visual system begins to program a saccade to the new location. These attentional movements are primary, and eye movements are secondary (Findlay & Walker, 1999). Perceptual and cognitive processing both affect saccadic release. First, a preattentive map of likely stimulus locations is made available to the attention allocation system. Second, stimulus locations are weighted so that attention is allocated to the stimulus location with the largest weight (Findlay & Walker, 1999). When we scan an object, how does the brain know where to scan? We now know that the brain will scan the areas that give it the most information. When scan patterns of eye movements were recorded, they found the eye spends more time on angles or corners of an object. With a face, it spends more time on the eyes and nose, as these areas are critical for identification (Deubel & Schneider, 1995). When a person is reading and is fixating on a word, he or she can subconsciously perceive information about the length and shape of the word in the periphery. This helps him or her to know where to move his or her eye on the next fixation (Hoffman & Subramaniam, 1995). This means that attention and saccades are not independent. Both attention and saccades are mediated by the same neural circuitry. That is, when one attends or moves his or her eyes to a location, a set of commands is sent to the brain structures, such as the superior colliculus, that are responsible for oculomotor control. The oculomotor hypothesis makes two predictions: (1) preparing to make a saccade to a location should produce attention enhancement at that location and (2) attending to a location should result in fast saccades to that location (Hoffman & Subramaniam, 1995).

Extensive behavioral research has been dedicated to testing the relationship between visual spatial attention and oculomotor functions and has highlighted both the concerted action between the two functions and the ability to dissociate between them. Recent brain-imaging studies have supported a neuroanatomical link between visual spatial attention and eye movements.

There is a strong relationship between the neural systems for covert attention and the sensorimotor systems that control the related overt behaviors. Visual spatial orienting tasks may be considered as covert analogues of oculomotor tasks. Attention, even when performed as a mental act with no overt manifestation, seems to draw upon the functional neuroanatomy of more basic sensory and motor processes for its instantiation. This is analogous to other cognitive functions, such as visual or motor imagery, which seem to be intrinsically bound to their perceptual and motor counterparts.

The precise nature of the intimate relationship between attention and sensorimotor systems remains to be resolved. Overlap in brain activations by different cognitive functions may represent two types of underlying functional anatomy:

1.   The functional distinction between the systems is very blurred, and overlapping areas are truly shared by both cognitive systems all the time. There may be enough complexity within such a shared system to allow for functional dissociations between covert attention and eye movement depending on demand posed by the environment.

2.   Brain areas are capable of multitasking, and the same anatomical areas can perform different functions at different times. Both of these possibilities require that the same neurons show specializations adept for both cognitive processes. Single-unit studies support the existence of neurons that contain both attentional and oculomotor specializations. The overlapping areas contain separate interdigitated pools of neurons that belong to the different cognitive processes, but contemporary brain imaging methods are unable to resolve the spatial separation between these neuronal populations (Nobre, Gitelman, Dias, & Mesulam, 2000).

Researchers in the early 1950s discovered that your eyes never stop moving, even when they are fixed on a single object, such as a letter. When the eyes fixate on something, as they do 80% of the time during waking hours, they still jump and jiggle imperceptibly, which is critical for vision and seeing. If you could somehow stop these miniature motions while fixating your gaze, a static scene would fade from view. The area of the scene that fades last is the area that gives the brain the most information. For 5 decades, a debate has raged about whether the largest of these involuntary movements, the microsaccades, serve any purpose at all. These microsaccades are helping us to understand the brain's code in creating conscious perceptions of the visual world. Animal nervous systems have evolved to detect changes in the environment because spotting differences promotes survival. Motion in the visual field may indicate that a predator is approaching. Unchanging objects do not generally pose a threat, so animal brains—and visual systems—did not evolve to notice them. This is why motion in our peripheral field is a strong stimulus for detection and attention. An unchanging stimulus leads to neural adaptation in which visual neurons adjust their outputs, such that they gradually stop responding. To stop adaptation, these involuntary eye movements shift the entire visual scene across the retina three to four times a second, forcing neurons into action and counteracting neural adaptation. Also, these little eye movements may help expose a person's subliminal thoughts. Even if your gaze is fixed, your attention can unconsciously shift about a visual scene to objects that attract your interest.

PREMOTOR THEORY

We have all seen the situation where we have worked with a child on one area, such as oculomotor, and other areas have improved. This was mentioned in the introduction with visual motor improvements after doing eye exercises. There is evidence for activation in the posterior parietal cortex associated with selective visual attention in relation to reaching behavior, saccadic behavior, and ocular fixation. This indicates the importance of the posterior parietal cortex in visuomotor control of these behaviors. On the basis of this and other physiological and neurobehavioral evidence, Milner (2006) proposed a premotor theory of selective spatial attention. According to this theory, which is explained in detail in Chapter 2, the mechanisms responsible for attention are intrinsic to the spatial coding associated with particular visuomotor systems. In other words, visual attention to a particular part of space is nothing more or less than the facilitation of particular subsets of neurons involved in the preparation of particular visually guided actions directed at that part of space. It has been found that neurons in separate parts of the premotor cortex are also linked respectively with ocular and manual movements, and it was found that single cells in the posterior parietal cortex were actively enhanced, prior to both saccades and to hand movements. One could interpret this finding as supporting the hypothesis that when one region of the visual field is selected, it is selected for all potential response systems equally (Milner, 2006). Another interesting note on Rizzolatti's theory is that of dealing with distracting visual stimuli on the performance of pointing movements. The effect of distraction on the performance of pointing movements is dependent on the location of the stimulus with respect to the starting position of the hand. When subjects raised their right hands, stimuli to the right of that hand were more distracting than stimuli to the left; the opposite pattern was seen when subjects used their left hands.

The acts of motor and attention cannot be separated. The premotor theory assumes that motor plans are in place before the motor movement. To give an example of this, they found that when a subject is cued to shift attention to another object after the saccadic eye movement has started to the first object, the trajectory of the eye movement is curved away from the new target. It still reaches the new target, but the first motor plan has interfered with the new motor plan, showing that the original motor plan had to be corrected in midsaccadic movement, an indication that visuomotor planning, attention, and eye movements are all interconnected and also that attention in one sensory modality can influence processing in another modality (Indovina & Sanes, 2001).

There is no doubt concerning the role of attention in saccadic and pursuit eye movements. Saccades require a shift of attention (Kowler, 1994), and pursuits require focused and sustained attention. These two eye movements are critical for any training program. When a person fixates on an object, the focused attention inhibits saccades. A saccade may be planned but not executed during a fixation (Anderson, 1989). When attention is engaged, the saccadic system is inhibited; when attention is disengaged, the saccadic system is released from this inhibition (Taylor, 1998). This is why children with poor attention usually have poor saccades during reading.

TRANS-SACCADIC MEMORY

Although we perceive the world as a continuous panorama (even with saccadic suppression), considerable evidence suggests that memory across eye movements (trans-saccadic memory) is severely limited. This implies that our impression of a unified and coherent visual environment is due to the contents of the individual fixations, rather than to any detailed mental image that is built up across saccades. It is estimated that only between three and six elements of a visual pattern are maintained in memory over a saccade. This shows that trans-saccadic memory is limited. It also appears that information near the saccadic target is more likely to be encoded (stored) into trans-saccadic memory than is other information around it. The question is, why is information near the saccadic target remembered better? Research suggests that this is because attention precedes the eyes to the saccadic target, and this increases the likelihood that letters (if looking at a letter string) near the target location will be encoded into trans-saccadic memory at the expense of other letters. Attention determines what information is encoded into memory (Schneider, 1998).

PRIMITIVE REFLEXES

Within the first few weeks of postnatal life, the primitive, postural reflexes (i.e., the tonic labyrinthine reflex [TLR] and the tonic neck reflex [TNR]) should be present. The stimulus that evokes the TLR is the earth's gravitational force. It acts on the neuromuscular system in such a manner that, when the head is prone, flexor muscles are facilitated, and when the head is supine, extensor muscles are facilitated. The asymmetrical TNR is elicited by stimulating receptors in the neck joints. When the head is turned to the right, so that the chin approximates the shoulder,

extensor tone is increased in the right arm and flexor tone is increased in the left arm. When the head is turned to the left, extensor tone is increased in the left arm and flexor tone in the right arm. As a child matures, these reflexes become integrated into the central nervous system, largely through inhibition as higher centers of the brain mature (Ayres, 1973). Some call these reflexes developmental reflexes, and persistence often indicates neurological dysfunction. A persistence of the TNR would contribute to poor pursuit eye movements, and persistence of the TLR would contribute to difficulties in visual perception (Wahberg, 2005). In fact, a persistent or reappearance may indicate brain damage. It is also thought that in severe cases, they inhibit certain motor abilities in cerebral-palsied children (Capute et al., 1984). Studies have shown that these residual primitive reflexes may be correlated with reduced saccadic accuracy. If these primitive reflexes remain after 6 months of age, they may hinder normal development of the postural reflexes and of oculomotor motility (Gonzalez, 2008). Development of the visual system depends first on the early presence of these reflexes and later on inhibition of both the TNR and TLR along with the Moro reflex (MR). The MR is an infant's response to auditory or visual stress. The MR and TLR are closely bound to the first months of life. They are of vestibular origin, and both can be activated either by stimulation of the labyrinth or by alteration of body position in space. If the MR remains too long, the infant will be hypersensitive in one or more of the sensorial channels, and the eyes will be attracted automatically toward any bright light, any movement, or any alteration in the visual field. Hence, this may lead to distractibility, poor balance and coordination, and oculomotor problems. A retained TLR may prevent complete development of the ocular reflex and the head right reaction. Balance will be adversely affected by poor visual information, and vision will be affected by poor balance. Research has shown that the TNR is the most predictive of a saccade-based interrelationship. Saccadic parameters also correlated with TLR. The study found a correlation between the remaining primitive reflexes and saccadic eye movements in fifth-grade children with reading problems. Primitive reflexes that are poorly integrated and persist may not allow the proper development of visually guided movement necessary for adequate visuomotor coordination and may interfere with development of higher-level visual spatial concepts.

COLOR VISION AND EYE MOVEMENTS

What is the purpose of our visual system? Originally, in the Cambrian period, it was light detection. This was later modified so we could detect motion and be warned about predators or help in finding food. We started out nocturnal and lived in a dark environment; however, as our ancestors became daylight animals, we developed cones for more detailed vision. Later, color vision was added so we could detail different fruits from leaves to help us identify food. To understand how our visual system has evolved, hold your finger at arm length and move it from the far periphery to the midperiphery. The far periphery was our very early vision that was mainly for light detection and detection of movement. This is a function of the rods. Now, slowly move your finger toward your central vision. You now will see that detail and color has been added. This is the result of the cones in our retina. This experience will take you through hundreds of millions of years of evolution. Throughout this book, we talk about two visual systems. Keep in mind the exercise that you just finished. The M system is the system mainly controlled by our peripheral vision and consists mainly of rods. This is also called the "where" system. The P system is mainly controlled by cones and is for detailed and color vision. This is also called the "what" system. Before we explain color vision in detail, it is important to get a clear understanding of eye movements. The sole purpose of eye movements is to move your eyes so the visual image focuses on the fovea. These eye movements are controlled by six muscles that act as antagonistic pairs. One pair is responsible for up-and-down movements of the eyes, one pair for side-to-side movements, and one pair for a rotational movement. The saccadic movement is the type of eye movement that is involved in reading, when you move your eyes across a line of print. A saccadic eye movement is a very rapid eye movement to an object or figure that the brain wants to further evaluate. During natural viewing conditions, a normal adult makes three to five saccades every second separated by periods of 200 to 300 msec during which the eyes do not make a movement. These periods are called fixations (Fischler, 1987). Saccadic eye movements are very fast with speeds of 1/25 to 1/50 of a second. What is amazing is that the brain does not just guess where to move the eyes; it knows the target in advance from the "where" system (rods) and then figures out how far and with how much effort it will take to move the eyes. The brain must monitor visual inputs from both eyes, so the command to move the eyes has information about final position, direction, and speed. It also has to take into account the elasticity of the orbital tissues, which tend to pull the eyes back to the center position. To make this even more difficult, it has been shown that the stiffness in the left eye is 11% greater if the eye is moved "out" rather than "in." It is also known that both eyes do not travel at the same speed. For example, the saccadic movements of the eye going from midline ("out") has a higher velocity, shorter duration, and is more skewed than the saccades of the fellow eye (moving in). As a result, the eyes diverge (turn out) as much as 3 degrees during horizontal (left to right) saccades. There also appears to be a postsaccadic drift so that the fovea of each eye is guided toward the target. The purpose of this drift is to correctly put the image of both eyes on their foveas at the same time. This procedure happens three to five times a second for your entire life. A child under 1 year of age usually needs more than one saccade to reach a target. After 1 year, he or she can do this in one movement. Most children who are 5 years old have difficulty performing accurate saccadic eye movements; however, this improves, so that most 7 year olds can perform them normally. This means that children in kindergarten do not have the eye movement skills to read correctly without losing their place as they read, and most first graders would also have difficulty with these movements.

Color is not actually a property of light or of the objects that reflect light. It is a sensation that arises within the brain (Goldsmith, 2006). Just as vision is a sensation in the brain, so is color. Most of us take our color vision for granted. We do not notice the incredible assortment of colors. It is remarkable that, for most human beings, any color can be reproduced by mixing together just three fixed wavelengths of light at certain intensities. This is called trichromacy and arises because the retina uses only three types of light-absorbing pigments for color vision. Although trichromacy is common among primates, it is not universal in the animal kingdom. Almost all nonprimate mammals are dichromats, with color vision based on just two kinds of visual pigments. Some birds, fish, and reptiles have four visual pigments and can detect ultraviolet light invisible to humans (Jacobs & Nathans, 2009). It was not until the early 1970s that we became aware that many vertebrates could see a part of the spectrum that was invisible to us (Goldsmith, 2006).

A common misconception that we first learned in school is that objects absorb some wavelengths of light and reflect the others and that colors we perceive "in" objects relates to the wavelengths of the reflected light. The three visual pigments responsible for our vision each absorb light from a particular region of the spectrum that is characterized by the wavelength it absorbs most efficiently. The short wavelength (S) pigment absorbs light maximally at wavelengths of about 430 nanometers (a nanometer is one billionth of a meter). The medium wavelength (M) pigment maximally absorbs light at approximately 530 nanometers (nms), and the long wavelength (L) pigment absorbs light maximally at 560 nms. This corresponds to hues that the typical human perceives: blue (470), green (520), and yellow (580 nms) (Jacobs & Nathans, 2009). When the pigment absorbs light (or to be more precisely, absorbs discrete pockets of energy called photons), the added energy causes the retina to change shape, triggering a cascade of molecular events leading to excitation of the cone cell. This excitation in turn leads to activation of retinal neurons, one set of which fires impulses in the optic nerve, conveying information to the brain. The more intense a light, the more photons are absorbed by the visual pigments, the greater the excitation of each cone, and the brighter the light appears (Goldsmith, 2006).

It has been proposed that primate color vision evolved in two steps. Ancient mammals were nocturnal, possessed a single M/L cone, and were monochromats (one color). The ancient form of color vision appeared when mammals acquired S cones, initially to enlarge their spectral sensitivity, and then developed the neural circuitry for blue-yellow color combinations (Kaas, 2004). This gave an advantage over dichromats in some environments. The colors of ripe fruit, for example, frequently contrast with the surrounding foliage, and dichromats were less able to see such contrasts because they had low sensitivity to color differences in the red, yellow, and green regions of the visual spectrum. An ability to identify fruit would likely aid the survival of the animal. It appears that trichromacy was at first only a female trait and later was transferred to males as well as females (Jacobs & Nathans, 2009).

Children who are colorblind can still see colors; however, they will often have a color-labeling problem. The most common defect is referred to as a red-green dichromat. They will confuse greens with reddish purples or with reds. Although red-green dichromats are essentially monochromatic for wavelengths beyond about 545 nm, they do remarkably well at labeling colors. This is especially true because they know what others call certain colors. They get into trouble assigning color labels to manufactured items, such as the pattern on a blouse or shirt, because they may not know how others would label the colors contained within the pattern. They know that others see an apple as red, but do not know how others see the stripes on a particular shirt. They also see a green traffic light as whitish. The majority of red-green defects are inherited and transmitted in an X-linked recessive fusion. Consequently, they are considerably more common in men than women, with a prevalence of 8.0 and 0.4, respectively (Schwartz, 2004).

Questions About Color and Children

1. Do color lenses improve reading?
2. Do colored overlays work?
3. Does color help AD/HD children?
4. Can color be used to improve attention?
5. Is a certain color better for print color?
6. Can a colored background help in attention?

Do Color Lenses Improve Reading?

Some theories state that a defective M pathway may be the cause of dyslexia in some children; therefore, can a certain colored lens that improves the M pathway help these children? This is a difficult question to answer with just yes or no. I proposed this question to a college professor: "What color lens would you use to stimulate just the M pathway?" His answer was, "Both M and P cells receive inputs from M and L cones. There is, therefore, no spectral stimulus that can be used to stimulate the M pathway that will not also provide input to the P cell pathway."

The term *scotopic sensitivity syndrome* (SSS) has been around for more than 20 years. It really took off when its author, Helen Irlen, went on the *60 Minutes Australia* program in 1985. The theory states that some children have a difficult time processing full-spectrum light efficiently, and this may affect the way they see the printed page. It states that a person who has SSS can experience any or all of its five factors: light sensitivity, inadequate background accommodation, poor print resolution, restricted span of recognition, and a lack of sustained attention. The self-test to see if you have SSS may be found in Table 1-1.

If you answered yes to three or more of these questions, then you might be experiencing the effects of SSS (Irlen, 1991). The problem with this syndrome is that all of these symptoms are usually caused by visually related problems. Most of these symptoms are caused by oculomotor problems or other visual areas that are easily corrected with vision therapy. Also, I wish it was that easy to help these children. There is no quick-fix cure for reading disabilities. In my experiences, I have not seen much benefit from tinted lenses in reading. What seems to help is not color as much as the luminance difference between print and background. The larger the difference, the easier it is for reading (Knoblauch, Arditi, & Szlyk, 1991; Legge & Rubin, 1986). That being said, let's go to the next question.

Do Colored Overlays Work?

When we get to the chapter on dyslexia, I will tell you that sometimes blue or gray overlays seem to help the M pathway. The theory is that a defective M pathway could be causing some reading problems, and if you can improve the M pathway, you can improve a child's reading. The M pathway is also the main pathway for attention. It appears that the M pathway attracts attention and the P holds attention. (Peripheral attracts, central vision holds.)

Can a color overlay (not an eyeglass lens that was discussed earlier) improve the M pathway, and if so, what color? A study in 1998 answered this question (Iovino, Fletcher, Breitmeyer, & Foorman). Previous research has shown that relative to white backgrounds, short wavelength (blue) backgrounds increase the processing rate of the M system, whereas long wavelength stimuli (red) decrease the processing rate (Breitmeyer & Williams, 1990; Edwards, Hogben, Clark, & Pratt, 1996). A sample consisting of 60 children and adolescents ranging from 8 to 18 years of age was used in the study. Participants read black-lettered text covered with either red, blue, or no overlay. The reading material included two standardized measures of achievement:

1. The word identification subtest of the Woodcock Reading Mastery Test—Revised (WRMT-R).
2. The Formal Reading Inventory—A reading comprehension task.

TABLE 1-1. Cross Section of the Human Eye

	YES	NO
Do you skip words or lines when reading?		
Do you reread lines?		
Do you lose your place?		
Are you easily distracted when reading?		
Do you need to take breaks often?		
Do you find it harder to read the longer you read?		
Do you get headaches when you read?		
Do your eyes get red and watery?		
Does reading make you tired?		
Do you blink or squint?		
Do you prefer to read in dim light?		
Do you read close to the paper?		
Do you use your finger as a marker?		
Do you get restless, active, or fidgety when reading?		

The results showed that the red overlays did not consistently impede or help. The blue overlays had a significant effect on reading comprehension but resulted in slower reading rates (Solman, Cho, & Dain, 1991). Improvement in reading comprehension with decreased reading rate may reflect the operation of other factors, such as increased attention to the text (Iovino et al., 1998). To give another side of the story, a study published in 2005 showed that reading-impaired children had significant gains in reading after wearing yellow filters for 3 months (Ray, Fowler, & Stein, 2005), the theory being that it improved the M pathway.

Does Color Help AD/HD Children?

Hyperactive children are viewed as being less tolerant of situations involving minimal stimulation, thus explaining their exacerbated symptomatology in overly familiar contexts. Added stimulation has been shown to be most beneficial for hyperactive children during those tasks that involve considerable repetition and monotony (sustained attention). Previous research had shown improved performance for young normal children by adding discriminative stimuli to letters (e.g., dots to b and p). This research did things such as widening the black or colored ink line of certain letter parts that had been documented to be important for legibility (e.g., closing tops of letters) in order to increase attention to this relevant letter detail. In a task that involved copying words, the added color greatly helped the AD/HD

children in the beginning, but by the second page of copying, the novelty had worn off, and the error rate was noted at their previous rate. It had no effect on the control group. It appears that color did initially help AD/HD adolescents perform better (Zentall, Falkenberg, & Smith, 1985).

Can Color Be Used to Improve Attention?

In normal children, this research showed that the P pathway (central vision) is capable of automatic attention capture. Hence, color vision not only aids target identification, but is also a strong aid for target detection and localization (Snowden, 2002). Therefore, color does seem to improve attention. In another study, it was found that by decreasing visual similarity between target and background items, there will be an improvement in performance for measures of reaction time. It was found that search time increased as a function of color size (number of colored items in the display) in comparison to using just one color. Therefore, using just one color (one time) helped in reaction time, but using too many colors slowed reaction time (Farmer & Taylor, 1980).

Is a Certain Color Better for Print Color?

Research has shown that the legibility of text was determined primarily by the luminance contrast between the text and the background rather than the specific color

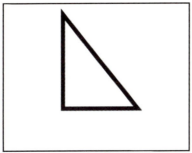

Figure 1-7. Base-left prism.

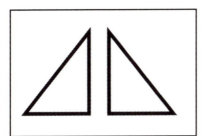

Figure 1-8. Base-in prism.

used. Therefore, except when the eye needs glasses, there is little evidence to suggest that wavelength should be an important variable for reading. On the whole, wavelength (color) only occasionally plays a significant role in reading. When it does, performance tends to be depressed either in red or blue and tends to be better in green and gray. These results were obtained by measuring observed reading rates for text composed of letters of different colors presented on a dark background (Legge, Parish, Luebker, & Wurm, 1990; Legge & Rubin, 1986).

Can a Colored Background Help in Attention?

It has been repeatedly demonstrated that processing at the global level interferes with local processing more than the local interfering with the global. In other words, you notice the overall shape of the object before you notice details in the object. The human M pathway is responsible for processing more global stimuli than the P pathway, which is more detailed stimuli. If a way could be found to decrease the global interference, it would be easier to detect and pay attention to the feature in which you are interested. Several studies have found that a red background decreases M processing and helps P. Therefore, if you want a child to more easily see and pay attention to a figure, a red background is better than white or green (Breitmeyer & Breier, 1994; Michimata, Okubo, & Mugishima, 1999).

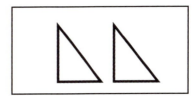

Figure 1-9. Base-left yoke prisms.

PRISMS

A prism causes light to change in direction. The change is termed *deviation*, and the amount of deviation is denoted by the prism power (strength). The direction the light is deviated is always opposite the base of the prism. Therefore, if you wanted to move a perceived image to the right, you would put the base to the left (Figure 1-7).

Because the image moves to the right, the child's eye will also turn right. We often use prism with strabismus patients whose eyes turn "in" or "out." For example, if you had a child whose eyes drifted "in," you would put base-out prism in front of each eye to move the light to where his or her eyes are deviated. This takes the stress off of the visual system by moving the light to where the child's eyes are drifting. Of course, to train this type of child, we would use base-in prism and train him or her to move his or her eyes "out" to help overcome the eyes turning in (Figure 1-8).

Most vision therapy deals with prisms that have the bases in the opposite direction to help train the eyes to move "in" or "out" to train binocular vision. OTs will not experience these types of prisms because prisms correct binocular problems and are prescribed by an optometrist. OTs will often see prisms with their patients but these will be yoked prisms. A yoked pair of prisms has their bases in the same direction called either base left, base right, base up, or base down (Figure 1-9). The goal of this type of prism is to shift the child's visual world either right, left, up, or down.

How prisms affect intersensory perception has been a subject of considerable interest. It is thought that when the body adapts to prism, it is because of a rearrangement of the eyes' control over the limbs and objects of manipulation (Cotter, 1995). For example, if a child has yoked prisms on and you throw him or her a ball, he or she will often miss catching it at first because the child is getting conflicting signals sent from the eyes and the rest of the body. After a short period of time, however, he or she will adapt to the prism and be able to catch the ball. This reorganization he or she is experiencing causes "learning." The brain had to learn to catch the ball when the visual signals were different than the kinesthetic and proprioceptive signals.

AMBIENT VISION

There are two separate visual processing systems. The first system has been called the focal process. Information is sent primarily to the occipital cortex for the purpose of seeing detail. If all we had was the focal process, the world would break apart into a mosaic of fragments. We would see only the lines, shadows, and shapes on a person's face, and although we would see clearly, we would not be able to recognize the relationship of all these details. We would only see parts, not whole objects. Approximately 20% of fibers from both eyes are delivered to the midbrain. Here, the visual process matches information with kinesthetic, proprioceptive, tactile, and vestibular information. This portion of the brain has been called the sensory motor feedback loop. It serves to organize spatial information about position and orientation. Information received particularly from the peripheral vision is matched up with these other sensory-motor processes for the purpose of developing concepts of midline, body position, and orientation. Once this is accomplished, a feed-forward phenomenon occurs. Information is relayed from the midbrain up to the occipital cortex, where it preprograms the higher-seeing areas to know how to look at visual information first spatially before focalizing detail. This is called the ambient visual process.

The ambient visual system is important for establishing the concept of visual midline. If the visual midline shifts, it will reinforce postural imbalances. Keep in mind that the ambient visual system, to a great extent, deals with our peripheral vision. Following a brain injury, cerebrovascular accident, multiple sclerosis, cerebral palsy, or autism, interference with function can often occur with ambient visual processing. When this occurs, information is received by the occipital cortex without spatial preprogramming. The ambient process has also been shown to reorganize visual function. Without this process, any movement will appear as detail and not only can become quite disturbing, it will directly interfere with our ability to maintain our spatial orientation. A person may find that any movement in his or her peripheral vision is overwhelming. It has been shown that sometimes a low amount of base-in prism with binasal occlusion (a vertical cover placed at the nasal part of each lens in glasses to force use of peripheral vision) re-established spatial organization in the ambient process, thereby influencing the wave form generated in the occipital cortex. There are a lot of optometrists who use base-down prism to treat such disorders as autism. However, base-down prisms are not a cure-all. We are all too smart to think that a prism will cure autism. Will it help? I think the jury is still out on this. Some people have had some success, while others have not seen any improvement.

VISUAL MIDLINE SHIFT

When an individual has a neurological problem that is affecting one side, the visual midline will shift, usually away from the affected side. In this case, the optometrist will prescribe prisms that can be used to counter the distortion of space caused by the injury and shift the midline to a more centered position. For example, if a person is leaning to the left and you want to center him or her, use base-left prism to shift his or her visual world right, thereby causing him or her to shift right. If a child constantly has his or her head down and you want to have him or her move his or her head up, put base-down prism in front of the child, and his or her visual image will shift up and cause him or her to move his or her head up.

EYE MOVEMENT AND ATTENTION

It is apparent that vision and action systems evolved together to enable successful interactions with the environment. The ability to extract information to guide goal-directed behavior, such as pursuit of prey or avoidance of predators, is fundamental to an organism's survival. Hence, massive evolutionary pressure has ensured that the most exquisitely efficient systems have evolved (Gazzaniga, 2004). One such system involves eye movements. You cannot separate eye movements and attention. Most early works studying links between attention and action have examined saccades. The premotor theory is based on two complementary ideas. The first is the notion that preparation of eye movements automatically involves shifts of attention. The second idea concerns the alternative relationship between attention and saccades; that is, orienting attention to a location automatically activates motor responses such as saccades to the location (even though no overt saccades need be produced). For example, one study showed that the trajectory of saccades evoked by stimulation of cells in the superior colliculus was influenced by the spatial location of the monkey's covert attention (Gazzaniga, 2004). There is a massive amount of information concerning attention and saccades (Bruce & Goldberg, 1985; Deubel & Schneider, 1995; Kingstone & Klein, 1993; Stelmach, 1997). These studies show that the process of making a saccade involves disengaging, moving, and re-engaging covert attention. There is no doubt that attention and motor programming go together. In fact, spatial attention can modify the trajectories of ocular saccades. The human visual system has two means to sample information from a visual scene—visual and attentional. Visual means moving the eyes to get the image in focus on the fovea. You can shift attention without moving your eyes, but you cannot make an eye movement without shifting attention (Kingstone & Klein, 1993;

Stelmach, 1997). It also appears that attention is required to select the information needed to determine the landing point of the eye movement (Deubel & Schneider, 1995). It does this by selecting the object of interest for perceptual processing and recognition. Without attention, there would not be any planned motor movement or any object recognition, and we would live in a very confusing world. If attention and motor programming go together, then it stands to reason that training one would also train and improve the other. This combination, I feel, has led to the success of many sensory integration (SI) and VT programs. Any therapy program should and must include a large proportion of oculomotor activities. Training the oculomotor system has the effect of activating many of the neurons in area 7 in primates (area 39 in humans) of the parietal lobe. These include fixation neurons and saccadic neurons. The parietal lobe, particularly area 7, contains a neural apparatus for the direction of visual attention to objects of interest and for shifting the focus of attention from one to another (Kawano, Sasaki, & Yamashita, 1984; Lynch, Mountcastle, Talbot, & Yin, 1977). This part of the brain is critical for spatial skills and eye movements and is stimulated with both vision therapy and SI therapy that involves eye movements and fixation training. It has also been shown that the parietal and prefrontal areas of the brain are critical for developing a child's inhibitory control. We often see that children who have attention problems have a difficult time inhibiting their responses. We see this with go-no-go training in which a child is trained to inhibit his or her response. The ability to suppress irrelevant information and actions becomes more efficient with age and develops from age 6 to 10 years. Children use the same neural activity as adults but are much less effective in inhibiting their responses. Activity in bilateral, ventral prefrontal cortex, the right prefrontal cortex, and the right parietal lobe increases during performance of go-no-go trials. These regions are involved in response inhibition (Durston, 2002). The parietal lobe is extremely important for most areas of oculomotor and other sensory functions. In fact, the parietal lobe should not be viewed as primarily a sensory or primarily a motor structure. Rather, it apparently occupies a location somewhere between these two points, integrating sensory information to be used for formulation of motor behaviors. Put quite simply, the area is involved in sensory-motor integration. This area has been known for years to be involved in the control of visual spatial attention (Giesbrecht, Woldorff, Song, & Mangun, 2003; Lynch et al., 1977). In fact, neuroimagery studies have shown regions of both the superior frontal cortex and the parietal cortex to be involved in spatial attention. Studies have shown the parietal cortex to be involved in saccadic eye movement, visual fixations, smooth pursuit eye movements, and visually guided hand projection movements (Robinson, 1978; Sakata, Shibutani, Kawano, & Harrington, 1985). The neurons in the posterior parietal cortex provide a

physiological mechanism underlying visual attention. The cells in this cortex are responsive to visual stimuli and are capable of dealing with visual events. They have a selective mechanism that provides a neurophysiological substrate of attention because it selects significant objects out of the environment (Robinson, 1978). Area 7 of the parietal cortex is also thought to provide information about the spatial location of objects, not their contour, orientation, or color. This region is thought to be involved in the combined actions of hand and eye within the immediately surrounding behavioral space and, more generally, with maintaining relations between internal bodily and external spatial coordinate systems. There is considerable evidence to suggest that this area (area 7), together with the cortical and subcortical areas with which it is linked, plays a role in direction of attention (Vandenberghe, Gitelman, Parrish, & Mesulam, 2001). It is, therefore, very important that any training program to improve attention stimulate this area of the brain. Activities such as spatial awareness, smooth pursuits, visual fixation, and saccadic eye movements must be a part of any training program. It is also important to know that visuospatial attention is relatively unaffected by age, and individuals up to 75 years of age can be helped (Greenwood, 1994).

CROWDING

Remember, there is a limit on how much we can see at one fixation. This is the result of the way the eye has evolved. The peripheral visual system (M) detects an object and directs our central vision (P) to evaluate the object.

If we think of a selection region as a region in space that has multiple objects that attract our attention, then the smallest selection region the brain can see and identify objects has to be at least five times the size of the smallest object we can see. This is if the light focuses directly on the fovea. If light focuses only 15 degrees away from the fovea (or 15 degrees in our peripheral vision), then the selection region has to be 30 times larger than the smallest object we can see. This is because of a condition called crowding. It is a reduction in acuity caused by surrounding spatial patterns (Schwartz, 2004).

Look at Figure 1-10. When we fixate the middle X of the middle row, the M to the right is easily identified. However, when we fixate the middle X of the top or bottom lines, the M is not easily identified due to the competition of other figures competing to be identified. This condition is worse if a child has amblyopia and reduced visual acuity. When we test a child who has amblyopia, we often use one letter at a time to find the true acuity. This condition is also worse when print becomes smaller and the letters are closer together. We see this often with children who have eye tracking problems and lose their place when tracking a horizontal line of print. Often, their reading becomes worse

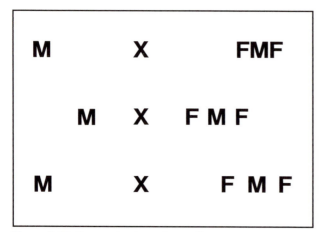

Figure 1-10. Demonstrations of crowding.

when they go from second grade to third grade because the print becomes smaller and closer together. In order to overcome this, the print would have to be larger than the normal print. Therefore, amblyopic children or children who have eye tracking problems should have larger and more widely spaced print. In the phenomenon of crowding, the inability to identify or even access the location of crowded items is more than just poor visual acuity. It implies a fundamental property for information the brain has stored and made available for selection. Objects available for identification are not stored as a picture. They are stored as a description. For example, a B would be a vertical line and two loops on the right. The problem comes when, because of crowding, the objects are close together and the brain does not know what to identify. If more than one item lies within the selection region, there may be no description of the combination stored in the brain that allows us to then break it down to access each constituent item individually. If two letters are in the selection region, for example, the result might be a description such as "letters," "some letters," or "some lines" depending on what is available. None of these allows us to recover the identities of the letters (Posner, 2004). Therefore, you can understand the confusion for a child who is just learning to read and who has poor eye tracking or visual scanning skills.

It has also been found that the lower visual field has better selection resolution and is better for attention than the upper. This is because the lower field is over-represented in the occipital parietal regions. The parietal areas that are involved for tracking and pursuit movements are closely linked to those for attention selection. A study showed that subjects could track four items with high accuracy if two of the targets were in the left field and two were in the right field. In fact, they were no less accurate in tracking two in each field than when tracking just two alone, either in the left or right field. This suggested that the targets in the separate hemifields did not draw on the same capacity. More importantly, when four targets were placed in the same field, either the left or right, performance plummeted. This implies that the capacity for tracking and the number of independent selection targets is limited within hemifields to about two per field (Posner, 2004). These studies show that, to help children's attention, you must not overcrowd the target area, and children may have better attention in the lower than upper visual field.

INERTIA

We have all experienced a young child watching TV and apparently ignoring everything around him or her. You get frustrated because you cannot get his or her attention. There now appears to be a reason for this type of behavior, and it is called attentional inertia. Most of the past studies with very young children were based on the child's ability to look at stimuli that were uninteresting. These studies showed that an infant's attention rapidly declines with repeated exposures to visual stimuli (habituation) and that young infants do not engage in visual attention for extended periods of time (Richards & Cronise, 2000). The key to these studies is that they used uninteresting stimuli. The results are completely different when interesting stimuli such as *Sesame Street* are used. These studies found that infants and young children became increasingly engaged with interesting visual stimuli within the course of a single look. In addition, over the course of a testing session, infants and young children may remain engaged with the stimuli, look durations do not necessarily decrease, and heart rate changes may occur (decrease). The inertia theory states that at the beginning of a look, attention is relatively unengaged. As the duration of a look increases, attention becomes progressively engaged. If a look survives beyond the first few seconds, attentional inertia begins to hold fixation toward the stimulus, and the probability of being distracted or looking away decreases, leading to extended looks. These studies have shown that during attention engagement, the infant or young child attends to objects in one part of the visual field and ignores others, whereas when attention is disengaged, the young child is responsive to the whole visual field. The attentional inertia model for television viewing is based on the hypothesis that each look consists of the aggregation of brief comprehension units of approximately 1 to 2 seconds in duration. According to this model, at the end of the first comprehension unit (about 1 second), attention engagement is relatively weak, resulting in a high level of looking away. The largest probability of looking away occurred in looks that had been in progress for 0 to 5 seconds before the distraction. Other studies have shown that distractors are less effective in interrupting looks to a television program if presented at least 15 seconds after the start of the fixation (Richards & Turner, 2001).

SUSTAINED INATTENTIONAL BLINDNESS AND ATTENTIONAL BLINK

"Your problem is that you see, but you do not observe," snapped Sherlock Holmes to his friend, D. A. Watson. The great English detective was making a point that often we do not pay attention to the obvious, even if it is right in front of us, because we are too interested in something else (Maslen, 2007).

> *It is a well-known phenomenon that we do not notice anything happening in our surrounds while being absorbed in the inspection of something; focusing our attention on a certain object may happen to such an extent that we cannot perceive other objects placed in the peripheral parts of our visual field, although the light rays they emit arrive completely at the visual sphere of the cerebral cortex.* (Reiso Balint, 1907, p. 1059)

Recent research on visual integration and change direction reveals that we are surprisingly unaware of the details of our environment from one view to the next. We often do not detect large changes to objects and scenes (changes blindness). Furthermore, without attention, we may not even perceive objects at all (inattentional blindness). Taken together, these findings suggest that we perceive and remember only those objects and details that receive focused attention.

We have all experienced a situation in which we are looking for someone in a crowd and cannot find him or her. You finally see the person, and he or she was directly in front of you moving his or her hand. My cousin did not notice the party decorations in his house when he came in from work. The entire living room was set up with balloons and party decorations, and he walked right through it. When we miss entire objects, this is called inattentional blindness. This happens because we perceive and remember only the objects and details that receive our attention. If we are attending to something else, we do not see what is right in front of us. It has been reported that observers often fail to notice large changes to objects or a scene from one view to the next, particularly if those objects are not the center of interest in the scene. Studies have shown that attention is necessary for change detection. For example, in one study, observers who were given directions by one person, later replaced by a different person, during an interruption did not notice it was a new person. It seems that without attention, visual features of our environment are not perceived at all (or at least not consciously perceived). In the most famous demonstration of inattention blindness, observers were to watch a video of a basketball game.

They were to attend to one team of players, pressing a key whenever one of them makes a pass, while ignoring the actions of the other team. After about 30 seconds, a woman carrying an open umbrella walks across the screen. (This was superimposed on the others so that all the events were partially transparent). She is visible for approximately 4 seconds before walking to the far end of the screen. The game then continues for another 25 seconds before the tape is stopped. Of 28 observers, only six reported the presence of the woman with the umbrella, even when questioned directly after the task. These cases led to the conclusion that observers often do not see unanticipated objects and events and that attention plays a critical role in perception and in representation. Without attention, we often do not see unanticipated events, and even with attention, we cannot encode and retain all of the details of what we see (Simons & Chabris, 1999).

CHANGE BLINDNESS

Studies have shown that relatively little visual information is preserved from one view to the next, which asks the question: Do we store a detailed visual representation in the brain from one view to the next? In order for the brain to form an accurate, stable representation of our visual world, we must somehow extract the invariant structure of the world from our everchanging sensory experiences. For example, as we view scenes in the real world, we move our eyes (saccades). Because we move our eyes and pause for fixations, objects in the world are projected onto different parts of the retina. Somehow, we integrate information across these fixations to achieve a stable representation. We must recognize that two consecutive views are of the same scene, even when the viewpoint or viewing angle differs. Studies have shown a large amount of "change blindness." Observers do not appear to retain many visual details from one view to the next. Somehow, visual integration in the real world must accommodate changes to our eyes, head, and body positions. In order for this visually to be integrated, stimuli presented in two different fixations must be integrated visually. That is, our visual system must determine that an object is the same even when it stimulates different areas of the retina on consecutive fixations (Simons & Levin, 1997). But, is the visual form of an object integrated across fixations? They have found the same results as change blindness across blinks when they changed the object being viewed very quickly (temporal change) (Luck, Vogel, & Shapiro, 1996). Visual scenes contain far more information than we can consciously perceive at any given instant. Information that does reach visual awareness is selected by an attentional system. However, our attentional capacities are limited, and as a result the cost of attention selection to a visual stimulus can be functional blindness to other unattended stimuli. Any distraction that the brain experiences because of its limited processing capacity to select targets among distractors will limit awareness of visual stimuli. The brain cannot and does not have the capacity to remember exact details from one fixation to the next. That would overload our processing capacities and, as William James said, would create a "blooming, buzzing state of confusion." In contrast, a system that only integrates the gist (and perhaps the layout and movement direction) from one view to the next would give the impression of stability rather than chaos (Simons & Chabris, 1999). By not preserving too much detailed information, the brain experiences continuity. An experiment was performed when observers had to read lines of text that alternated case with each letter (some upper- and some lowercase). During some saccades, every letter in the sentence changed case, so that the visual form of every word was different. Surprisingly, when the changes occurred during eye movement (so they did not detect them), subjects almost never noticed the changes. That is, the subjects not only failed to integrate the visual form of the letters from one instant to the next, they could not even tell that the visual form was changing. Apparently, the information integrated across fixations during reading is not contingent on the precise visual form of the word (Simons & Chabris, 1999).

What does this information tell us about children?

1. Attention is critical. Even short periods of daydreaming or having your mind on something else such as a toy or older children texting will cause a failure to notice important events.

2. We fail to notice changes in scenes that do not produce motion on the retina. Therefore, use something like hand movements to direct attention or change your position. Do not just stand still or sit—get up and "move."

3. When observers are not searching for a change, they usually do not detect a change. So, inform them to be aware that a change is coming.

4. People tend to notice changes in events that pertain to what they are expected to see. If they expect to see a construction worker with a hard hat, then they will notice a construction worker without a hard hat. If a child expects to see and remember a toy with a certain feature, then he will remember a toy without that feature. In the case with the upper- and lowercase letters, they did not notice the change; however, if suddenly some of the letters were in color (e.g., red), then a change would be noticed.

5. To keep attention or to direct attention, use something entirely different from what is expected, such as color, movement, or verbally directing attention. Never assume the child has noticed the change. If he or she was daydreaming, he or she might have missed the entire gist of why you are showing him or her.

VISUAL ACTIVITIES

Binasal Occlusion

Area: Ambient vision

Materials: Glasses (or just a frame) with strips of tape in the nasal position of each lens. Try to put the tape close but not over the patient's pupil.

Procedure: The child should wear the binasal glasses for 2 hours a day to build up his or her peripheral vision.

Saccadic Memory

Area: Visuospatial memory

Materials: Pen light

Procedure: Stand in front of the child and have him or her fixate on your nose. Then, take your pen light and move it to two to four different positions and flash it once. The child is not to move his or her eyes until you tell him or her to. When you say move, he or she is to remember the locations of where you flashed the pen light and then move his or her eyes to those locations and then back to your nose. Start with two positions, and then work up to five or six.

Antisaccade

Area: Executive function

Materials: Two pen lights

Procedure: Stand in front of the child while holding two pen lights. The child is to stand by, fixating on your nose. Tell him or her that when you flash one of the pen lights once, he or she is to quickly move his or her eyes to the pen light and then back to your nose. If you flash one of the pen lights twice, he or she is to quickly move his or her eyes to the other pen light (the one not flashed) and then back to your nose.

SUMMARY AND ATTENTION TIPS

1. Smooth pursuit training—This is the ability to follow a moving target. This should be a part of all SI training and is initially done one eye at a time and then binocularly.

2. Saccadic fixation—This should follow smooth pursuit training. It involves having the child fixate between stationary targets, such as two pencils. This should be started one eye at a time and then binocularly.

3. If a child uses his or her right hand, he or she is faster finding a target on his or her right side.

4. A child will more likely be faster at picking up an object with his or her right hand if the object is oriented to the right.

5. Motion or movement stimulates attention.

6. A peripheral target will dominate over a central target for attention.

7. When a child raises his or her right hand, stimuli to the right side are more distracting than stimuli to the left.

8. Retention of primitive reflexes of TLR, TNR, or MR may not allow proper development of visually guided movement necessary for adequate visuomotor coordination and visuospatial concepts.

9. Blue overlays may improve comprehension.

10. Improve attention to a certain letter by adding a dot above it or by making it a different color.

11. Search time increases with the number of different colors you use. Too many colors slows reaction time.

12. Legibility of text is determined by the luminance contrast between the text and the background, rather than the specific color of ink used.

(continued)

SUMMARY AND ATTENTION TIPS (CONTINUED)

13. Processing at the global level interferes with local processing more than the local interfering with the global. You notice the overall shape of an object before you notice details. If you decrease global interference, the child will be able to pay more attention to details.

14. A red background makes it easier for a child to pay attention to the figure on the paper compared to a white or green background.

15. Train peripheral vision using binasal occlusion to force peripheral vision.

16. Training eye movement helps to train attention.

17. Train areas that affect the parietal cortex to improve attention. These are pursuits, saccades, and peripheral training.

18. Eye tracking improves with larger and more widely spaced print.

19. Lower visual field is better for attention. A child will have poorer attention in upper field.

20. The capacity for tracking objects is limited to about two per visual field.

21. A child is less distracted from watching TV if the distraction is presented at least 15 seconds after the start of the fixation.

22. Even short periods of daydreaming or having your mind on something else such as a toy or older children texting will cause a failure to notice important events.

23. We fail to notice changes in scenes that do not produce motion on the retina. Therefore, use something like hand movements to direct attention or change your position. Do not just stand still or sit—get up and "move."

24. When observers are not searching for a change, they usually do not detect a change. So, inform them to be aware that a change is coming.

(continued)

SUMMARY AND ATTENTION TIPS (CONTINUED)

25. People tend to notice changes in events that pertain to what they are expecting to see. If they expect to see a construction worker with a hard hat, then they will notice a construction worker without a hard hat. If a child expects to see and remember a toy with a certain feature, then he or she will remember a toy without that feature. In the case with the upper- and lowercase letters, they did not notice the change; however, if suddenly some of the letters were in color, (e.g. red), then a change would be noticed.

26. To keep attention or to direct attention, use something entirely different from what is expected, such as color or movement.

REFERENCES

American Optometric Association. (1995). Care of the patient with strabismus: esotropia and exotropia. *Optometric Clinical Practice Guideline.* St. Louis, MO: Author.

Anderson, R. A. (1989). Visual and eye movement functions of the posterior parietal cortex. *Annual Review of Psychology, 12,* 377-403.

Ayres, J. (1973). Sensory integration and learning disorders. Torrance, CA: Western Psychological Services.

Breitmeyer, B. G. & Breier, J. I. (1994). Effects of background color on reaction time to stimuli varying in size and contrast: inferences about human channels. *Vision Research, 34*(8), 1039-1045.

Breitmeyer, B. G. & Williams, M. C. (1990). Effects of isoluminant-background color on metacontrast and stroboscopic motion: interactions between sustained (p) and transient (m) channels. *Vision Research, 30*(7), 1069-1075.

Bruce, C. J. & Goldberg, M. E. (1985). Primate frontal eye fields. I. single neurons discharging before saccades. *Journal of Neurophysiology, 53*(3), 603-635.

Capute, A. J., Palmer, F. B., Shapiro, B. K., Wachtel, R. C., Ross, A., & Accardo, P. J. (1984) Primitive reflex profile: a quantitation of primitive reflexes in infancy. *Developmental Medicine and Child Neurology, 26,* 375-383.

Cave, K. R. & Bichot, N. P. (1999). Visuospatial attention: beyond a spotlight model. *Psychonomic Society, Inc., 6*(2), 204-223.

Ciuffreda, K. J. (2002). The scientific basis for and efficacy of optometric vision therapy in nonstrabismic accommodative and vergence disorders. *Optometry, 73*(12), 735-762.

Colombo, J. (1987). The stability of visual habitation during the first year of life. *Child Development, 58,* 474-487.

Colombo, J. (1996). Four-month-olds recognition of complementary—contour forms. *Infant Behavior and Development, 19,* 113-119.

Colombo, J. (2001). The development of visual attention in infancy. *Annual Review of Psychology, 52,* 337-367.

Colombo, J. (2004). The developmental course of habituation in infancy and preschool outcome. *Infancy, 5*(1), 1-38.

Cooper, J. (2000). Convergence insufficiency: incidence, diagnosis, and treatment. *Journal of the American Optometric Association, 11*(13), 82-89.

Cotter, S. (1995). *Clinical use of prisms.* Philadelphia, PA: Mosby Publications.

Deubel, H. & Schneider, W. X. (1995). Saccade target selection and object recognition evidence for a common attentional mechanism. *Vision Research, 36*(12), 1827-1837.

Dillon-Crunly, J. (1991). Evolution of the eye and visual system. New York, NY: The MacMillan Press Ltd.

Durston, S. (2002). A neural basis for the development of inhibitory control. *Developmental Science, 5*(4), F9-F16.

Edwards, V. T., Hogben, J. H., Clark, C. D., & Pratt, C. (1996). Effects of a background on magnocellular functioning in average and specifically disabled readers. *Vision Research, 36*(7), 1037-1045.

Eliot, L. (1999). *What's going on in there?* New York, NY: Bantam Books.

Farah, M. (2000). *The cognitive neuroscience of vision.* Malden, MA: Blackwell Publishers, Inc., U.S.A.

Farmer, E. W. & Taylor, R. M. (1980). Visual search through color displays: effects of target-background uniformity. *Perception and Psychophysics, 27*(3), 267-272.

Findlay, J. M. & Walker, R. (1999). A model of saccade generation based on parallel processing and competitive inhibition. *Behavioral and Brain Sciences, 22*(4), 661-721.

Fischler, M. (1987) *Intelligence: the eye, the brain, and the computer.* Upper Saddle River, NJ: Addison-Wesley Publishing Co.

Gazzaniga, M. (2004). *The cognitive neurosciences iii.* Cambridge, MA: MIT Press.

Giesbrecht, B., Woldorff, M. G., Song, A. W., & Mangun, G. R. (2003). Neural mechanism of top-down control during spatial and feature attention. *Neuroimage, 19*(3), 496-511.

Goldsmith, T. (2006). What birds see. *Scientific American, July,* 69-75.

Gonzalez, S. (2008). The correlation between primitive reflexes and saccadic eye movements in 5th grade children with teacher-reported reading problems. *Optometry and Vision Development, 39*(3), 140-145.

Goodale, M. A. & Humphrey, G. K. (1998). The objects of action and perception. *Cognition, 67,* 181-207.

Greenwood, P. (1994). Attentional disengagement deficit in non-demented elderly over 75 years of age. *Aging and Cognition, 1*(3), 188-202.

Heijden, V. (1992). *Selective attention in vision.* New York, NY: Routledge.

Hoffman, J. E. & Subramaniam, B. (1995). The role of visual attention in saccadic eye movements. *Perception and Psychophysics, 57*(6), 787-795.

Horwood, A. (2003). Too much or too little: neonatal ocular misalignment frequency can predict later abnormality. *British Journal of Ophthalmology, 87*(9), 1142-1145.

Indovina, I. & Sanes, J. N. (2001). Combined visual attention and finger movement effects on human brain representations. *Experimental Brain Research, 140*(3), 265-279.

Iovino, I., Fletcher, J. M., Breitmeyer, B. G., & Foorman, B. R. (1998). Colored overlays for visual perception deficits in children with reading disability and attention deficit/hyperactivity disorder. *Journal of Clinical and Experimental Neuropsychology, 20*(6), 791-806.

Irlen, H. (1991). *Reading by the colors.* New Hyde Park, NY: Avery Publishing Group, Inc.

Jacobs, G. H. & Nathans, J. (2009). The evolution of primate color vision. *Scientific American, 300*(4), 56-63.

Kaas, J. (2004). The primate visual system. *Methods and New Frontiers in Neuroscience.*

Kawano, K., Sasaki, M., & Yamashita, M. (1984). Response properties of neurons in posterior parietal cortex of monkey during visual-vestibular stimulation I. Visual tracking neurons. *Journal of Neurophysiology, 51*(2), 340-351.

Kingstone, A. & Klein, R. M. (1993). Visual offsets facilitate saccadic latency: Does predisengagement of visuospatial attention mediate this gap effect? *Journal of Experimental Psychology, 19*(6), 1251-1265.

Knoblauch, K., Arditi, A., & Szlyk, J. (1991). Effects of chromatic and luminance contrast on reading. *Journal of the Optical Society of America, 8*(2), 428-439.

Kowler, E. (1994). The rule of attention in the programming of saccades. *Vision Research, 35*(13), 1897-1916.

Lawson, K. (1992). Maternal behavior and infant attention. *Infant Behavior and Development, 15,* 209-229.

Legge, G. E. & Rubin, G. S. (1986). Psychophysics of reading, iv. Wavelength effects in normal and low vision. *Journal of the Optical Society of America, 3*(1), 40-51.

Legge, G. E., Parish, D. H., Luebker, A., & Wurm, L. H. (1990). Psychophysics of reading, xi. Comparing color contrast and luminance contrast. *Journal of the Optical Society of America, 7*(10), 2002-2010.

Leigh, J. (1983). *The neurology of eye movements.* Philadelphia, PA: F.A. Davis Company.

Luck, S. J., Vogel, E. K., & Shapiro, K. L. (1996). Word meanings can be accessed but not reported during the attentional blink. *Nature, 383,* 616-617.

Lynch, J. C., Mountcastle, V. B., Talbot, W. H., & Yin, T. C. (1977). Parietal lobe mechanisms for directed visual attention. *Journal of Neurophysiology, 40*(2), 362-389.

Lyon, R. (1996). *Attention, memory and executive function.* Baltimore, MD: Paul H. Brookes Publishing Co.

Marcois, R. (2005). Capacity limits of information processing in the brain. *Phi Kappa Phi Forum, 85*(1), 30-33.

Maslen, G. (2007). Search for the center of attention: The eyes have it. *Brain in the News, 14*(7).

Michimata, C., Okubo, M., & Mugishima, Y. (1999). Effects of background color on the global and local processing of hierarchically organized stimuli. *Journal of Cognitive Neuroscience, 11*(1), 1-8.

Milner, D. A. (2006). *The visual brain in action.* New York, NY: Oxford University Press.

Motter, B. C. & Mountcastle, V. B. (1981). The functional properties of the light-sensitive neurons of the posterior parietal cortex studied in waking monkeys: Foveal sparing and opponent vector organization. *Journal of Neuroscience, 1*(1), 3-26.

Nakayama, K. (1990). The iconic bottleneck and the tenuous link between early visual processing and perception. Vision: coding and efficiency. In C. Blakemore, ed. *Vision: Coding and Efficiency.* Cambridge, UK: Cambridge University Press; 441-422.

Nash, J. M. (1997, February). Fertile minds. *Time Magazine.* Retrieved from http://www.time.com/time/magazine/article/0,9171,985854,00.html.

Nelson, L. (2005). *Pediatric ophthalmology.* Philadelphia, PA: Lippincott Williams & Williams.

Nobre, A., Gitelman, D. R., Dias, E. C., & Mesulam, M. M. (2000). Covert visual spatial orienting and saccades: overlapping neural systems. *Neuroimage, 11*(3), 210-216.

Patel, N. (2004). The use of frequency doubling technology to determine magnocellular pathway deficiencies. *Journal of Behavioral Optometry, 15*(2), 31-35.

Posner, M. (2004). *Cognitive neuroscience of attention.* New York, NY: The Guilford Press.

Ray, N. J., Fowler, S., & Stein, J. F. (2005). Yellow filters can improve magnocellular function: Motion sensitivity, convergence, accommodation, and reading. *Annals of the New York Academy of Sciences, 1039,* 283-293.

Richards, J. E. & Cronise, K. (2000). Extended visual fixation in the early preschool years: look duration, heart rate changes, and attentional inertia. *Child Development, 71*(3), 602-620.

Richards, J. E. & Holley, F. B. (1999). Infant attention and the development of smooth pursuit tracking. *Developmental Psychology, 35*(3), 856-867.

Richards, J. E. & Turner, E. D. (2001). Extended visual fixation and distractibility in children from six to twenty-four months of age. *Child Development, 72*(4), 963-972.

Robinson, L. (1978). Parietal association cortex in the primate: Sensory mechanisms and behavioral modulations. *Journal of Neurophysiology, 41*(4), 910-932.

Sakata, H., Shibutani, H., Kawano, K., & Harrington, T. L. (1985). Neuro mechanisms of space vision in the parietal association cortex of the monkey. *Vision Research, 25*(3), 453-463.

Saxon, T. F., Frick, J. E., & Colombo, J. (1997). A longitudinal study of maternal interactional styles and infant visual attention. *Merrill-Palmer Quarterly, Jan,* 48-66.

Schall, J. (1999). Neural selection and control of visually guided eye movements. *Annual Review of Neuroscience, 22,* 241-259.

Schneider, W. (1998). *Mechanisms of visual attention: A cognitive neuroscience perspective.* Oxfordshire, UK: Taylor & Francis, Inc.

Schwartz, S. (2004). *Visual perception.* New York, NY: McGraw Hill Companies.

ScienceDaily. (2000, April). Ophthalmologists discover relationship between eye condition and attention deficit hyperactivity disorder. Retrieved from http://www.sciencedaily.com/releases/2000/04/000417095552.htm

Simons, D. J. & Levin, D. T. (1997). Change blindness. *Trends in Cognitive Sciences, 1*(7), 261-267.

Simons, D. J. & Chabris, C. F. (1999). Gorillas in our midst: sustained inattentional blindness for dynamic events. *Perception, 28*(9), 1059-1074.

Slater, A. M. (1998). *Perceptual development.* Oxfordshire, UK: Taylor & Francis, Inc.

Smith, F. (1994). *Understanding reading.* Mahwah, NJ: Lawrence Erlbaum Associates Publishers.

Snowden, R. J. (2002). Visual attention to color: parvocellular guidance of attentional resources. *Psychological Science 13*(2), 180-184.

Solman, R. T., Cho, H. S., & Dain, S. J. (1991). Colour-mediated grouping effects in good and disabled readers. *Ophthalmic and Physiological Optics, 11*(4), 320-327.

Steinman, B. A., Steinman, S. B., & Lehmkuhle, S. (1995). Visual attention mechanisms show a center-surround organization. *Vision Research, 35*(13), 1859-1869.

Steinman, B. A., Steinman, S. B., & Lehmkuhle, S. (1997). Transient visual attention is dominated by the magnocellular stream. *Visual Research, 37*(1), 17-23.

Stelmach, L. (1997). Attentional and ocular movements. *Journal of Experimental Psychology, 23*(3), 823-844.

Taylor, T. (1998). The disappearance of foveal and nonfoveal stimuli: decomposing the gap. *Canadian Journal of Experimental Psychology, 52*(4), 192-199.

Trobe, J. (2001). *The neurology of vision.* New York, NY: Oxford University Press.

Vandenberghe, R., Gitelman, D. R., Parrish, T. B., & Mesulam, M. M. (2001). Location or feature based targeting of peripheral attention. *Neuroimage, 14,* 37-47.

Wahberg, T. (2005). Can replicating primary reflex movements improve reading ability? *Optometry and Vision Development, 36*(2), 89-91.

Wetherford, M. (1973). Developmental change in infant visual preferences for novelty and familiarity. *Child Development, 44*, 416-424.

Zentall, S. S., Falkenberg, S. D., & Smith, L. B. (1985). Effects of color stimulation and information on the copying performance of attention problem adolescents. *Journal of Abnormal Child Psychology, 13*(4), 501-511.

Zipser, D. & Andersen, R. A. (1988). A back-propagation programmed network that simulates response properties of a subset of posterior parietal neurons. *Nature, 331*, 679-684.

SUGGESTED READING

Anderson, T.J., Jenkins, I. H., Brooks, D. J., Hawken, M. B., Frackowiak, R. S., & Kennard, C. (1994). Cortical control of saccades and fixation in man: a pet study. *Brain. 117,* 1073-1084.

Tucker, M. & Ellis, R. (1998). On the relations between seen objects and components of potential actions. *Journal of Experimental Psychology, 24*(3), 830-846.

Attention

We all take attention for granted; however, without it, we could not function. Our ancestors would not have survived because they would not have had any warning about predators. You would live in a completely scrambled, disorganized world in which you could not function. You would not be able to control motor actions such as eye or hand movements, and your environment would appear to be a kaleidoscope of confusion. You would not be able to tell if features in an object were part of that object or were connected to another object. Activities such as driving a car would be impossible. Looking at a page of print would appear to be a scrambled, disorganized maze of lines and curves. There would be no long-term memory because your short-term working memory is connected and driven by attention. Animals also have attention, but humans are different in that our attention is connected to top-down (cognitive) functions, not just bottom-up (lower brain areas) as in animals (Wolfe, 1994). Without top-down attention, we could cease to be human.

The neurons of the central nervous system are engaged in the following three operations:

1. Reception of sensory signals from outside and from within
2. Planning and execution of motor acts
3. Intermediary processing interposed between input and output

We all think of numbers 1 and 3 above as the main functions of the central nervous system; however, it is number 2 that has been the main driving force of the central nervous system throughout our human history. This also appears to be the main function of our visual system.

In the grand scheme of things, our brains solved the problem of attention by creating two visual pathways—one to peripheral vision (M system) and the other to central vision for further evaluation (P system). The M system alerts, and the P system identifies. If this system was not in place, the brain would be overloaded by all of the sensations it renews every second.

The brain and visual system are bombarded with stimuli. Synaptic activity is staggering: 10 quadrillion (10^{16}) neural connections per second. The nearly 1 million ganglion cells in the retina of the eye compare visual signals received from groups of half a dozen to several hundred photoreceptors, with each group interpreting what is happening in a small portion of the visual field. To build a computer to do the same processing as the brain would require it to duplicate a neural network of a trillion (10^{12}) neurons connected by 10 quadrillion (10^{16}) synapses (Kennedy, 2006). Something has to help the brain organize this vast amount of information, and this is attention. At the psychological level, attention implies a preferential allocation of processing resources and response channels to events that have become behaviorally relevant. At the neural level, attention refers to alterations in the selectivity, intensity, and duration of neuronal responses to relevant events (Mesulam, 1981). The work of attention is part of everyday experience. Orientation, exploration, concentration, and vigilance are positive aspects of attention, whereas distractibility, inpersistence, confusion, and neglect reflect attentional deficits. There is a strong relationship between attention and perception, memory, motor, and problem solving. It is what makes us human. While animals also have attention, it is our ability to add cognition to attention that separates us

Lane, K. A. *Visual Attention in Children: Theories and Activities* (pp. 29-60).
© 2012 SLACK Incorporated.

from them. To understand this, we need to talk about being human.

WHAT IS IT LIKE TO BE A HUMAN?

The following is taken from *The Cognitive Neurosciences III*, Chapter One:

The lack of detailed and reliable maps of human and ape cortex makes it difficult to compare the subdivisions of higher-order cortex across species; however, humans clearly did modify the internal organization of certain cortical areas, evolving distinctive patterns of compartmentalization and distinctive neuronal phenotypes. In addition, humans appear to exhibit greater degrees of hemispheric asymmetry than other primates.

To be sure, nearly everyone acknowledges at least one specialization of the human brain: its enormous size. Yet, it is by no means clear that we can account for our cognitive and behavioral capacities as a single consequence of brain expansion. We have no well-developed theory to explain how the tripling of brain volume in the human lineage in the 5 to 8 million years since humans last shared a common ancestor with the African apes relates mechanistically to our capacity for language, which is uniquely human, nor to our more general capacity for symbolic representation, nor to our ability to represent certain kinds of mental states. Humans do not merely think better than other animals; we think differently.

There is, then, ample reason to suspect that there is more to human brain evolution than just brain enlargement. Most of the difference in brain size between humans and great apes is accounted for by the expansion of the cerebral cortex. It has usually been supposed that this increase was not global but rather involved certain regions more than others, specifically the classical "association" areas of the parietal, temporal, and frontal cortices. Given its role in higher-level cognitive functions, much attention has been paid to the possibility that the frontal cortex, and in particular the prefrontal subregion, was differentially enlarged during human evolution.

The frontal lobe as a fraction of total cortical volume (about 35%) is at most marginally larger in humans than in the great apes. Some have concluded that the view that humans have an unusually or disproportionately large frontal lobe is mistaken and have suggested that the expansion of frontal cortex is not a hallmark of human

evolution. Whereas apes have brains on the order of 350 to 500 g, humans' brains average about 1,300 g. When we compare body size to brain size, we have far more brain than we should have.

The question is, was this brain expansion global, affecting all areas equally or nearly so, or was there differential expansion of particular regions? Two areas that can be readily identified in all primate species and measured with some confidence are the primary visual area V1 (also called striate cortex), Brodmann's area 17, and the primary motor area (M1). It is instructive that the absolute sizes of both V1 and M1 are very similar in great apes and humans. Thus, the primary cortical areas of humans are the absolute sizes one would expect for an ape of our body size. It is the higher-order associational areas that underwent expansion in humans.

It seems very likely that brain enlargement during human evolution involved primarily the disproportionate expansion of higher-order cortical areas, including the prefrontal cortex, which in humans comprises by far the largest portion of the frontal lobe. We can suppose that expansion was not limited to the prefrontal portion of the frontal lobe but also involved the higher-order parietal, temporal, and occipital cortices. The question is, was the evolutionary enlargement of the human brain accompanied by the appearance of new cortical areas? If areas really do have narrow functional commitments, it makes sense that evolution would instantiate new functions by adding new areas to the cortex rather than by disrupting pre-existing functions.

As sensible as this seems, there is at present no good evidence that humans do, in fact, possess uniquely human cortical areas.

In addition to the lack of direct evidence for new, human-specific cortical areas, there is a growing sense that some human-specific functions are represented in areas that have similar structures in other primates.

More recently, it has become clear that Broca's area in humans represents nonlinguistic movements of the hands as well as the mouth and that the same is true of the presumed Broca's area homologue (similar structure) in monkeys. Finally, the ventral premotor cortex of a monkey contains so-called mirror neurons, neurons that respond when an animal either performs a particular movement or views the performance of the same movement, and Broca's area in humans has been shown to be activated under similar task conditions (Figure 2-1).

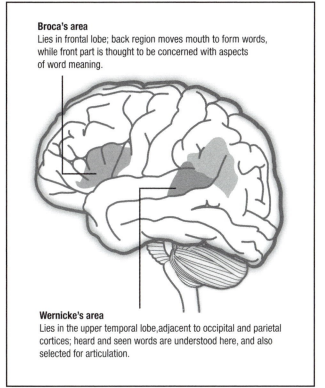

Broca's area
Lies in frontal lobe; back region moves mouth to form words, while front part is thought to be concerned with aspects of word meaning.

Wernicke's area
Lies in the upper temporal lobe, adjacent to occipital and parietal cortices; heard and seen words are understood here, and also selected for articulation.

Figure 2-1. Location of Broca's and Wernicke's areas.

The case has also been made that nonhuman primates possess homologues of posterior language areas, specifically Wernicke's area and the supramarginal and angular gyri. Although the argument is somewhat less well developed than that for Broca's area, the form of the argument is the same: homologies between human and nonhuman areas based on similarities in location within the cortical mantle (relative to better established areas), similarities in architectonic (same type of architecture) appearance, and similarities in nonlinguistic functions. Human cognitive specializations are not limited to language. Behavioral and neuropsychological evidence suggests that humans have specialized ways of representing the behavioral interactions of physical objects, such as the manner of action of tools on other objects in the environment and specialized representations of the manual actions involved in tool use. These functions probably involve portions of the superior temporal cortex in the case of object interactions and subdivisions of posterior parietal cortex and ventral premotor cortex in the case of tool manipulation. There is, however, no evidence that the emergence of these new functions entailed the emergence of new cortical areas; in fact, two of the areas that are crucially involved in manipulation, the ventral intraparietal (VIP) area and the posterior ventral

premotor (F4) area, are well-known in macaque monkeys. In this instance, as in the case of language, there is some indication that the emergence of functional specialization was accompanied by hemispheric specialization rather than the evolution of a new area; tool manipulation activates the cortex of the left hemisphere whether the manipulations are made with the right or the left hand. Given the evidence summarized above, it is clear that we need to take seriously the possibility that evolution has modified the functions of the human brain at least in part by modifying the organization of existing areas rather than (or in addition to) adding new cortical areas.

Homo sapiens have been referred to, with justice, as the "the lopsided ape." One of the strangest things about humans is that for most activities that involve the use of a hand, a large majority of the members of our species will spontaneously use the right hand, which is mainly under the control of the left hemisphere. In contrast, while individual apes and monkeys may show a preference for one hand or the other in a particular activity, the preference is typically modest, and some may prefer to use a different hand for a different activity. Other aspects of human function are also strongly lateralized. In a large majority of humans, the left hemisphere carries out most of the neural functions involved in language. The right hemisphere is uniquely involved in aspects of visuospatial attention in humans, and, as a consequence, lesions of the right hemisphere are far more likely to result in hemispatial neglect than are lesions on the left. In macaque monkeys, in contrast, lesions of either hemisphere are about equally effective in producing neglect. The strong population bias for left hemisphere control over the hand and language in humans suggests that our lopsidedness is the result of natural selection for genes that influence the functional commitments of each hemisphere. There is one neural domain, however, for which we have enough information to begin to frame some hypotheses about human functional specialization, and that is the visual system.

The central-most part of the human retina is virtually free of short wavelength (S) cones, which is not the case in Old World and New World monkeys. The large, parasol class of retinal ganglion cells (which project to the magnocellular [M] layers of the lateral geniculate) have much larger dendritic fields in humans than in macaques, although the dendritic fields of midget cells (which project to the parvocellular [P] layers of the geniculate) have similar dimensions in macaques and humans. These anatomical differences suggest that humans should be more sensitive in the long-wavelength part of the spectrum than macaques and that humans and macaques should have different sensitivities to stimuli that activate the M pathway.

There is evidence for evolutionary change in the extrastriate cortex as well, changes that also involve the M pathway and the dorsal (or parietal) processing stream, which receives strong inputs from the M pathway and is involved in processing information about motion.

Humans also had several foci of activation in the posterior parietal cortex that were not found in macaques under the same viewing conditions. These results could be interpreted in several ways. Humans might possess additional visual areas in the parietal cortex that are absent in macaques. Alternatively, macaques and humans might possess the same complement of parietal areas. If the latter is true, we might expect that monkeys do not extract information about the three-dimensional characteristics of objects in quite the same way that humans do. This is not surprising, given the evidence that humans represent object properties and interactions in ways that differ from nonhuman primates. These results provide additional evidence that functional organization of the dorsal visual stream was modified in hominoid and/ or human evolution. This area is critical for our understanding of attention (Gazzaniga, Michael S., ed., The Cognitive Neurosciences III, third edition, 1200 word extract from pages 1-15., © 2004 Massachusetts Institute of Technology, by permission of The MIT Press.)

DORSAL AND VENTRAL PATHWAYS

The concept of dual pathways was mentioned in Chapter 1; however, due to its importance, it needs to be explained more in detail. There is a large body of evidence that shows that vision for perception and vision for action are mediated by two different pathways. The human visual system does not construct a single representation of the world for both visual perception and visual control for action. Instead, vision for perception and vision for action appear to depend on separate neural mechanisms that would be differentially affected by neurological damage. There is the ventral stream (P), which arises from the primary visual cortex and projects to the inferotemporal cortex, and a dorsal stream (M), which arises from the primary visual

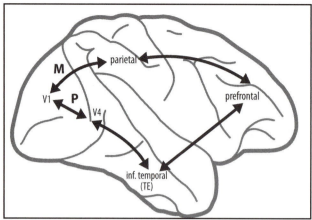

Figure 2-2. Ventral stream (P) and dorsal stream (M).

cortex but projects instead to the inferior temporal cortex (Figure 2-2).

One system (P) deals mainly with an object's features and the other (M) with the object's location in space. The P and M systems are not exactly the same systems as the ventral and dorsal systems. The ventral and dorsal systems are part of the P and M systems and start at the lateral geniculate nucleus. The transformations carried out by the M system (dorsal stream) deal with moment-to-moment information about the location and disposition of objects in egocentric (in relation to ourselves) coordinates and thereby mediate the visual control of skilled actions, such as manual prehension directed to those objects (Goodale & Haffenden, 1998) and eye movement to those objects.

The M system directs movement to the object, and the P system helps to identify it. The perceptual representations constructed in the P (ventral) stream are part of a high-level cognitive network that enables us to select a particular course of action with respect to objects in the world. The visuomotor network in the M system is responsible for programming the particular movements (eyes and hand) that are selected for action (movement). While similar (but not identical) visual information about an object's size, local orientation, and location is available to both systems, the two systems perform different functions (Brown, Moore, & Rosenbaum, 2002; Goodale & Haffenden, 1998). It is the M system with which we are most concerned when we talk about visual attention. It is also the system that has shown the greatest enhancement in evolution. By improving this system, we can improve visual attention. To stress the different functions of the two systems, the following story will help you to understand their functions.

This is the case of D.F., a young woman who developed a profound visual form of agnosia following carbon monoxide-induced anoxia. Even though D.F.'s "low-level" visual abilities were reasonably intact, she could no longer recognize common objects on the basis of their form or even the faces of her friends and relatives, nor could she identify the simplest of geometric shapes. If an object was placed in her hand, of course, she had no trouble identifying it by touch, and she could recognize people from their voices. Remarkably, however, D.F. showed strikingly accurate guidance of her hand and finger movements when she attempted to pick up the very objects she could not identify. Thus, when she reached out to grasp objects of different sizes, her hand opened wider midflight for larger objects than it did for smaller ones—just as it does in people with normal vision. Similarly, she rotated her hand and wrist quite normally when she reached out to grasp objects in different orientations, and she placed her fingers correctly on the boundaries of objects of different shapes. In other words, D.F.'s visual system was no longer able to deliver any perceptual information about the size, shape, and orientation of objects in the world to help identify them (P system). Yet, at the same time, the visuomotor systems in D.F.'s brain that controlled the programming and execution of visually guided actions remained sensitive to those same object features (M system).

There is no doubt that action upon an object requires that the location of the object be encoded. The cells in the posterior parietal region have this property. The neuronal properties of the posterior parietal cortex qualify it as the prime mediator of visuospatial attention. Many cells, especially in area 7A, are modulated by switches of attention to different parts of the visual field (Goodale & Milner, 1992). However, it would be wrong to assume that spatial attention is only controlled by the posterior parietal cortex. It is known that neurons in many parts of the cortex, including area V4 and the inferotemporal region within the ventral stream (P), are also known for attentional modulation.

The two systems of both the dorsal and ventral streams are parallel operations that control our everyday lives. Each system has evolved to transform visual inputs for different functional outputs. One is for action, and one is for perceptual identification. They are under the control of our attentional system, and neither would function properly without attention. Both of these systems are discussed extensively throughout this book.

The parietal cortex is the termination point of the dorsal stream. It performs a command function for hand and eye movements exploring the visual and somatosensory environment. Its neurons provide holistic command signals for the motor system and are active during saccadic and pursuit eye movements, and there are also fixation neurons (Corbetta, Miezin, Dobmeyer, Shulman, & Petersen, 1991; Robinson, Goldberg, & Stanton, 1978). It is also extremely important in several areas and not just spatial attention. Research has found the existence of a right frontoparietal network for sustained and possibly selective attention and a left frontoparietal network for the phonological loop component of working memory (Coull, Frith, Frackowiak, & Grasby, 1996). Parietal regions were consistently activated during tasks involving attention, spatial perception and imagery, working memory, spatial

episodic encoding (related parts), episodic retrieval, and skill learning. According to the working memory interpretation, parietal regions are involved in the storage of verbal information in working memory. This idea is consistent with evidence that left posterior parietal lesions can impair verbal short-term memory (Cabeza & Nyberg, 2000). It appears that the parietal cortex, especially the right side, is the site for interactions between different attentional processes (Cabeza & Nyberg, 2000). Its phylogenetic expansion rivals that of the frontal lobe. The posterior parietal cortex is situated at the confluence of visual, auditory, somatosensory, and vestibular unimodal areas. It is well positioned to mediate the type of sensorimotor and cognitive integration that is needed for spatial attention. It is involved in convert visuospatial attention, tactile exploration, oculomotor search, auditory target detectors, visually-guided, reaching-guided saccades, and mental reactivation of spatial maps. The neurons of the parietal cortex can be said to represent the extrapersonal world according to the motor output needed for grasping and exploring behavior. Some of the neurons can also use proprioceptive information related to head position to create a body-centered representation and vestibular information in order to create a world-centered representation (Mesulam, 2000).

The parietal cortex is equally as important as vestibular areas in any sensory integration program. The child who has the poor spatial and visual motor skills is in need of remediation in this area. To achieve this, any sensory integration program must include oculomotor activities along with vestibular activities. Using combinations of vestibular and saccadic fixations is a critical element in helping a child with sensorimotor and spatial problems.

RIGHT VERSUS LEFT HEMISPHERE

The right hemisphere is dominant in the control of, among other things, our sense of how objects interrelate in space. This is different from the right visual field (Figure 2-3). The left hemisphere of the human brain controls language. It also controls the remarkable dexterity of the right hand.

Biologists and behavioral scientists generally agree that right-handedness evolved in our ancestors as they learned to build and use tools about 2.5 million years ago. Right-handedness was also thought to underlie speech. They felt that the left hemisphere simply added sign language to its repertoire of skilled manual actions and then converted to speech. The right hemisphere was thought to have evolved by default into a center for processing spatial relations after the left hemisphere became specialized by handedness. There is now more research that supports the view that specialization of each hemisphere in the human brain was already present in its basic form when vertebrates emerged about 500 million years ago. The more recent specializations (like speech) of the brain hemispheres evolved from the original functions by the process of evolution. Those with this view feel that the left hemisphere of the vertebrate brain was originally specialized for the control of well-established patterns of behavior under ordinary and familiar circumstances. The right hemisphere was the primary seat of emotional arousal and was first specialized for detecting and responding to unexpected stimuli in the environment. It took primary control in potentially dangerous circumstances that called for rapid reaction; otherwise, control passed to the left hemisphere. In other words, the left hemisphere became the seat of self-motivated behavior, sometimes called top-down control. The right hemisphere became the seat of environmentally motivated behavior or bottom-up control (like reaction to a dangerous animal). The processes that direct more specified behavior—language, tool making, spatial interrelations, face recognition, and the like—evolved from those two basic controls (Macneilage, 2009). The right hemisphere is the critical hemisphere for the regulation of the attentional matrix. This is based on several sources. First, simple reaction times to ipsilateral (same side) stimuli are faster with the left hand (left hand-left side is faster). Second, patients with right hemisphere lesions are more likely to have bilateral deficits in reaction times. Third, in split brain, patients' vigilance is more effective when the task is being mediated by the right hemisphere. Fourth, patients with right hemisphere damage show less physiological arousal to sensory stimulation (as measured by galvanic skin responses) than patients with equivalent damage to the left hemisphere (Mesulam, 2000; Posner, 2004).

There is evidence that maintenance of the alert state is dependent upon the right-hemisphere mechanism and also that it is closely tied with attention. These two facts both suggest the hypothesis that a norepinephrine (NE) system arising in the locus ceruleus may play a critical role in the alert state. Studies in rats have shown that lesions of the right cerebral hemisphere but not the left hemisphere lead to depletion of NE on both sides. These studies support the idea that NE pathways provide the basis of maintaining alertness and that they act most strongly on the posterior attention systems of the right cerebral hemisphere (Lynch, Mountcastle, Talbot, & Yin, 1977; Posner & Petersen, 1990).

In humans, the right hemisphere "takes in the whole scene," attending to the global aspects of its environment rather than focusing on a limited number of features. That capacity gives it substantial advantages in analyzing spatial relations. Memories stored by the right hemisphere tend to be organized and recalled as overall patterns rather than as a series of single items. In contrast, the left hemisphere tends to focus on local aspects of its environment. Evidence for the global-local dichotomy in humans was brought to light by an experiment involving brain-damaged patients. They were asked to copy a picture in which small copies of

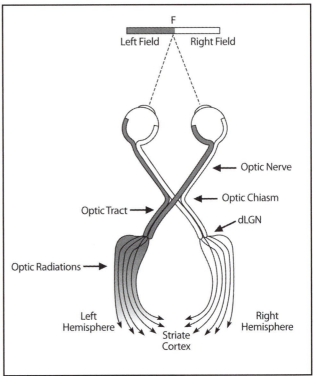

Figure 2-3. Right and left visual fields.

the upper case letter H have all been arranged to form the shape of a large capital H. Patients with damage to the left hemisphere often make a simple line drawing of the H with no small H letters included, while patients with damage to the right hemisphere see the H letters unsystematically all over the page (Macneilage, 2009).

These studies concerning the right hemisphere all seem to stress its importance in attention. We, therefore, need to do activities that stress this hemisphere to help improve attention. They would include using the left hand or foot, blocking the left visual field with occluders on glasses (Figure 2-4), or training saccadic and smooth pursuit eye movements. Also, when you are teaching the child, try to stay more on his or her left side, which will be processed more by his or her right hemisphere and will keep him or her more alert.

The right cerebral hemisphere is normally the more specialized for spatial representation. In touching pairs of nonsense shapes simultaneously, one with the right hand and one with the left hand, the one that was touched with the left hand is usually identified more accurately than that touched by the right hand.

Control of the attentional matrix by prefrontal and parietal cortices displays a pattern of right hemisphere specialization. Thus, sustained and divided attention tasks in any sensory modality elicit a greater activation in the right posterior parietal and prefrontal cortices. Furthermore, the posterior parietal or prefrontal lesions that give rise to confusional states are almost always located in the right hemisphere. Also, the ability to develop and maintain our

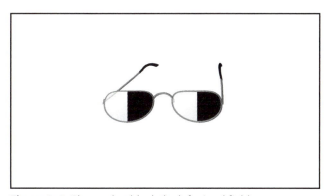

Figure 2-4. Glasses that block the left visual field.

alert state depends heavily upon the integrity of the right cerebral hemisphere. This has led to the notion that all spatial attention is controlled by the right hemisphere and right hemisphere damage causes difficulty with alerting. Performance vigilance tasks are also more impaired with right rather than left lesions (Posner & Petersen, 1990).

Numerous studies have demonstrated a specialized role for the right hemisphere in directed attention. These findings are based on three assumptions:

1. The intact right hemisphere may contain the neural apparatus for attending to both sides of space, although the preponderant tendency is for attending to the contralateral (opposite) left hemisphere (Facoetti, Paganoni, & Lorusso, 2000).

2. The left hemisphere is almost exclusively concerned with attending to the contralateral right hemisphere.

3. More synaptic space is devoted to attentional functions in the right hemisphere than in the left, so that most attended tasks involving either hemisphere will generate greater activities of the right hemisphere (Vidyasagar, 2001).

There is a slight tendency of the average person to pay more attention to events on his or her left side because the right hemisphere contains the mechanisms needed to maintain an alert state (Posner & Petersen,1990).

Neglect is a common and disabling syndrome following right hemisphere strokes. Patients with spatial problems often feel as if the left side of their world does not exist, appearing oblivious to stimuli falling toward the contralesional side. Neglect can be demonstrated by pen and paper tests. Patients with neglect after right hemisphere damage typically mark only some of the targets toward the left, missing leftward targets even with unlimited time.

A further difference from primary sensory loss is illustrated by a component present in many (but not all) neglect patients: perception extinction. Patients with extinction can usually perceive a unilateral stimulus (opposite side) presented alone toward the affected side but miss the same stimulus when it is presented concurrently with another stimulus near the ipsilesional side (affected side). The deficit seems to arise when two stimuli must compete for attention. Extinctions may reflect a pathological bias in spatial attention, possibly combined with some reduction in overall capacity. Much progress with understanding extinction has stemmed from relating it to constraints on attentional competition in the normal brain (Gazzaniga, 2004). It has been shown that patients with right parietal lesions frequently bisect lines too far to the right and fail to report left-most letters in a letter string. However, these effects are attentional and not in the recognition process itself. Evidence for this is that they can frequently be corrected by cueing the person to attend covertly to the neglected side. The cues appear to provide time for the damaged parietal lobe to disengage attention and thus compensate for the damage. It is also possible to compensate by substituting a word instead of a random string of letters. Patients who fail to report the left-most letters of a random string will often report correctly when the letters make a word. If cues work by directing attention, they should also influence normal performance. Cues presented prior to a letter string do improve the performance of normals for nearby letters, but cues have little or no influence on the report of letters that make words. Blood flow studies of normal humans show that an area of the left ventral occipital lobe is unique to strings of letters that are pseudowords or regular words. This visual word form area appears to operate without attention and thus confirms other data that recognition of a word may be automated as not to require attention, whereas the related tasks of searching for a single letter in a letter string do rely on attention. Automated word recognition would only apply to normal readers. Most first-grade readers only average a couple of letters at a time as they read words, and dyslexic readers are also processing one or two letters at a time; therefore, in these cases, attention is critical for word recognition. An inefficient M pathway to the right parietal lobe is often shown by poor spatial skills when the child has to draw the face of a clock with the numbers in the correct spatial position. The result is similar to a neglect patient because, often, all the numbers are on the right side of the clock (Figure 2-5).

Drawing the face of a clock is a good quick test to give a child to determine if an M system is deficient.

Another interesting study showed that speech produces lateralized interference on activities of the right hand but not the left hand. Because speech is produced in the left side of the brain and right-hand movement is controlled by the left side, the two can interfere with each other. It would, therefore, be inefficient for a right-handed person to talk and draw at the same time (Sheliga, 1995).

AREAS OF ATTENTION

Attention can be divided into the following five areas:

1. Focused attention—Basic responding to stimuli (e.g., head turning to auditory stimuli)

2. Selective attention—Freedom from distractibility (Sohlberg, 2001)

3. Divided attention—Ability to respond to two tasks simultaneously

4. Sustained attention—Vigilant maintenance of attention over time during continuous activity (Sohlberg & Mateer, 1987)

5. Shifting attention—The ability to shift rapidly to another area for attention

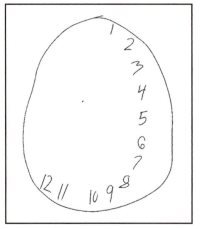

Figure 2-5. Neglect patient.

Focused Attention

This is the ability to respond discreetly to specific visual, auditory, or tactile stimuli. Focusing attention to a stimulus is similar or equivalent to increasing the intensity of that stimulus (Braun, Koch, & Davis, 2001). Therefore, focused attention is extremely important. It is the first order of attention and must be accomplished before any of the other attention areas can be activated. It is the first of the attentional factors of (1) focus—execute, (2) sustain, (3) encode, and (4) shift. It involves spatial orienting and depends on the posterior attentional systems, which include the posterior parietal lobe, the superior colliculus, and the lateral pulvinar nucleus. In order to have focused attention, the person has to be in an alert state. This is accomplished by activation of the midbrain reticular formation and of thalamic intralaminar nuclei (Kinomura, Larsson, Gulyás, & Roland, 1996). Many processes that help control focused attention are so rapid and automatic that the person is not consciously aware of these processes. There is abundant evidence that visual processes can flow automatically into actions such that actions can be evoked with little or no conscious intention to act.

Pre-Cueing to Improve Attention

It has been demonstrated that a spatial cue can increase the efficiency of processing visual targets. The reason is a shift of covert attention. There are many cues that can be used to direct attention. These include the brightening of a box around the areas where the target will appear, the onset of a dot, a horizontal line beneath the position where the target will appear, and a combination of target orientation and color. The greatest enhancements of visual processing occur closest to the cue. It is commonly believed that the spatial pre-cue directs attention to the probable location and produces some localized enhancement in perceptual efficiency regardless of whether the cued target appears alone or with some distractors. These cues are usually used directly before the onset of the desired target for identification. The reason why the pre-cue is so effective is the limited

pool of processing resources that can be distributed across a spatial region that varies in size. Perception processing is done in parallel within the region, with the quality of processing dependent on the amount of capacity devoted. The rate of processing is assumed to be faster with more capacity. When a target location is unknown, resources are evenly distributed across all spatial regions. On the other hand, when the target is indicated by a valid location pre-cue, more of the limited resources can be allocated to this region in advance, thus speeding up the processing. Experiments have clearly shown that the person's knowledge about where in space a stimulus will occur affects the efficiency and speed of detection. When trying to locate a target, knowledge about possible location in finding a target is more important than knowledge about its shape or form. Also, we do not have to use the central part of our vision (the fovea) to improve attention. Attention can be likened to a spotlight that enhances the efficiency of detection of events within its beam. Unlike when acuity is involved, the effect of the beam is not related to the fovea. A person's assumption that the fovea is closely coupled to attentional systems is a correlation he or she carries over from everyday life. It is usually appropriate because we move our eyes to those things in which we are interested. However, the fovea has no special connection to attention (Shiu, 1994). It is the M (peripheral) system that directs attention to the P (central vision) for it to identify the target. Because the visual cortex is organized by spatial position, orienting can be viewed as the selection of a position in space (Posner, 1980, 2004).

To improve a person's or child's ability to quickly attract his or her attention to an object, the most important aspect of helping him or her is to find a way to have him or her quickly locate the point in space where the object is located. Experiments do this by using cues that occur briefly before the target appears. In the real world, we cannot do this. However, cues can still be used (e.g., a laser pointer flashed at a particular point in space, underlining a word or letter with a colored line, an arrow pointing to the location you want him or her to look). Anything that you can think of to direct the child's attention in space will speed up his or her reaction time to the desired target. One experiment used large and small letters to direct attention. When the subjects attended to the large letters, they were more accurate in their attention. The use of small and large letters is a method of directing attention (Posner & Petersen, 1990).

With foveal attention, disruption is caused by nearby objects or letters. The disruption diminishes as the nearby letters are moved outward away from the target letter. It appears that the area that is best for focused attention is 1 degree (or about four letter positions on a page of print). Keep the focused areas of attention free from distractors—letters or objects. If you want to maximize a child's focused attention, keep distracting nearby letters or objects at least one degree away from the target letter. This is called angle of foveal vision (Wickens & McCarley, 2008).

The Visual Lobe and Useful Field of View

Unless a target object is conspicuous enough to be detected with global parallel processes, search will require serial scanning with focal attention. Exactly how focused, though, is focal attention? In other words, how big is the visual lobe? The visual lobe is also called the useful field of view. This is the area surrounding the point of regard from within which information is processed at each fixation. This is not to be confused with the angle of foveal vision and is often larger than the 4-degree angle visually associated with the fovea. As might be expected, the exact size of the visual lobe varies with stimulus characteristics and task demands. In general, the visual lobe is smaller when the target is smaller, inconspicuous, or appears embedded among distractors than when it is large, salient, or appears by itself. The visual lobe also tends to be smaller in older rather than younger adults and shrinks when the observer is placed under high levels of stress or cognitive load.

The size of the visual lobe affects search performance because it determines how carefully the observer must scrutinize the search field. A large visual lobe enables the observer to process a greater portion of the image with each gaze, ensuring that fewer eye movements will be required to blanket the field. Accordingly, visual lobe size is correlated with search efficiency. The good news is that the visual lobe can be expanded through training. In one example, workers who did industrial inspections were successfully trained to increase visual lobe size compared to untrained workers (Wickens & McCarley, 2008).

Selective Attention

This area of attention refers to the ability to maintain a behavioral or cognitive set in the face of distracting or competing stimuli. Individuals with deficits at this level (e.g., AD/HD children) are easily drawn off task by extraneous, irrelevant stimuli. These can include external sights, sounds, or activities as well as internal distractions (worry,

etc.). Examples of problems at this level include an inability to perform a task in a stimulating environment (Sohlberg, 2001). However, before there is a need not to be distracted, the individual has to decide what part of the environment he or she will select and direct his or her attention to it. The question is, what are the units of attentional selection? Does attention select spatial locations, feature dimensions, or whole objects or groups?

Location-Based Selections

Evidence that location often serves as the unit of attention selection comes from behavioral studies showing greater interference from distractors appearing near a target stimulus compared to those appearing further away (Gazzaniga, 2004; Kastner, De Weerd, Desimone, & Ungerleider, 1998). The one central resource for which stimuli compete seems to be the receptive field. Studies have confirmed that attentional effects of area V4 in the brain are much larger when target and distractors compete within the same receptive field than in any other configuration. If the desired targets compete for a response, then response time increases. If, however, a top-down clue (higher-brain areas) such as "the target will be in the center of the board" is given first, then there is less interference from other targets.

Feature-Based Selections

Behavioral studies in humans indicate that it is possible to select visual information by feature dimensions such as color or motion and that such feature-based selection enhances activation of cortical areas specialized for processing that feature. For example, subjects performed a color discrimination task on two separate moving dot arrays. The neural response in area V4 to the dot array that was not the target was higher when it was the same color as the target dot array, indicating that by being the same color, it would interfere with the target selection.

Object-Based Selections

Studies show that objects function as units of attention selection. A subject's attention will be drawn first to a complete object if it is in a mix of different features, such as color. Objects function as the units of attention selection over and above any tendency to select features or locations even when the task requires only selection of a single visual attribute. It is faster to find a known object, such as a square, than a color or line orientation.

Even when the target selection is guided by top-down control, the ability to find a target is still dependent on bottom-up stimulus factors, especially the visual similarity of targets to nontargets. For example, in Figure 2-6, the target is a large white vertical bar. This target is much harder to find in Figure A where each nontarget shares two properties with the target than in B where only one property is shared (Desimone, 1995). Also, a single inverted letter in Figure C is easier to find among upright letters than in D when you had to find the single upright letter. This is due to novelty

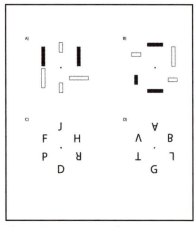

Figure 2-6. Example of top-down and bottom-up stimulus factors.

bias as the result of long-term memory. It is easier to find the inverted letter among familiar letters than the opposite. This implies that multiple objects have parallel access to memory and that familiarity is a type of object feature that can be used to bias attention compilation. Your attention is going to be drawn to something that is familiar. For example, in a noisy room, your attention can be attracted by the sound of one's own name spoken nearby. Similarly, long practice with one set of visual targets makes them hard to ignore when they are subsequently made irrelevant. Thus, the top-down selection bias of a current task can sometimes be overturned by information of long-term or general significance (Desimone, 1995). A child's attention, for example, will be drawn to his or her mother in a room full of people instead of paying attention to the teacher.

The importance of selectivity becomes clear when one considers the severe capacity limitations that characterize humans—we can only be conscious of a small part of the information that is picked up by the eyes as they scan a scene. Our ability to make visually guided actions is similarly limited to one of a few objects at a time. Without selective attention, we would not be able to function. During visual perception and recognition, our eyes move and successively fixate at the most salient parts of an image. Simultaneously, the mechanism of visual attention chooses the next eye position using the information extracted from our peripheral vision. Thus, our eyes actively perform problem-oriented selection and processing of information from the visible world under the control of visual attention (Paletta, 2007). The question is, then, what can be encoded (taken and stored) from each selected region? Many studies have shown that only the features of the target object are selected initially and not the features of other objects even though they are at the same location. Subjects were asked to track the features of one or both targets taken from *Principles of Visual Attention* by Bundesen and Habekost (2008), as they changed their orientations, colors, and bar widths over time. The subjects could keep track of the features of one of the two objects, accurately reporting any abrupt changes in two properties (the target's orientation and color). However, they could not track the properties of both objects at the same location even though they still had to report only the changes in two features (the orientation of one and the color of the other). These results suggest not only that the information available at a location is limited to the features of the target object but also that only one object can be selected at a given location (Desimone, 1995; Posner, 2004).

All of these studies show the severe limitations of our attentional system. We were not developed to identify several objects at a given location. This is why selected attention is one of the biggest problems with dyslexic children. If their attention is not completely on the reading material, then the reading material does not get processed, and their comprehension and reading speed suffer.

One of the best ways to help children is to limit the number of competing features. Studies have shown an increase of 50 msec in target detection time for each similar nontarget added to a display. Crowded printing is going to slow down a young child's reading speed. This is called biased competition. Some kind of short-term description of the information the brain uses to find the target is in short-term memory to help against biased competition, so that it will only be looking for that particular target. For example, in finding the letter "b," the brain knows that a "b" has a loop at the lower right side. This short-term description has been called the attentional template. It is one aspect of working memory. Thus, the time it takes to find the target may be independent of the number of nontargets if the nontargets are not similar to the target. If they are similar, then more targets add to the time to find the real target (Desimone, 1995).

Divided Attention

Divided attention requires a person to engage in more than one attentional task at a time. We have already stressed that we were not developed to do this, and it is very difficult to share our attention. An experiment was conducted to show the difficulty of making judgments on two different objects. Subjects were presented with small displays, each consisting of two overlapping objects (a box with a line struck through) (Figure 2-7).

The task was either (a) to report one aspect of one of the objects (e.g., the tilt of the line), (b) to report two aspects of one of the objects (e.g., tilt and texture of the line), or (c) to report one aspect of one object and one aspect of the other object (e.g., the tilt of the line and the size of the box). It was found that the performance in condition (c) was inferior to the performance in conditions (a) and (b). There is a real negative difference when a person has to attend to two or more objects rather than one. It seems that different features of the same object can be recognized without interference, but features of different objects cannot (Bundesen

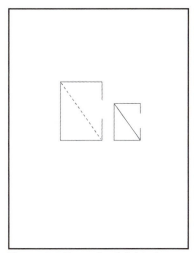

Figure 2-7. Example of divided attention.

& Habekost, 2008). This is a direct result of visual attention and is the result of the design of the eye and the fovea being the area that light has to focus. This need to focus attention to attain maximal sensitivity explains why it takes longer to find an object mixed with a lot of other similar objects. The person has to use serial visual processing and attend to each object in sequence rather than look at all of the objects at the same time.

While multitasking with two things at once is difficult, science now knows that multitasking with three things is extremely difficult. Research has shown that humans have a hard time making choices between more than two things, and previous work has indicated that people like binary choices, or decisions between two things. They have difficulty when decisions involve more than two choices.

When faced with three or more choices, subjects do not appear to evaluate them rationally; they simply start discarding choices until they get back to a binary choice. This is because, when faced with two tasks, a part of the brain known as the medical prefrontal cortex (MFC) divides so that half of it focuses on one task and the other half on the other task. This division of labor allows a person to keep track of two tasks pretty readily, but if you add a third, things get difficult.

A number of different metaphors have been used to describe the manner in which attention is distributed in visual space. One such metaphor is that attention is like a spotlight and acts in the same way as a spotlight might be used to illuminate an actor on a stage. All events within the spotlight are processed, whereas the events that fall out of the spotlight beam are ignored. Some have suggested that visual attention is like a zoom lens on a camera. Thus, attention can either be focused on a small region of space or alternatively focused on a large region of space. Models that employ these metaphors assume that attention cannot be simultaneously allocated to noncontiguous areas of the visual field (Schneider, 1998). The following are some

examples of situations when a person can attend to one part of the visual field but also discriminate visual information in another part:

- Essentially, visual search appears to be serial (one at a time) for targets and nontargets that exhibit highly similar features or if feature differences among nontargets are large enough to obscure any differences between targets and nontargets. Within a spatial range, similar visual features mask each other, and this effect is compounded in a dense or crowded visual location. A stimulus that is very easy to detect is called a "pop-out" stimulus, in that it possesses a feature (color, shape, motion, etc.) that is locally unique (i.e., is not found in other stimuli nearby). It has been estimated that the visual world is represented by approximately 30 visual cortical areas and that neurons in these areas encode a wide variety of visual information. An important component of the interactions between these neurons is inhibition between stimuli. For example, in area V1, the response of 80% of orientation-selective neurons to a bar of the preferred orientation is suppressed when similarly oriented bars are presented nearby. In the middle temporal area (MT), the responses of 40% of direction-sensitive neurons to dots moving in the preferred direction are suppressed when nearby dots move in the same direction. As a result of this inhibition from outside the receptive field, the visual cortical response to a given stimulus is attenuated when similar stimuli are present in the visual field. Attention is critical to counteract the inhibition.

- Visual responses to a stimulus are stronger when the stimulus is relevant to the behavior (e.g., when the child is carrying out a visual task with respect to the stimulus rather than where the stimulus is merely viewed passively). For example, a child will pay closer attention to and find a colored pencil when he or she knows he or she is going to use that pencil rather than just find a colored pencil.

- An object that is considered to be a "pop-out" object does not require attention because there are no competing objects. In Figure 2-8A, you do not need much attention to notice the X; however, in Figure 2-8B, you need attention to find the central X. In Figure 2-9, the F in the bottom row is easier to find than in the top row. It is possible that attention modulates visual responses indirectly by suppressing surrounding inhibition at the attended location. This would allow attention to protect the response to attended stimuli. Therefore, to improve a child's attention to the desired object, do not clutter the visual field with similar objects.

- As discussed earlier, one way to manipulate the distribution of attention across a visual field is visual cueing. Cueing effects are maximal at the cued locations and decrease with increasing distance from

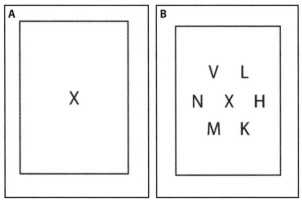

Figure 2-8. (A) Example of pop-out target. (B) Example of competing targets.

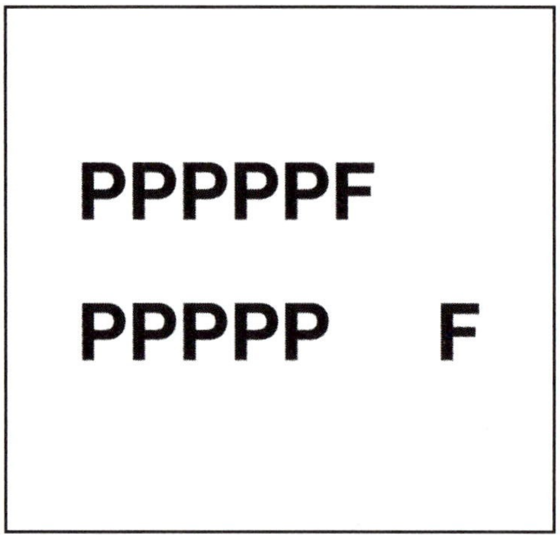

Figure 2-9. Example of pop-out target in bottom row.

that location. Cueing can enhance performance dramatically. It is more effective if the cue is presented directly before you want the child's attention to the object. For example, if you want the child to look at an object, use a laser pointer and flash the object directly before you want him or her to find it. You do not need to keep the pointer on. Just a quick flash will direct his or her attention to the desired location.

- Significantly shortened attentional dwell times were obtained when two stimuli were presented simultaneously rather than sequentially. This is the result of the idea that visual attention operates during the time of the stimulus, rather than later when the stimulus has already been committed to visual memory. A study showed that when four numerals were presented either simultaneously or in rapid succession (in this case followed by a mask), subjects were better able to identify and remember the numerals that were presented simultaneously. This suggests that attention can more readily be divided between simultaneous rather than sequential stimuli. Therefore, if you want a child to remember four numbers, it is better if you put all four numbers on a sheet of paper rather than to show him or her the numbers one at a time.

- All experiments have shown that not all tasks require visual attention in equal amounts. In particular, pop-out targets appear to be a privileged kind of visual stimulus, the detection of which requires relatively little attention even when the pop-out is outside the person's visual focused area. If you want the child to detect two stimuli simultaneously, make the one in his or her peripheral vision unique. The peripheral target will not require much attentional effort.

- Studies show that complex figures such as letter identification will not be discriminable outside the attentional focus. You can discriminate visual form, but not detail, outside the attentional focus. It appears

that parallel attentional mechanisms contribute certain types of information to the observer's visual experience (Parasuraman, 2000). To put it another way, your peripheral vision can contribute to the visual experience as long as it fills the role of a pop-out target. You can identify a target's color, orientation, and location in your peripheral vision, but not the target's fine details, such as connecting lines or other detailed parts. For example, when you read, your peripheral vision identifies shapes and spacing between words, not the identity of words. When several stimuli are in your peripheral vision, the most that can pop out simultaneously is two. Do not expect a child to pay attention to more than two targets in his or her peripheral vision, and do not expect him or her to quickly identify them.

Sustained Attention

Sustained attention is the ability to maintain a consistent behavioral response during continuous or repetitive activity (Sohlberg, 2001). Attention deficit disorder is an excellent example of a malfunctioning of this system. Sustained attention is the opposite of attention shifting and is a situation in which subjects must maintain an attentive state for minutes or longer. It is also called vigilance. Radar operators in a darkened room often perform normally for 1 hour or longer before they begin to slow the vigilance decrement that is seen as the hallmark of this attentional system. Clinical interest in this form of attention is high because deficits in it occur in many disorders, including epilepsy, closed head injury, hyperactivity, neglect, and schizophrenia (Parasuraman, 2000).

The development of smooth pursuit and saccadic eye movements is closely related to the development of sustained attention. Smooth pursuit eye movements continue to develop through infancy and childhood into adulthood.

At birth, a reflexive saccade system, relatively unaffected by attention, dominates the control of eye movement. This explains the predominance of saccadic tracking of stimuli during the first 6 to 8 weeks. After about 2 months, instead of a reflexive system, the smooth pursuit and saccadic eye movement systems involve areas of the brain, such as the posterior parietal cortex and medial temporal areas that are affected by attention (Richards & Holley, 1999). Most of the children that I have seen have very poor pursuit movement at age 5 but become much better as they get older. Poor pursuit movements are a sign of poor attention and are very common with dyslexic children.

Vigilant attention can be impaired though administration of drugs (e.g., clonidine) that inhibit noradrenaline release. One study showed that noradrenaline suppression in humans led to vigilant attention lapses, but also showed that this effect was much attenuated when the participants were exposed to loud white noise while performing the task. Another study showed that clonidine-induced noradrenergic suppression impaired vigilant attention performance much more if the task was familiar than when it was unfamiliar (Gazzaniga, 2004).

Arousal has been defined as "some level of nonspecific neuronal excitability" (Gazzaniga, 2004). The English word for arousal is generally translated as *vigilance* in French and *vigilanz* in German. It refers to a general state of wakefulness (Parasuraman, 2000). If our mind wanders, we are not in an alert state. On the average, students have reported that their minds wandered four to five times in a 45-minute session. Each of us has billions of neurons in our head. Yet, we find it difficult to stay focused for more than a few minutes during even the easiest tasks, despite the fact that we make mistakes whenever we drift away. Some people now find that mind wandering is not useless mental static. It may allow us to work through some important thinking. Our brains process information to reach goals, but some of these goals are immediate while others are in the future. Somehow, we have evolved a way to switch between handling the here and now and contemplating long-term objectives. It may be no coincidence that most of the thoughts that people have during mind wandering have to do with the future (Zimmer, 2009). The problem, of course, is when our mind wandering can put us in a dangerous situation, such as going through a stop sign or, in the case of children, not learning in the classroom. The ability to suppress irrelevant information and actions becomes more efficient with age. There is definitely a decrease with susceptibility to interference with age, and the ability to override a salient response develops with age. There is continued maturation of circuitry underlying the development of inhibitory control from ages 6 to 10 (Durston, 2002).

It has recently been proposed that there are three interacting networks mediating different aspects of attention: a posterior attention system composed of parietal cortex, superior colliculus, and the pulvinar that is concerned with spatial attention; an anterior system centered on the anterior cingulate in the medial frontal lobe that mediates target detection and executive control; and a vigilance system consisting of the right frontal lobe and brainstem nuclei, principally the noradrenergic nucleus locus coerulus (LC). It is also suggested that the vigilance system was right lateralized due to greater innervation of the right hemisphere by ascending noradrenergic pathways (Aston-Jones, Chiang, & Alexinsky, 1991; O'Connor, 2003; Parasuraman, 2000; Pardo, Fox, & Raichle, 1991; Robertson, Tegnér, Tham, Lo, & Nimmo-Smith, 1995; Sturm et al., 1999).

There is a strong connection between vigilant attention on the one hand and the activity of the noradrenaline system on the other hand. There is also strong evidence that noradrenaline has a stronger right than left hemisphere innervation, giving support to a particularly close relationship between the vigilant attention system and noradrenaline activity. The Yerkes-Dodson law proposes that any task will have an optimal level of arousal below and beyond which performance will decline and that this optimal level is lower in challenging tasks than in routine tasks. Stress can improve performance on routine and nondemanding tasks, but the same levels of stress can impair performance on more complex and demanding tasks (Gazzaniga, 2004). The right inferior parietal cortex has a role in the routine semiautomatic maintenance of sustained vigilant responding, whereas the right dorsolateral prefrontal cortex has a more "executive" role in maintaining the vigilant state. One hypothesis for what this executive role involves might be to engage/initiate the vigilant state based on a dynamic assessment of the optimal arousal level of motor performance to task demands.

Shifting Attention

The ability to rapidly shift your visual attention from one object to another requires saccadic eye movement and involves attention. Tests show that, within the frontoparietal networks that control saccadic generation, the frontal eye fields are critical for planning the saccades and the parietal cortex is critical for the disengagement of attention. Although saccadic programming includes covert shifts of spatial attention to the upcoming target location, "shifting attention" refers to the process of disengaging the mechanisms responsible for object identification so they can be used elsewhere (Heijden, 2004).

The preparation of eye movements automatically involves shifts in attention, and most evidence now supports a link between attention and eye movements (Gazzaniga, 2004). An example of how this system works is best explained by discussing reading and eye movements. At the beginning of an eye fixation, attention is focused on the word centered on the fovea. When lexical access of that word is complete, or when the present criteria of processing of that word are reached, attention shifts or moves to the next word. This shift of attention automatically initiates the programming of an eye movement to fixate the new attended location. In this situation, the completion of processing provides the signal for shifting attention, and the shift of attention initiates the programming of the saccadic eye movement (Heijden, 2004). The practicing of saccadic eye movements in training is also practicing the shifting of visual attention. When a child has to use saccadic eye movements to differentiate objects, the shift of attention always precedes the actual eye movement. An example of this is a concept called trans-saccadic memory. This states that information near the saccadic target is more likely to be encoded into trans-saccadic memory than other information in the display. The reason is that attention preceding the eyes to the saccadic target increases the likelihood that letters near that location could be encoded (Schneider, 1998). You can see from this that a child with poor attention would have poor comprehension. The child would lose some visual information as he or she moves his or her eyes across a line of print because of a decrease in attention to the word he or she is trying to read.

THEORIES ON ATTENTION

Wilhelm Wundt is typically given credit for having developed the first experimental psychology laboratory in 1879. At the end of the 19th century, it was argued that attention is essential for visual perception. However, it is William James' (1890-1950) views on attention that are probably the most well-known of the early psychologists. His definition of *attention* is widely quoted. According to James,

> *It is the taking possession by the mind in clear and vivid form of one of what seems several simultaneously possible objects or trains of thought. Focalization, concentration of consciousness are of its essence. It implies withdrawal from some things in order to deal effectively with others.* (Johnson & Proctor, 2004, p. 11)

The idea that concentrating one's attention on a particular object, sensation, or thought increases its mental clarity and vividness goes back at least to the beginnings of experimental psychology (Downing, 1988). There are, however, numerous theories on how attention is organized and how it functions. I am going to describe in detail two of the most-researched theories (1) the Premotor Theory of Attention and (2) the Feature Integration Theory (FIT) Before we discuss these theories, the following is a list of other theories on attention.

1. Selection for action view—According to this view, attentional limitations should not be attributed to a limited capacity resource or mechanism. Instead, the limitations are byproducts of the need to coordinate action and ensure that the correct stimulus information is controlling the intended responses. A recent application of this approach is the Executive-Process/Interactive Control (EPIC) model, which attempts to account for limitations in multiple-task performance in terms of strategic factors rather than in terms of structural capacity limitations (Johnson & Proctor, 2004).

2. Lower arousal versus upper arousal—Variables that negatively affect the state of arousal, such as time on task, noise, sleeplessness, and alcohol, reduce accuracy. Variables that are associated with a higher level of arousal, such as performance incentives and testing at a later time of day, improve performance. It has been found that children who have low basic arousal are impulsive. About 70% of these children (or adults) can be successfully treated with a stimulatory substance. When a person is given a stimulant, his or her arousal level is heightened. In turn, he or she becomes more selective and, therefore, less distractible. He or she also becomes less impulsive because impulsivity is strongly related to the capacity to inhibit undesired tendencies. It has also been found that sleepiness during the day is linked to AD/HD behavior, and children who snore face nearly double the risk of being inattentive and hyperactive. Caffeine improved the performance of high-impulsivity subjects, presumably by increasing their arousal to a more optimal level, whereas the performance of the low-impulsivity subjects was worse with caffeine, presumably because their arousal levels were already optimal (Johnson, 2004).

3. Filter theory—This theory hypothesized that attention operates to select information at an early precategorical level based on attributes such as the location of the stimuli or basic perceptual features, such as pitch or loudness. According to filter theory, a selective filter protects the information-processing channel from being overloaded by too much information. This filter, which is not for basic stimulus characteristics, such as location, color, pitch, or loudness, allows only some information to enter the system and excludes the rest. For example, when driving a car along a crowded street, one is usually able to concentrate on the traffic sign boards (which can be distinguished by location, color, or shape) and ignore signboards and other advertisements along the wayside (Johnson & Proctor, 2004).

4. Late selection view—This theory suggests that selection does not occur on the basis of an early selection filter but only after stimuli have already been identified. This view shows that attention is not needed to perceptually process and identify items, but it is needed to create a more durable representative of this information. That is, information that is not explicitly attended will be seen or heard, but this

information will decay rapidly in the absence of attention and will not reach the level of conscious perception (Johnson & Proctor, 2004).

5. Object versus location based—Visual objects can be described as the combination of simpler visual features (color, motion, orientation, texture, disparity, and location). Visual objects are encoded (stored) into object-centered representations that are derived from earlier stages of processing-related feature analysis. Blood flow studies have shown that directing attention toward features of objects independently of location significantly modulates activity in the visual system. Selective enhancement of blood flow occurs in extrastriate visual regions specialized in feature or object analysis when these features or objects are in the focus of attention.

Observers can attend to a location in an empty field, which is an example of space-based selection. Alternatively, an observer can attend to the location of an object. In that case, attention is distributed over the object and moves with the object, suggesting that the object, rather than an unrelated set of locations or a region of space, can be a unit of selection. The focus of attention typically changes every 200 to 300 msec, in conjunction with the execution of saccadic eye movements, but covert shifts of attention can occur independently from such overt shifts. Attention to an object produces selective increases of an activity in specialized processing regions of the ventral or object-oriented visual system. While the source of spatial modulation is the superior parietal cortex, the activity is sensitive to location information and to integration across features (Parasuraman, 2000). Therefore, it seems that attention to features or to objects amplifies relevant information in specialized processing regions of extrastriate visual regions. Regions in the superior parietal cortex select locations and object locations for focal processing stimulating activity in ventral (P) regions are related to object processing.

Experiments have shown that when deciding which theory, object, or location is more important for attention, attention is directed to perceptual objects that are formed by grouping visual elements, thus supporting object-based theories of attention and verifying the vital role of perceptual organization in visual selection (Yantis, 1992).

6. Theory of visual attention (TVA)—This theory states that selection of attention precedes on the basis of different stimulus features. Two things are selected simultaneously (a perceptual item and a categorization for item) and selection is seen as a choice among categorization of perceptual inputs. In this theory, location is a feature of an item just like color, form, and so on. The categories used in the theory can be basic qualities such as "red," "round," or "top-left corner" and can be applied to each feature of the stimulus. Attention to the object is then most likely to be allocated to meaningful pertinent information (Johnson, 2004). In essence, TVA describes a computational system that does the tasks of filtering and pigeonholing sensory input from a (front end) visual system and controls parameters from a high-level executive system. The filtering mechanism selects inputs while pigeonholing classifies the selected inputs (Bundesen & Habekost, 2008).

7. Early versus late selection—According to the late view on attention, the entire visual array is perceptually analyzed preattentively to a high level including identification of objects. Attention then selects a subset of this highly processed information for further analysis and response planning. In contrast, the early selection view holds that only rudimentary perceptual processing is carried out preattentional, and focused attention is necessary for objects' recognition and many other aspects of perceptual analysis.

Current literature indicates that attention can affect information processing even at the first stages of visual processing but that, under some task conditions, selection may be shifted to later processing stages. In terms of what attention selects, it can select regions of space, stimulus features, or whole objects (Gazzaniga, 2004).

8. The integrated competition hypothesis—This hypothesis rests on three general principles:

o Many brain systems—sensory and motor, cortical and subcortical—are activated by visual input. Within many and perhaps most of these systems, activations from different objects compete. A gain in activity for one object is accomplished by a loss in activity for others.

o Though competition takes place in multiple brain systems, it is integrated between systems. As a winning object emerges in one system, it also tends to become dominant in others. The general idea in this model is that, directly or indirectly, units responding to the same object in different modules support one another's activity, whereas units responding to different objects compete.

o Competition can be directed on the basis of relevant object properties. Undoubtedly, there are enduring or bottom-up biases toward objects that are moving or are bright, large, and so on. But, in general, it must be possible to select any kind of object for control of behavior, depending upon the task demands. It is suggested that task-specific selection is controlled by top-down neural priming. Suppose that a person is told to search for objects of a particular color. Units responding to that color are primed in one or more systems within which color is coded. Objects of the desired color then gain a competitive advantage in the primed system. In accord with the previously stated principles, as the object gains control in the primed system, it tends also to take control of others. The end result should be generalized ascending of the desired object in multiple systems, making its different properties concurrently available.

According to the integrated competition hypothesis, there is no localized system responsible for visual attention; even functional components have no distinct localization. Instead, selection of objects for the control of action arises through cooperation and competitive activity across multiple brain systems. At the same time, the hypothesis imposes severe limits on parallelism (doing two things at once). Integration severely restricts the ability of multiple brain systems to work concurrently on different tasks (Friedman-Hill, Robertson, & Treisman, 1995). For example, it is difficult to study and listen to music at the same time, regardless of what the child says.

Premotor Theory of Attention

Those of us who work with children on a daily basis realize the importance of motor training. When a child plays and exercises large muscles or pursues games and hobbies that build fine motor skills, he or she is strengthening motor synapses that are next-door neighbors to the neurons that manage mental behaviors, including attention (Healy, 1999). Brain mechanisms of attention were originally derived from evolutionary pressure on an animal to select one out of a set of appropriate actions. The ability to quickly choose one action pattern to be carried out to the exclusion of others confers considerable selective advantage. Possessing such an ability makes it possible to achieve a goal that would otherwise be interfered with by the attempt to undertake two actions simultaneously (Edelman, 1992). The main motor area that is critical for attention is eye movements. The premotor theory of attention states that attention allocation requires preparation of eye movements. There are no specific attention circuits and no part of the brain that is entirely devoted to attention. As far as spatial attention is concerned, it is the consequence of cooperative action of various pragmatic maps (for oculomotor, reaching, walking). In man, because of the strong development of foveal vision and the neural mechanisms for foveation, a central role in spatial attention is played by maps that code space for programming eye movements.

This proposal is known as the premotor theory (Sheliga, 1995). Evidence in favor of premotor theory derives from neurophysiological studies showing that those structures that are involved in spatial attention are also involved in motor planning. Studies have shown that when subjects have to redirect attention across the horizontal or vertical meridian, they have to pay an extra cost with respect to when they have to move attention. This is difficult to account for if attention is not related to motor programming, while it is easy to understand when one accepts the proposition that oculomotor programming underlies attention orientation.

There is no doubt that, in humans, the central role in spatial attention is played by circuits that code space for the programming of eye movements. Space is coded in a series of parietofrontal circuits working in parallel. There are three functional aspects of these circuits that are worth noting. First, none of them contain anything that resembles a spatial multipurpose map. Second, in each of them, spatial information is elaborated for specific motor purposes. Third, space is not coded identically in various cortical areas. The coordinate frame in which space is coded depends on the motor requirements of the effectors that a given circuit controls. Given this strict link between space coding and action programming, the premotor theory of attention postulates that spatial attention is a consequence of an activation of those cortical circuits and subcortical centers that are involved in the transformation of spatial information into action. Its main assumption is that the motor programs for acting in space, once prepared, are not immediately executed. The condition in which action is ready but its execution is delayed corresponds to what is introspectively called spatial attention. In this condition, two events occur: (1) There is an increase in motor readiness to act in the direction of the space region toward which a motor program was prepared, and (2) the processing of stimuli coming from that same space sector is facilitated. There is no need, therefore, to postulate an independent control system. Attention derives from the mechanism that generates action (Craighero, Fadiga, Rizzolatti, & Umiltà, 1999).

Several subcortical regions also contribute to attentional processing. The pulvinar nucleus of the thalamus may participate in the modulation of activity in visual cortices to enable filtering of irrelevant distractors. Also, evidence suggests that the cerebellum also plays a role in attention. Research has shown that the cerebellar cortex participates in the rapid sequential changes and adjustments of neural activity in order to proceed from one activity to another. The neocerebellum's participation in attention arises from the need to predict, prepare for, and adjust to imminent information acquisitions, analysis, or action. There is numerous evidence that the cerebellum supports memory for complex sensorimotor skills (Le, Pardo, & Hu. 1998).

Numerous studies have established that attention and eye movements are closely related. For example, during the preparation of a saccade, the selection of a location is controlled by the oculomotor system. Also, preparing eye movement toward a location enhances the visual processing of stimuli presented at the same location (Corbetta et al., 1991).

To further demonstrate the importance of preprogram eye movements, it has been shown that attention is oriented to a given point when the oculomotor preprogram for moving the eyes to this point is ready to be executed. Attentional cost is the time required to erase one ocular program and prepare for the next one. Several experiments have demonstrated that an observer is faster and more accurate in responding to a stimulus when it appears in an expected location than in an unexpected one (Rizzolatti, Riggio, Dascola, & Umiltá, 1987). This is because the oculomotor program has been prepared, and then the brain has to change it if it changes to an unexpected location. When a person attends to a given location in space, a program for a shift in gaze to that location is prepared. For example, when attention is primed to the right side, the eyes, although still directed at fixation, are "implicitly" shifted to the right. This facilitates the sensory centers located on that side, which, in turn, facilitates detection of stimuli located in that region of space (Schneider, 1998). Although shifts of attention are usually accompanied by overt eye and body movements, focal attention can also be aligned covertly in the absence of movements of the head or eyes. This supports the notion that attention allocation in space leads to an activation of oculomotor movement in spite of eye immobility; therefore, if the person thinks the eye movement is left, there will be a shift of space representation to the left before the eye moves. A conducted experiment had the person think the next eye movement was to the right horizontal target but was changed at the very last second to a vertical movement to the top right instead of what the brain thought was going to happen to the right horizontal. The result was a deviation slightly to the left for the vertical eye movement. This was the result of the erroneously remapped eye position. This error caused the slight contralateral deviation. This experiment proved that the eye plans in advance when it knows the intended eye movement.

The mechanism of visual attention chooses the next eye position using the information extracted from the retinal periphery. Thus, the eyes actively perform problem-oriented selection and processing of information from the visible world under the control of visual attention (Paletta, 2007). One study showed a sharp increase in reaction time to nonattended stimuli located across the vertical meridian, relative to nonattended stimuli, located in the attended hemifield at the same distance from the focus of attention. It has been shown that attention spreads over the entire visual hemifield and that the vertical meridian acts as a barrier that separates the attended from the nonattended region. There is no obvious reason why attention movements should be slowed down when crossing the vertical meridian unless some neural constraints are introduced. That may be the crossing of the corpus callosum (Rizzolatti

et al., 1987). These studies may explain why we often see a flick or tremor as a child's eyes move across midline. It may also mean that placing objects that you want them to quickly grab or identify should stay in one meridian and not have them spaced all over the visual area you are using. Also, the premotor theory stresses the importance of motor training. These premotor programs are the result of motor experience, especially oculomotor.

The stimulus-response compatibility (SRC) paradigm states that subjects make speeded choice responses based on the value of a stimulus property. This indicates that mapping properties that the stimulus and response share are faster than mappings that do not match such properties. In the simplest case, assigning a left response to left stimuli and right response to right stimuli results in shorter response latencies than does the reverse mapping. For example, moving an object to the left that is in the left field of vision is faster than moving the same object to the right. The evidence from SRC supports the view that certain action-related properties of a stimulus generate automatic response codes, at least with information about spatial location. Although of primary importance, location is only one of many object properties (stored information about the object) that are relevant to potential actions. Size, shape, and orientation all contribute to an object's affordances and are also processed together with spatial locations in the dorsal visual pathway. Cells that are responsive to quite specific action-related properties of objects, such as grip type and stimulus orientation, can be found stored in the parietal and motor areas. The question is, when you reach and grasp an object, is the information about the required preshaping of the hand produced from scratch at the moment the intention is formed or is some information already represented? With respect to the planning of eye movements, there is evidence that eye movement plans are selected from already an existing repertoire of motor signals. Selecting movement plans from an already existing repertoire of motor signals has advantages both in terms of execution time and perhaps, more importantly, in terms of making available the actions required in a given environment (Tucker & Ellis, 1998). Practice is important after all.

Object grasping is a highly complex motor behavior that requires the capacity to configure the hand according to the shape of a potentially limitless number of known and unknown objects. The physical characteristics of objects, such as size, shape, and orientation, must be visually perceived and used to select the most appropriate hand shaping. One possible way the brain can compute this visuomotor transformation is to automatically link the object representation (its visual properties) to a specific, predetermined grasping movement. It would be beneficial to select the appropriate motor program from an already existing repertoire of motor programs rather than generate a new one.

In the posterior parietal cortex, which belongs to the dorsal stream, neurons are sensitive to visual characteristics of the objects that are to be grasped. Each region within the posterior parietal cortex projects to separate regions within the premotor areas of the frontal lobes where movements are programmed. Thus, the dorsal stream (M pathway) performs the sensorimotor transformations required for visually guided actions, such as grasping a specific object. If size and orientation of a to-be-grasped object are processed by the dorsal stream, it is conceivable that such visual primes invoke stored information about the nature of the object, which, in turn, might determine the action program initiated with respect to the object. Research has also shown that the mere presentation of visual objects automatically evokes object-related motor responses.

Neuropsychological findings have led to the notion that there are two independent routes from seen objects to action: one route that is mediated by the visual activation of semantics (functional knowledge about objects) and a second route that is mediated solely by visual information derived from the objects. The direct route is thought to operate through associations between stored visual representations of objects and learned actions. The stored visual representations would belong to a structural description system, separate from semantic memory. Studies have shown that normal people possess strong associations between objects and the actions commonly carried out with them. People's knowledge about the movements underlying functional interactions with objects are incorporated with cognitive representation of objects. Knowledge about objects and their functions can trigger an appropriate hand shape, and the required configuration could be primed before the onset of reaching (Craighero et al., 1999). This is the basis of the premotor theory.

Premotor plans of action are essential to our everyday lives. The brain registers events via the sense organs almost immediately, but it takes up to half a second to become conscious of them. In order to generate effective responses in a fast-changing environment, the brain must plan and execute movement-by-movement actions unconsciously. It takes up to 400 msec for the brain to process incoming information to the stage where it may become conscious. It takes a similar length of time to prepare the body for action. So, if we waited to be conscious of a sight or sound before starting to respond to it, our behavior would lag almost a second behind the events to which we are responding. By the time we leapt out of the way of a speeding car, it is likely to have run us over. The brain speeds up our physical responses by fast-tracking sensory information to the motor planning areas along an unconscious pathway. A visual stimulus such as a moving object prompts neural activity that works out where it is in relation to the body. Various parts of the occipital and parietal cortex between them calculate the object's shape, size, relative motion, and trajectory. This information is then brought together and used to form an action plan. The chosen response is largely learned; for example, a skilled athlete is likely to catch or hit a speeding ball while an unpracticed player might miss it. The following is an example of how a professional tennis player might return a serve. Unlike novice players, professionals do not have to think consciously about each muscle movement because practice has turned the relevant action sequences into automated motor programs that are stored and run unconsciously.

- 0-msec—Attention: The player's brain prepares for action by focusing attention on his or her opponent. If the player is familiar with the opponent's playing style, his or her brain will register the movements made by the opponent as he or she serves and will compare them with previous observations to help predict where the ball will land. Attention to such cues may speed up reactions by 20 to 50 msec.

- 70-msec—Body memory: The ball is not yet consciously visible to the player, but, unconsciously, his or her brain is already planning the actions he or she must make to return it. The visual information from the opponent's movements activates the player's parietal cortex, which in turn calls up relevant procedural memories. These are learned actions—such as how to return a serve—that have become encoded as automatic motor programs.

- 250-msec—Action plan: The receiving player's brain brings together the information that has been registered so far to construct a response to the fast-approaching ball. This plan is held in the premotor areas, which lie just in front of the motor cortex. This is like a rehearsal stage, allowing action to be played out as a pattern of neuronal activity without affecting the muscles.

- 285-msec—Conscious thought starts: The player's brain becomes consciously aware of the ball moving away from the opponent's racket, but his or her brain has already (unconsciously) predicted its real-time position and, providing the two information streams do not clash, the player is likely to think he or she sees the ball where it is (Carter, 2009).

- 355-msec—Sending signals: The action plan held in the premotor cortex is transmitted to the motor cortex. The neurons on this strip of the brain connect via the spine to skeletal muscles. The sequence of limb movement is controlled by the cerebellum.

- 500-msec—Conscious act: If the player's conscious perception of the ball's trajectory differs markedly from his or her earlier, unconscious prediction, he or she may veto the earlier action plan and start to construct an alternative or try to adjust the current plan. It takes another 200 to 300 msec, however, to incorporate the new conscious information into a

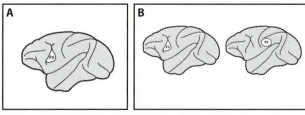

Figure 2-10. (A) Region F5. (B) Areas F5 and PF.

revised action plan, and by then the ball has traveled too far for any player to be able to return it.

Mirror Neurons

As is the case of many great discoveries, the mirror neuron system was first observed while Rizzolatti and his colleagues were studying something completely different. In the late 1980s, he and his colleagues had identified neurons in the macaque monkey's premotor cortex, which responded when the monkey performed specific actions, such as grasping a peanut. While investigating the specificity of the responses of neurons using single-unit electrophysiology in region F5 (Figure 2-10A) of the premotor cortex, the experimenter noted that certain neurons would respond not only when the monkey, for example, grasped the peanut, but also when the monkey observed the experimenter grasping the peanut. Likewise, another neuron would respond both when the monkey put the peanut in its mouth and when the monkey observed the experimenter putting the peanut in his or her mouth. Four years later, in a paper in the journal *Brain*, these neurons were dubbed "mirror" neurons as their response to observed actions appeared to "mirror" the response to performed actions. It is proposed that mirror neurons fundamentally mediate the mapping of one dimension (vision or auditory) in a brain map onto a completely different dimension (motor). Thus, the mirror neurons in the motor system remap a visual representation of observed actions onto the observer's motor representation (Gallese, Fadiga, Fogassi, & Rizzolatti, 1996). In a similar sense, language processing may involve a remapping of visual and auditory representations onto motor representations. Also, social processes such as empathy might involve a remapping of visual representations into limbic and premotor brain regions in order to have an embodied representation of mental states (Pineda, 2009). For example, you can see your friend crying, so you raise your hand to put it on his or her shoulder.

An interesting side note to mirror neurons is that many now feel they instigated language development (Rizzolatti, 1998). The development of the human lateral speech circuit may be a consequence of the fact that the precursor of Broca's area was endowed, before speech appearance, with a mechanism for recognizing actions made by others. This mechanism was the neural prerequisite for the development of interindividual communication and finally speech. It is suggested that, at a certain stage, a brachiomanual communication system evolved, complementing the orofacial one. This development greatly modified the importance of vocalization and its control. Whereas during the closed orofacial stage, sounds could add very little to the gestural message (e.g., orofacial gesture "be scared"), the orofacial gesture plus vocalization could relay "be more scared." Their association with gestures allowed them to assume the more open, referential character that brachiomanual gestures had already achieved. An object or event described gesturally (e.g., large object—large-gesture or arms; small object—tiny opening of the fingers) could now be accomplished by vocalization. If identical sounds were constantly used to indicate identical elements (e.g., large object—large opening of the mouth, vowel "a"; small object—tiny opening of the mouth, vowel "i"), a primitive vocabulary of meaningful sounds could start to develop.

In primates, three brain areas have been particularly associated with the perception of the action of other individuals: the superior temporal sulcus (STS), area PF of the inferior parietal lobule, and area F5 of the ventral premotor cortex (Figure 2-10B).

Two of these areas (PF and F5) have been shown to contain neurons called "mirror" neurons. It has been shown that these neurons respond during the execution of particular actions, even if the monkey or person cannot see him- or herself perform the action (e.g., because he or she closed his or her eyes). Second, they respond during the observation of another individual who performs similar actions (Pineda, 2009).

Recent studies have found that a certain, as yet unknown, proportion of mirror neurons are active both when moving and when watching movement. Neurons in the premotor cortex concerned with planning to move the legs are activated when you watch a person run. In other words, when you see someone doing something, in your brain, you do it, too. However, in order to mirror another action, the sight of the action must "resonate" with a motor program that the brain has already learned (Carter, 2009). For example, if you had never learned to run, watching someone else run would not activate your mirror neurons for leg movements. To mirror another's actions, the brain must know how it feels to do it. For example, to mirror expert dance moves, you would have to have some idea of how to go about doing them, even if you could not produce them perfectly.

Two movements may be identical but may signal very different things in different contexts. Human mirror neurons seem to take this into account. When a person sees another person picking up a cup in order to drink from it, a different set of neurons are activated from those that light up at the sight of a person making the identical movement but in the context that suggests they are clearing the cup away. Hence, the observer's brain does not just generate a faint idea of what the other person is doing with his or her body, but also an echo of his or her intention in doing it. This allows us to get a glimpse of another individual's plans and thought processes without consciously having to work it out (Carter, 2009).

The actions that most commonly activate mirror neurons are grasping, holding, and object manipulation. The mere presentation of visual objects, including interesting stimuli such as food items, sight of faces, or body movement, is ineffective in activating mirror neurons (di Pellegrino, Fadiga, Fogassi, Gallese, & Rizzolatti, 1992; Gallese et al., 1996; Pesaran, Pezaris, Sahani, Mitra, & Andersen, 2002). The neurons that are discharged in response to the sight of a hand approaching and grasping an object are grasping neurons. The neuron's discharge begins during hand shaping and continues until the hand leaves the stimulus. Placing neurons (manipulation) discharge when the person moves a stimulus toward a plane or a support. Holding neurons are activated when a person observes a stimulus being held by another person.

These studies are very interesting in that a person's neurons that control his or her motor planning can be activated by the observation of another person doing a certain motor act. It has to be stressed that the person has to have had the motor experience that he or she is observing. You cannot program a child's premotor neurons by showing him or her a motor action that he or she has never experienced. What is interesting, though, is such actions as hand and finger placement around a cup or a pencil might stimulate the child's neurons that had learned this task originally but had learned it incorrectly. Taking the time to show the child the correct way to do a motor activity he or she is doing incorrectly and making sure he or she is paying attention to your examples might be an effective way to improve motor actions.

Feature Integration Theory

The feature integration theory put forward by Treisman and Gelade (1980) assumes that features receive a sort of preferential processing. In this model, features such as color, orientation, spatial frequency, brightness, and direction of movements are assumed to be registered early, automatically, and in parallel across the visual field. In this sense, all of the elemental bits of information present in a display (patches of color, line segments, etc.) are also present in the early stages of information processing. Feature information must then be combined in order to recreate the objects in the display. This process of "gluing" features back together is assumed to require attention, and attention is allocated on the basis of spatial location. More specifically, selection takes place on the basis of a master map of locations, which contains all locations where features have been detected. Each location within the master map has access to the feature maps (which indicate whether a specific feature is present at that position) created during the early parallel

processing of the feature information. Focusing attention at a position automatically activates the features that are present at the attended position (Treisman & Paterson, 1984; Prinzmetal, Presti, & Posner, 1986). These features are then assembled into a temporary object file. Finally, features in the object file are compared with representations of objects in memory (the object frame). Identification takes place when the object file matches an object frame. The feature integration theory includes a number of feature maps for each basic dimension, and attention is required to combine features into objects. However, attention might be needed to combine different values of the same feature as well. For example, "purple" is subjectively a combination of blue and red. Feature maps within a dimension such as color might be limited in number and by the fact that purple has to be constructed as a conjunction of blue and red. The finding that search for a purple target is much less efficient (slower) when the distractors are red and blue as compared to when there are other colors matched for similarity suggests that the number of feature maps with a stimulus dimension may indeed be limited (Johnson & Proctor, 2004). When attention is divided, subjects often report many illusory conjunctions (combinations of features) by recombining features for the wrong objects present in the display (Treisman, 1990). This could easily be the case with children claiming that letters from different words overlap as they read. Poor attention is causing a conjunction illusion. A skilled reader who is processing the entire word in a parallel fashion would not experience an illusion conjunction, but an unskilled reader who is attacking the word in a serial fashion could experience this if his or her attention is divided.

Experiments show that conjunctions involving size give the fastest search rates, those involving color were next, motion third, and those involving orientation were quite slow. There was a strong correlation between the ease of conjunction search and the ease of segregating the same displays to allow the perception of groups. For example, in Figure 2-11A, the different targets are organized in groups. This makes it easier to find the desired target. The brain in this case only has to scan three choices; however, in B, because there are no groups, only undivided targets, the brain has to scan 15 targets. By grouping some of the targets, the search time was decreased. Also, search rates for known targets are faster than unknown targets, and it is much more difficult to find a conjunction target among four different types of distractors than among two. All of these examples stress the importance of an uncluttered space for a child to quickly find the desired target.

In one experiment, it was found that a search for a circle with a slash among circles without slashes was parallel (fast and subconscious). A search for a circle without a slash among circles with slashes was serial and was affected by display size (Figure 2-12).

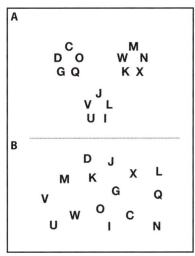

Figure 2-11. (A) Example of grouping. (B) Example of no grouping.

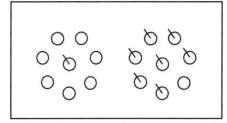

Figure 2-12. Circles with and without slashes.

The question is why is it easier to find a target with an added feature compared to finding a target without a feature? It appears that the brain considers an added feature as a "pop-out" (parallel processing). It is easy to find, but to find a target without a feature (serial processing) is difficult. This would indicate that if you ask someone to find a target with a certain feature among many similar targets, this is easier to do than asking a person to find the target without a certain feature among similar targets (Treisman, 1982).

There are several assumptions in the feature integration theory:

- The visual search assumption says that visual search allows us to define a target either by its separate features or by their conjunction (combinations). If we can detect features with no attention (parallel), the search for targets defined by its features (e.g., red or vertical) should be affected very little by variations in the number of distractors in the display. Lateral interference and acuity limits should be the only factors tending to increase search times as the display size is increased. In contrast, we assume that focal attention is necessary for the detection of targets that are defined by a combination of properties. Such targets should, therefore, be found only after a serial scan of varying numbers of distractors.

- Illusory conjunctions are the result of time being too short for the search or because attention is divided or directed to other objects. The features of the unattended objects appear "free floating" with respect to one another. In vision, subjects sometimes wrongly recombine words presented successively in the same location.

- Identity and location—If focused attention is prevented, the location of the object would be a separate operation from identifying it. If we have correctly detected and identified a particular object, we must first have located it in order to focus attention on it and integrate its features. Thus, location must precede identification for conjunctions (objects with two or more features).

- A visual search for a conjunction of three features (e.g., color, size, shape) is faster than a conjunction with only two features (e.g., color, size) (Wickens & McCarley, 2008).

The role of focal attention in integrating separable features appears to hold not only with arbitrary pairings of colors and shapes or with unfamiliar faces but also with highly familiar stimuli, like letters. There is a greater risk of conjunction error with similar letters that share separable features, which could be interchanged to form different letters. A target letter R in a background of P and B distractors is found more easily than a target R in a background of P and Q distractors where the R could be formed by conjoining the P with a diagonal slash from the Q (Treisman, 1990). Although long-term familiarity with letters seems not to eliminate the conjunction effect, specific practice in particular search tasks may help. They eventually learn a set of disjunctive features that distinguish targets from distractors (Schmidt, 2002). It would appear from this that children would make fewer errors of letters and words running together if the same font was used throughout school from elementary to high school.

Selective spatial attention, memory for the target, object-based attention over large areas of the visual field, and identification of the target are all required in visual search for a target, and those components are commonly associated with dorsal, parietal (spatial attention), memory, and identification visual areas. Neurological patients with damage to either the parietal or temporal visual areas show deficits in attention and visual search (Ashbridge, Walsh, & Cowey, 1997).

UNLIMITED CAPACITY THEORY

Not everyone feels that there is limited capacity in the visual system. For example, the limited capacity conception had its origin in auditory theories. Broadbent's first and most fundamental principle for auditory information processing was that "a nervous system acts to some extent as a single communication channel, so that it is meaningful to regard it as having a limited capacity." For auditory information processing, this view is possibly correct; however, is it the same for visual processing? It was suggested that there is no reason whatsoever to assume that one or another limited capacity system is built into the visual information processing system. For the capacity issue, neither the amount of information nor the size of the brain is of any relevance. Of relevance is only the amount of information picked up by the receptors in the senses relative to the information-processing capacity of the brain. For vision, there is not very much reason to assume that the brain cannot deal with the information provided by the eyes. The eyes function as a very efficient information filter. There are, for instance, only three different types of cones for coding all wavelength information, and detailed spatial information is only registered in a small central region of the eye (the fovea). The brain, however, has quite a capacity for visual information processing. The visual brain is a diverging system, not a converging one, and billions of cells are available for processing the visual information presented by the 2 million neurons in the retina. This view states that our completely detailed, subjectively experienced visual world is an automatic consequence of (adequate) visual stimulation and not a two-stage system that first processes some information subconsciously and then picks an area for detailed processing. Selection is needed because of the diverse and incompatible response tendencies that may be instigated at any one time or to avoid the behavioral chaos that would result from an attempt to simultaneously perform all possible actions (Heijden, 1996). This view of unlimited capacity is opposite of the limited capacity view that we most often see in research and should be considered as an alternative viewpoint.

Most models hold that the early stages of the visual system process all locations in parallel but are capable of extracting only a limited amount of information from the visual input. Subsequent processes can perform other more complex tasks but are limited to one or perhaps a few spatial locations at a time. Information gathered by the parallel front end is used to restrict the deployment of the limited-capacity processes to those parts of the visual field most likely to contain items of interest. The control of this deployment can be exogenous (external), based on properties of the visual stimuli, or endogenous (internal), based on the demands of the person's visual system. These are not mutually exclusive. Deployment can be based on the subject's wish to look for a specific visual stimulus (Wolfe, 1989). As an example of this, it has been shown that subjects were more likely to scan visual displays horizontally and to a lesser extent vertically or diagonally. This is because subjects tend to search a visual display in a manner consistent with their reading habits (i.e., from left to right and top to bottom). When the required target was not placed in the upper left quadrant, the search times were long. For young subjects before they learned to read, it was found that search times were shortest when the target was placed central (Johnson & Proctor, 2004). Also, the human visual system has evolved a specialized processing focus for moving across a visual scene. A search for a target that has more than one feature is always searched in series unless it is much larger or has something that causes it to stand out (pop-out effect) (Koch & Ullman, 1985). It is much easier for a child to find the red square if the others are different colors. Also, if all of the targets have several features (e.g., color, orientation), the child has to focus each target in sequence (serially) (Nakayama & Silverman, 1986; Wolfe, 1989). Targets with more than one feature are always searched serially.

BINDING

The visual system is composed of many distinct areas, each processing a different set of visual attributes, such as motion, color, or orientation. Our perception, however, is not a random collection of features but of stable unified objects. Because color and object configuration are processed in different brain areas, it is the timing that determines if a color goes with the object. When both object and color areas are activated, the brain knows that it is the areas that are activated at the same time that belong to the same object. Studies have shown that the parietal lobes may play an important role in integrating individual features into stable object representations (Le et al., 1998). These results are important because the task of feature integration has been ascribed to visual attention. The feature integration theory states that features are detected preattentively and in parallel across the visual field, but their integration into single objects requires focused attention to each object's location in turn. Taxing attentional reserves, whether by short exposures, dual tasks, or some type of brain damage, can result in miscombinations of features or illusory conjunctions. Numerous data suggest that the parietal lobe may play a critical role in the proper working of the attentional mechanisms involved in the integration of features (Schneider, 1998). Limiting the resources available for visual processing through increased loads and/or reduced time leads observers to erroneously associate basic features present in the image into objects that do not exist (Paletta, 2007). The mechanism that helps to accomplish binding is

TABLE 2-1. PARALLEL VERSUS SERIAL SEARCH	
PARALLEL	*SERIAL*
Tilted line in vertical lines	Vertical line in tilted lines
Curved line in straight lines	Straight line in curved lines
Converging lines in parallel lines	Parallel lines in converging lines
Closed circle in circles with gap	Circle with gap in closed circles

attention. Attention is the glue that holds features together to form objects. Attention to spatial locations in normal human brains is necessary to properly bind the features of objects. Feature binding could, therefore, be disrupted by attentional overload or inaccurate spatial information (Friedman-Hill et al., 1995; Vidyasagar, 2001). Visual features of each object are integrated by a focal attention mechanism. The boundaries of the attention mark the edges of a specific area, and the features that are present in that area are integrated. Binding works in the following way. First, focal attention is used to mark a specific area. The boundaries of the focus of attention serve as the markers of the boundary of the area. After that, the attention mechanism glues together the various visual features that are within that area. An important aspect is the flexible focus of attention: the focus can expand or shrink like a spotlight (Cohen & Ivry, 1989). Illusory conjunctions between two objects outside the area of attention are formed only when the objects (or letters) are adjacent (as in reading). When the distance is large between the objects, the tendency for conjunctions is less. Inside the area of attention, all of the features are conjoined. The perceptual system "recognizes" the presence of an object (i.e., a particular conjunction of features) inside the area of attention and only the presence of individual features (not completed objects) outside the area of attention. It takes attention to glue the features together to form an object. This is one reason poor visual attention can cause a beginning or dyslexic reader to misname a word. A good reader would process it in parallel as a single unit, while a poor reader processes the word serially, and poor visual attention would cause letter movement or word substitutions due to guessing.

Illusory conjunction (confusion between objects with similar features) is more frequent in the following conditions:

- When exposures are brief and focused attention to each object is prevented
- Search for an object is slower when finding an absence of a feature
- The targets are close together (e.g., letters are close together in words)
- If attention is overloaded (dividing your attention)

- More errors occur in orthographic units (words)
- With objects that have similar features
- Poor visual acuity
- When the subject fixates centrally and the target is in his or her peripheral vision (Treisman, 1996, 1998)

As we have said, objects that can be identified in parallel without having to serially search each of their features are much easier to find in a search. An example of this is a human face, which can be seen as a global whole without requiring serial processing of each feature. Table 2-1 gives you an idea of what would be easy to find (parallel—no attention) and what would be difficult to find (serial search) and would require attention.

Evidence for a parietal role in spatial attention comes from a study of positron emission tomography (PET) activation. Continuous attention to motion, color, or shape gives enhanced activity in different extrastriate areas, but tasks that require active shifting of attention between locations give rise to activity in superior parietal areas. Parietal areas were also active in a task requiring feature binding (conjunction search) (Corbetta & Shulman, 1998; Treisman, 1990). This again points to the suggestion that training this area of the brain by doing activities that required shifting of eye movements or other parietal activities is critical in a child's development. Many studies have shown the importance of the parietal lobe in attention (Anderson, 1988, 1997; Batuev, Shaefer, & Orlov, 1985; Bisley & Goldberg, 2003; Cohen & Anderson, 2002; Connolly, Andersen, & Goodale, 2003; Corbetta, Miezin, Shulman, & Petersen, 1993; Corbetta, Shulman, Miezin, & Petersen, 1995; Coull et al., 1996; Culham, 2004; Darian-Smith, Johnson, & Goodwin, 1979; Farah, Wong, Monheit, & Morrow, 1989; Friedman-Hill et al., 1995; Friedman-Hill, Robertson, Desimone, & Ungerleider, 2003; Goodale & Milner, 1992; Hyvarinen & Poranen, 1974; Mirsky, Anthony, Duncan, Ahearn, & Kellam, 1991; Mountcastle, Andersen, & Motter, 1981; Neville & Lawson, 1987; Petersen, 1994; Posner, Walker, Friedrich, & Rafal, 1984, 1987; Robinson et al., 1978; Sakata, Shibutani, & Kawano, 1983; Selemon & Goldman-Rakic, 1988; Sieroff, 1988; Steinmetz, 1995; Vidyasagar & Pammer, 1999; Wojciulik & Kanwisher, 1999). One final note on binding again stresses the importance of attention.

The integrated-competition model offers an alternative framework for addressing the binding problem. In this view, directing attention to one of an object's features produces a competitive advantage for the object in the neural module encoding that feature, which is then transmitted to the modules encoding the other features of the object. The resulting activation of the entire network of specialized modules would then underlie the binding of features into a unified perceptual object (Schoenfeld et al., 2003). So by focusing attention on one feature, the other features are also easier to identify. This stresses the importance of proper and accurate saccadic eye movements, especially during reading. If the eye fixates on the wrong word, then the wrong features would be activated, which would then slow down the whole reading process.

GROUPING

When a set of line segments appears simultaneously in the visual field, they can be organized in a number of different ways by the perceiver. In one case, the segments can be perceived as independent, ungrouped, and belonging to different objects or figures. In a second case, the line segments can act as place holders where positions indicate salient points on a unitary figure, as when a group of stars forms a discernible constellation. In a third case, the position, orientation, and shape of the line segments interact to form a unitary group. The notion that groups can be regarded as attentional units agrees with Gestalt claims about perceptual groups; however, the Gestalt psychologists thought they were held together by electrical field action instead of attention as we know today. Grouping is important because the way figures are grouped will determine how much attentional demand will be needed. The Gestalt principles that are still followed today are the following:

1. Proximity—Components in close spatial proximity tend to be grouped together.

2. Similarity—Components that are similar in appearance tend to be grouped together.

3. Continuity—Components that follow a continuous contour tend to be grouped together.

4. Closure—Gaps between contours tend to be filled in.

5. Common fate—Components that move in the same direction or at the same speed will be grouped together (Johnson & Proctor, 2004).

These are mentioned because to improve a person's attention to a specific area, the presence of a group would draw his or her attention to the desired area. In another illustration, if you want a person to quickly attend to a particular object, the presence of a group would possibly distract him or her as his or her attention will be drawn to the group. To give an example of this, in a particular experiment, participants were to decide if a T or an F was presented among distractors. It was found that performance was worse when the target letter was clustered into the same group as the distractors than when it was not. In following the effect of continuity, when the target letter F was placed near the line of distractors, the subjects found it harder to find because they felt it was part of the group. It was easy to find when the F was to the side of the distractors.

Another illustration is when you want a person to quickly find a particular letter when there are other letters in the target area. A letter that needs to be found quickly should be placed a distance from the others so that it is not perceived as being connected with the other letters. Spatial proximity refers to the distances between the objects. The reaction time decreases as the spatial separation between the target and the other object increases. An example of chromatic proximity is that there is a tendency for items with the same color to be grouped together. Search for a single target is much easier if the target is a different color than the rest of the display (Johnson & Proctor, 2004).

INFANTS AND YOUNG CHILDREN

The development of the ability to orient both the eyes and attention in infancy is dependent on the stage of development of the brain. For example, visual orienting is contingent on the emergence of functioning of cortical oculomotor pathways between the ages of 2 and 3 months. Up to about 6 months of age, volitional control of eye movements develops as infants become increasingly able to inhibit automatic saccades, produce anticipatory saccades, and delay making planned saccades. Covert shifts of visual attention first emerge around 4 months of age. However, the ability to direct and sustain attention continues to develop into childhood. Infants have a tendency to look at stimuli that are especially attractive, being novel, dynamic, or colorful (Johnson & Proctor, 2004). For the first 4 months, attention is drawn to objects with greater light-dark contrast, those with a moderate number of edges, and those that move. At this age, novelty becomes more important for directing attention as infants attend less, or "habituate," to repeated stimuli (Lyon, 2005).

There are four major developmental transactions in early attention as reflected, in part, by infants and young children's patterns of looking at the external world. In the first transition at 2 to 3 months, infants' scanning shifts from fixation of external contours of objects toward fixations of internal features. The first transitional period begins a time of close social interaction between the parent and infant, involving mutual gaze and often positive effects. It also coincides with the emergence of the orienting/investigative system of attention. After an increase in looking at stationary visual displays during the first 3 months, looking times generally decrease from 3 months to the end of the first year. At approximately 5 months of age, infants are able to reach for and grasp objects.

A second major developmental shift occurs around 9 months of age. Now, infants appear to be able to remember past events with only a few cues available to support the memory. Changes during the 9- to 12-month period have been associated with development of the dorsolateral prefrontal cortex.

At 18 to 24 months, another major transition occurs. By late in the second year, the child can act on representations of events and can use language and other symbolic processes.

Finally, it is suggested that the second attention system continues to be consolidated throughout the preschool years with an enhancement around 4 years in the ability to inhibit actions on instruction from self or others. There is a leap in the child's ability to voluntarily direct attention to those aspects of the environment that are relevant to the task at hand and to inhibit responses to perceptually salient, but irrelevant, aspects. Thus, the child is better able to participate in structured, rule-governed tasks, which may require waiting for instructions (Ruff, 1996).

The reason that an infant looks at objects for a long time and to explain why the time decreases after 3 months has been found to be due to the infant being more efficient at encoding than when he or she was younger. It appears that older infants need less familiarization time to encode visual stimuli than younger infants. The reason why younger infants spend more time processing information is because of their tendency to process local features over global configurations. Infants with briefer looking patterns show evidence of a global-to-local shift in attention as familiarization increases (Posner & Petersen, 1990).

It has been well-known for 40 years that postnatal experience plays a critical role in determining the structure and function of the central nervous system and that early experiences tend to have a disproportionate degree of influence on mature function. Thus, it is reasonable to assume that early differences in attention may play a similar role in structuring the central nervous system and long-term development. We can delineate three different ways in the relationship that attention in infancy and early childhood to mature cognitive function can be conceptualized:

1. Early attention may be taken as a manifestation of later function. This has been widely investigated as an indicant of general intellectual function in predicting developmental outcome.

2. Clearly, attention mediates the types of experience that organisms will have.

3. A less obvious potential role of attention in long-term cognitive outcome lies in the direct effects that attention exerts on the brain per se. The evidence strongly suggests that the act of attending changes brain activity. For example, it modulates synchronous neural firing, and it enhances the neural activity of areas that correspond to the object or object properties being attended to. It is possible that these direct, physical, and typically short-term consequences of attention may cause disproportionate effects on the structure and function of the brain when they occur repetitively or for extended durations during early development (Posner & Petersen, 1990).

The visual tracking of a moving stimulus in the newborn has two characteristics. First, it is saccadic or step-like in manner, as opposed to the smooth manner of pursuits in adults and older children. Second, the eye movements always lag behind the movement of the stimulus. Newborns more readily direct their attention temporal, as opposed to in the nasal visual field.

Around 1 month of age, infants show obligatory attention; that is, they have a great deal of difficulty disengaging their gaze from a stimulus in order to look elsewhere. At about 2 months of age, infants begin to show periods of smooth visual tracking, although their eye movements still lag behind the movement of the stimulus.

One line of evidence that visual attention is critical for normal cognitive development comes from the significant correlations that have been reported between components of visual attention in early infancy and subsequent measures of temperament and intelligence. Specifically, a number of laboratories have reported significant correlations between measures such as the extent of preferential looking to a novel stimulus (when paired with a familiar one) as subsequent IQ measures at school age.

One hypothesis as to why an infant might fixate an object longer than another is that the magnocellular (M) system is slower in development than the parvocellular (P). Information processing in infants whose M system has been even further delayed would thus be slower to process visual stimuli and would be more inclined to attend and encode detailed rather than global aspects of the stimulus. Thus, such infants are less able to disengage their attention from the stimulus concerned, and they therefore show longer looking times (Parasuraman, 2000).

The debate is still going on as to fixation times of infants and later IQ scores. Do infants take a long time looking at an object because they do not understand or remember it, or are they really smarter and just taking more time analyzing the object?

One question is, are newborns capable of perceiving visual patterns? Infants clearly attend to both color and form. Four-month-olds seem to process color and form as separable components and not as compounds.

Multidimensional visual stimuli can be perceived in a compound (conjunction) manner by infants who are 4 or 5 months old. When considering how infants process objects, first realize that infants younger than 2 months scan visual stimuli less extensively than infants older than 2 months. Second, it has been suggested that young infants are biased toward scanning the external contours of stimuli. Much evidence suggests that such scanning patterns (and the distribution of attention that such scanning patterns presumably reflect) affect stimulus identification/ recognition performance. For example, infants who scan less extensively do not perform as well on stimulus recognition probes. Infants who look for longer durations have been shown to rely on local elements or features in visual stimuli recognition (Colombo, 2001).

Evidence from three particular areas of infant cognitive function can be brought to bear on endogenous (developing from within) attentional functions in infancy.

The first of these areas comes from shifts in visual attention in which two simultaneously presented stimuli are alternately inspected. The novelty-familiarization paired comparison is a fundamental technique to study infant cognition. The infant is exposed (familiarized) to a stimulus and then presented with a choice between fixating the familiarized stimulus or a novel one. Most often, when paired stimuli are presented to either side of midline, infants will alternately fixate the two stimuli. Such interstimulus shifting occurs at a relatively rapid rate, and the rate is affected by stimulus similarly. As a result, intrastimulus shifting has been taken to reflect an active and purposeful comparison of the paired stimuli and thus fits with the endogenous nature of these forms of attention. Interstimulus shifting is more common and faster in older infants than in younger infants.

A special form of interstimulus shifting is spontaneous alternation, which is a pattern in which the subject systematically alternates the position to which motor responses (reaching or searching) are made across trials. This pattern of responding depends on location memory for the previous choice in guiding the next choice and on the subject's ability to resist repeating a response to a spatial location when the response to that location has just been previously rewarded. As a result, spontaneous alternation has been taken as a measure of response inhibition in children. Such attention has traditionally been attributed to the function of higher brain areas, including the hippocampus, thalamus, and frontal lobes. Eighteen-month-old children readily show spontaneous alternation on a reaching task, but 6 month olds do not.

A second area of research relevant to the development of endogenous visual attention concerns the ability to inhibit attentional shifts. One way to test this is to have infants inhibit or suppress saccades to the appearance of peripheral targets. The frontal cortex is involved in the inhibition of saccades to peripheral stimuli. Voluntary suppression of such saccades may be taken as evidence of endogenous attentional function. Four month olds can learn to inhibit orienting to the peripheral target under such conditions. It therefore seems possible for infants to inhibit a saccadic response to a cue by 4 to 6 months of age.

Functional assessments of sustained attention have been obtained in infants as young as 8 weeks, and there is considerable evidence that there are significant changes in the amount, depth, and frequency of sustained attention from 3 to 6 months. The ability to sustain a vigilant state was present in the youngest age group at 5 months (Colombo, 2001).

The percentage of children who could do a relatively simple go-no-go vigilance task (e.g., press a key when a certain letter is shown and ignore it the rest of the time) increases from just 27% of children between 3 years and 3 years 5 months of age to 100% of children 4.5 years of age and older.

The development of the ability to orient both eyes and attention in infancy is dependent on the stage of development of the brain. For example, visual orienting is contingent on the emergence of functioning of cortical oculomotor pathways between the ages of 2 and 3 months up to about 6 months of age. Covert shifts of visual attention first emerge around 4 months. Many studies show that children are more sensitive to interfering information than adults. Younger children (6 to 8 years) are more sensitive to the spatial separation of two stimuli when they are required to ignore one spatially distinct stimulus in order to make a judgment about another than are older children (9 to 11 years). That is, they show more interference than older children when the stimuli are closer together. When the judgment requires attending to both stimuli, younger children are hurt more by a greater spatial separation.

Children (6 to 8 years) experienced more interference when the elements were closely spaced than older children (9 to 11). Older children and adults are often reported as being able to shift their attention more rapidly than younger children (Pearson & Lane, 1990). It was observed that younger infants took longer to covertly shift their attention to peripheral targets, whereas they were almost as fast as adults to shift to targets very close to fixation. This indicates that it is the speed of shifting rather than the latency to elicit a covert shift that improves with age.

Mothers and Child Care

The one area that everyone seems to agree on is the importance of the mother's interaction with the young child. There is a strong relation between aspects of infants' home environment and their intellectual and language development during the preschool years. There is evidence that children's early cognitive development is associated with such family environmental factors as the language stimulation available to the child, the responsivity of parents, the emotional support by parents, the number of stimulating toys and objects available, the extent to which the home is organized and safe, and the variety of out-of-home experiences provided to the child (Bradley & Caldwell, 1984).

Joint attention is an important component in the development of a child's lexical acquisition. Children of mothers who direct the child's attention rather than be with the child learn fewer object labels and have a weaker vocabulary. Specifically, object labels provided for objects during periods of joint attention (mother and child both looking at and interacting with the object) were learned more often than object labels provided when such objects were just brought into the child's focus of attention by the mother. Children who engaged in long periods of parent attention had a larger vocabulary. It is possible that mothers who facilitate the infant's own active attention to the objects are helping their infants to learn more, to be more competent, and to take more pleasure in their own mastery of objects and problems. These mothers not only explain the object but often take the infant's hands to go through the appropriate manipulation of the objects. Inattention of the infant is often demonstrated by dropping and throwing the objects. This was greatly decreased by the joint attention shown by the mothers.

Families who engage in behaviors to encourage children's cognitive and language development, such as direct teaching, reading to children at bedtime, explaining events, carrying on give-and-take-conversations, and providing children with stimulating and enriching experiences, have children who are more successful in school. Children who lack such experiences often fall behind both academically and in measures of language ability. In addition, parental warmth and responsiveness, as well as the use of gentle guidance and support as opposed to power (assertive and harsh discipline), have been associated with better cognitive functioning. Data from the National Institute of Child Health and Human Development (NICHD) found that not only family environment predicted children's ability to regulate their attention by the preschool years, but also that attention processes, in turn, predicted achievement, language, and social outcomes for these children. It is essential that children be able to discern what stimuli are relevant to a task at hand and then maintain focus on those relevant stimuli. They must develop the ability to ignore irrelevant stimuli and to inhibit the tendency to respond hurriedly to and be distracted by these stimuli (NICHD, 1999, 2000).

The past 25 years have shown a dramatic change for the experiences of the younger children in the United States. In 1975, 37% of married women with children younger than age 6 were employed; by 1998, the rate of employment for this group of women had risen to 64%. Employment rates for married mothers of infants younger than 2 have increased even more from 31% in 1975 to 67% in 1998. About 5% of preschoolers with employed mothers are cared for by their mothers at work, but the remainder regularly spend time being cared for by someone other than their mothers. Families with the lowest nonmaternal income were the most likely to place infants in care before the age of 3 months (NICHD, 2001). In contrast, infants from families with the highest maternal and nonmaternal incomes tended to start care between 3 and 5 months. The higher the mothers' earnings, the more hours the infants spent in nonmaternal care. However, the higher the nonmaternal (father's) earnings, the fewer hours they spend in care. The more positive care occurred when children were in smaller groups. The guidelines from the American Academy of Pediatrics for child-staff ratios are 3:1 at 6 and 15 months, 4:1 at 24 months, and 7:1 at 36 months. Groups sizes of six at 9 and 15 months, eight at 24 months, and 14 at 36 months are considered normal. The caregiver training should be formal, post–high-school training in child development, early childhood education, or a related field at all age levels. At 24 months, children who had experienced higher quality care reported few behavior problems by their mothers. When children spend more hours in childcare, mothers were less sensitive in their interactions with their children, and children were less positively engaged with their mothers. Children attending childcare centers and childcare homes had more ear infections and upper respiratory illnesses than children cared for at home, especially during the first 2 years. One of the most important results of studies in early childcare is that the worst possible situation is low-quality nonmaternal care and changing care arrangements numerous times. These result in an increased risk of insecure attachment when combined with less maternal sensitivity. At 15 months of age, children who experienced more changes in care arrangements and maternal insensitivity were at heightened risk. All of this gives a dim view of childcare centers; however, if a child is in a good childcare center by age 2, these children often do better on measures of cognitive and language development than children in other forms of care. Experience with group care (settings with at least three other children not counting siblings), whether in centers or childcare homes, made some difference in several social emotional outcomes at ages 2 and 3. The number of times children change care arrangements appears to affect children. At age 2, experience with more childcare arrangements was associated with a higher number of behavior problems; however, this was not found for children at age 3. Therefore, it is critical for children younger than 3 to have stability in care. The most important factor is the family relationship. Family influences are consistently better predictors of children's outcomes than early care experiences alone (NICHD, 2000, 2001). Studies have shown that, taking all of this into account, if a child has a good stable home and the childcare centers are good, then a child in the first 3 years can do well in a childcare situation (NICHD, 2003).

Interaction between the child and adults may be crucial to the development of the ability to direct attention voluntarily. When an adult directs a young child's attention stimuli of interest by alternating the stimulus characteristically in some way, this develops the child's voluntary attention. By about 4 years of age, children develop the ability to scan their environment actively, rather than being drawn by the novelty or salience of a stimulus. This internally driven attention is believed to be established by 5 or 6 years of age (Lyon, 2005).

I have noted many of the previous comments in 30 years of dealing with home schooled and public schooled children. More times than not, the home schooled children are much better behaved in the reception area than the children in public schools. This is not to say that home schooling is the way to raise a child. It does indicate that the relationship between the child and the mother is critical. The more time a mother can spend with her child, giving him or her positive feedback and encouragement, the better the results.

TIPS FOR INFANT ATTENTION

Newborns will prefer to look at the following:

- Patterned rather than unpatterned
- Horizontal rather than vertical gratings (stripes)
- Moving rather than stationary stimuli
- Three-dimensional rather than two-dimensional
- Curvilinear in preference to rectilinear patterns
- Objects in the frontoparallel plane rather than those at an angle
- High-contrast rather than low-contrast stimuli
- Objects at an optimal size (where this is usually the larger of two objects)
- Face-like in preference to non–face-like stimuli
- During the first 4 months of life, a baby should begin to follow movement with his or her eyes and reach for things, first by chance and later more accurately, as coordination and depth perception begin to develop. To help, use a nightlight or dim lamp in a baby's room. Move the crib and your child's position in it frequently. Keep reach-and-touch toys within his or her focus at about 8 to 12 inches. Talk to the baby as you walk around the room. Alternate right and left sides when feeding, and have a mobile above and outside the crib (American Optometric Association, 2005).

- Between 4 and 8 months, a baby should begin to turn from his or her side to use his or her arms and legs. Eye movement and eye/body coordination skills should develop further, and both eyes should focus equally. You should enable the baby to explore different shapes and textures with his or her fingers. Give the baby the freedom to crawl and explore. Hang objects across the room. Play "pat-a-cake" and "peek-a-boo" with the baby (American Optometric Association, 2005).

- From 8 to 12 months, a baby is now mobile and crawling or walking. He or she will begin to use both eyes together and grasp and throw objects with greater precision. Do not force early walking! Crawling is important in developing eye-hand-foot-body coordination. Give the baby stacking and take-apart toys, and provide objects he or she can touch, hold, and see at the same time.

- From 1 to 2 years, a child's eye-hand coordination and depth perception should continue to develop, and he or she will begin to understand abstract terms. Encourage walking; provide building blocks, simple puzzles, and balls; and let him or her explore indoors and out.

- Pursuit training should be part of every attention training program. For young children, use faces for targets.

- The development of the ability to orient both eyes and attention in infancy is dependent on the stage of development of the brain. For example, visual orienting is contingent on the emergence of functioning of cortical oculomotor pathways between the ages of 2 and 3 months up to about 6 months of age. Covert shifts of visual attention first emerge around 4 months. Many studies show that children are more sensitive to interfering information than adults. Younger children (6 to 8 years) are more sensitive to the spatial separation of the two stimuli when they are required to ignore one spatially distinct stimulus in order to make a judgment about another than are older children (9 to 11 years). That is, they show more interference than older children when the stimuli are closer together. When the judgment requires attending to both stimuli, younger children are hurt more by a great spatial separation.

SUMMARY AND ATTENTION TIPS

1. Use combinations of vestibular and oculomotor activities in your SI program.

2. Train the right hemisphere by having the child raise his or her left hand and left foot or use occluders on glasses to block the left visual field.

3. Take time to show a child the proper way to do a motor act to stimulate his or her mirror neurons to plan the same motor act (e.g., the proper way to grasp a pencil).

4. For pursuit training with young children, use faces for targets.

5. A right-handed person has more difficulty talking and writing than a left-handed person.

6. Spatial pre-cues can increase the efficiency of processing visual targets, such as a box around areas where the target will appear, the onset of a dot, a horizontal line beneath the position where the target will appear, and a combination of target orientation and color to direct the child's attention to the target. You can also quickly flash a laser pointer to the target and pre-cue the child's attention to it.

7. There is a greater risk of identification error with similar letters that show features, which can be interchanged to form different letters. A target R in a background of P and B distractors is found more easily than a target R in a background of P and Q distractors.

8. For young children who have reading problems, keep the font type the same in all of their reading materials.

9. It is faster to find the target in the upper left quadrant for children who know how to read. For those who do not yet know how to read, it is faster to find the target when it is in the center.

10. Reaction times to same-side stimuli are faster with the left hand (left side) than the right hand (right side).

(continued)

SUMMARY AND ATTENTION TIPS (CONTINUED)

11. You will keep the child's attention if you stay in his or her right hemisphere. Stand slightly to his or her right.

12. Have the child draw the face of a clock to see if he or she has poor spatial skills related to the M pathway.

13. Keep the focused area free from distractors. On a page of print, do not have letters closer than 1 degree (four letter positions on a page of normal print).

14. Dyslexic children need big and widely spaced print.

15. Do focused attention activities first in your attention program.

16. Make targets a different color than other objects in its area.

17. Novelty bias says that it is easier to find something that we are not used to seeing than something we are used to seeing. For example, it is easier for the child to find an inverted letter in familiar letters than the opposite.

18. You cannot pay attention and identify the features of two objects at the same time.

19. The more similar the targets, the longer the search time.

20. Responses to a stimulus are stronger when the stimulus is relevant to the child. For example, he or she is going to use the object he or she is trying to find.

21. It is easier to remember four objects presented at the same time than one right after the other.

22. In order for a child to quickly detect two stimuli, have one in his or her peripheral vision.

23. You can identify a target's color, orientation, and location in your peripheral vision but not details of the target.

24. A child cannot pay attention to more than one target in his or her peripheral vision.

(continued)

SUMMARY AND ATTENTION TIPS (CONTINUED)

25. Keep the objects you want the child to find in one meridian (e.g., right lower instead of all over the visual area).

26. It is faster to do a left response to a left-side stimulus or a right-side stimulus. For example, moving an object to the left that is in the left field of vision is faster than moving the same object to the right.

27. Fastest search times are for larger objects, followed by colored objects, followed by moving objects, and finally orientation differences.

28. It is faster to find the desired target if it is in one of several groups of targets instead of individual random targets.

29. It is easier to find a target with an added feature compared to finding a target without a feature.

30. Pop-out features do not require attention, whereas focal attention is necessary when a visual area has to be searched each item at a time, as when the target is defined by a combination of properties. For example, a large red square is faster to find than a square that has two features, such as orientation and color.

31. A visual search for an object with three features is faster than for an object with only two. For example, it is easier to find a target defined by color, size, and shape than just color and size. Pop-up targets are different. They usually only have one feature such as color, and they are the fastest to find in a search.

REFERENCES

American Optometric Association. (2005). *Infant's vision.* Retrieved from http://www.aoa.org/x4738.xml.

Anderson, R. (1988). Visual and visual-motor functions of the posterior parietal cortex. *Neurobiology of Neocortex,* 285-295.

Anderson, R. A. (1997). Multimodal integration for the representation of space in the posterior parietal cortex. *Philosophical Transactions of the Royal Society B: Biological Sciences, 352*(1360), 1421-1428.

Ashbridge, E., Walsh, V., & Cowey, A. (1997). Temporal aspects of visual search studied by transcranial magnetic stimulation. *Neuropsychologia, 35*(8), 1121-1131.

Aston-Jones, G., Chiang, C., & Alexinsky, T. (1991). Discharge of noradrenergic locus coeruleus neurons in behaving rats and monkeys suggests a role in vigilance. *Progress in Brain Research, 88,* 501-520.

Batuev, A. S., Shaefer, V. I., & Orlov, A. A. (1985). Comparative characteristics of unit activity in the prefrontal and parietal areas during delayed performance in monkeys. *Behavioural Brain Research, 16*(1), 57-70.

Bisley, J. W. & Goldberg, M. E. (2003). Neuronal activity in the lateral intraparietal area and spatial attention. *Science, 299,* 81-85.

Bradley, R. H. & Caldwell, B. M. (1984). The relation of infants' home environments to achievement test performance in first grade: a follow up study. *Child Development, 55*(3), 803-809.

Braun, J., Koch, C. & Davis, J. L. (2001). *Visual attention and cortical circuits.* Cambridge, MA: MIT Press.

Brown, L. E., Moore, C. M., & Rosenbaum, D. A. (2002). Feature-specific perceptual processing dissociates action from recognition. *Journal of Experimental Psychology, 28*(6), 1330-1344.

Bundesen, C. & Habekost, T. (2008). *Principles of visual attention: linking mind and brain.* New York, NY: Oxford University Press.

Cabeza, R. & Nyberg, L. (2000). Imagine cognition II: an empirical review of 275 PET and fMRI studies. *Journal of Cognitive Neuroscience, 12*(1), 1-47.

Carter, R. (2009). *The human brain.* New York, NY: D.K. Publishers.

Cohen, A. & Ivry, R. (1989). Illusory conjunctions inside and outside the focus of attention. *Journal of Experimental Psychology, 15*(4), 650-663.

Cohen, Y. E. & Andersen, R. A. (2002). A common reference frame for movement plans in the posterior parietal cortex. *Nature Reviews, 3*(7), 553-562.

Colombo, J. (2001). The development of usual attention in infancy. *Annual Review of Psychology, 52,* 337-367.

Connolly, J. D., Andersen, R. A., & Goodale, M. A. (2003). FMRI evidence for a parietal reach region in the human brain. *Experimental Brain Research, 153*(2), 140-145.

Corbetta, M., Miezin, F. M., Dobmeyer, S., Shulman, G. L., & Petersen, S. E. (1991). Selective and divided attention during visual discriminations of shapes, color and speed: functional anatomy by positron emission tomography. *The Journal of Neuroscience, 11*(8), 2383-2402.

Corbetta, M., Miezin, F. M., Shulman, G. L., & Petersen, S. E. (1993). A PET study of visuospatial attention. *The Journal of Neuroscience, 13*(3), 1202-1226.

Corbetta, M. & Shulman, G. L. (1998). Human cortical mechanisms of visual attention during orienting and search. *Philosophical Transactions of the Royal Society B, 353,* 1353-1362.

Corbetta, M., Shulman, G. L., Miezin, F. M., & Petersen, S. E. (1995). Superior parietal cortex activation during spatial attention shifts and visual feature conjunction. *Science, 270,* 802-805.

Coull, J. T., Frith, C. D., Frackowiak, R. S., & Grasby, P. M. (1996). A fronto-parietal network for rapid visual information processing: a PET study of sustained attention and working memory. *Neuropsychologia, 34*(11), 1085-1095.

Craighero, L., Fadiga, L., Rizzolatti, G., & Umiltà, C. (1999). Action for perception: a motor-visual attentional effect. *Journal of Experimental Psychology: Human Perception and Performance, 25*(6), 1673-1692.

Culham, J. (2004). Functional neuroimaging of visual cognition: attention and performance. New York, NY: Oxford University Press.

Darian-Smith, I., Johnson, K. O., & Goodwin, A. W. (1979). Posterior parietal cortex: relations of unit activity to sensorimotor function. *Annual Review of Physiology, 41,* 141-157.

Desimone, R. (1995). Neural mechanisms of selective visual attention. *Annual Review of Neuroscience, 18,* 193-222.

di Pellegrino, G., Fadiga, L., Fogassi, L., Gallese, V., & Rizzolatti, G. (1992) Understanding motor events: a neurophysiological study. *Experimental Brain Research, 91,* 176-180.

Downing, C. J. (1988). Expectancy and visual-spatial attention: effects on perceptual quality. *Journal of Experimental Psychology, 14*(2), 188-202.

Durston, S. (2002). A neuro basis for the development of inhibitory control. *Developmental Science, 5*(4), F9-F16.

Edelman, G. (1992). *Bright air, brilliant fire.* New York, NY: Basic Books.

Facoetti, A., Paganoni, P., & Lorusso, M. L. (2000). The spatial distribution of visual attention in developmental dyslexia. *Experimental Brain Research, 132*(4), 531-538.

Farah, M. J., Wong, A. B., Monheit, M. A., & Morrow, L. A. (1989). Parietal lobe mechanisms of spatial attention: modality-specific or supramodal. *Neuropsychologia, 27*(4), 461-470.

Friedman-Hill, S. R., Robertson, L. C., & Treisman, A. (1995). Parietal contributions to visual feature binding: evidence from a patient with bilateral lesions. *Science, 269,* 853-855.

Friedman-Hill, S. R., Robertson, L. C., Desimone, R., & Ungerleider, L. G. (2003). Posterior parietal cortex and the filtering of distractors. *Proceedings of the National Academy of Sciences, 100*(7), 4263-4268.

Gallese, V., Fadiga, L., Fogassi, L., & Rizzolatti, G. (1996). Action recognition in the premotor cortex. *Brain, 119,* 593-609.

Gazzaniga, M. (2004). *The cognitive neurosciences iii.* Cambridge, MA: MIT Press.

Goodale, M. A. & Milner, A. D. (1992). Separate visual pathways for perception and action. *Trends in Neurosciences, 15*(1), 20-25.

Goodale, M. A. & Haffenden, A. (1998). Frames of reference for perception and action in the human visual system. *Neuroscience & Biobehavioral Reviews, 22*(2), 161-172.

Healy, J. M. (1999). *Endangered minds.* New York, NY: Simon & Schuster.

Heijden, V. (1996). Two stages in visual information processing and visual perception. *Visual Cognition, 3*(4), 325-361.

Heijden, V. (2004). *Cognitive neuroscience of attention.* New York, NY: The Guilford Press.

Hyvarinen, J. & Poranen, A. (1974). Function of the parietal associative area 7 as revealed from cellular discharges in alert monkeys. *Brain, 97,* 673-692.

Johnson, A. & Proctor, R. W. (2004). *Attention: theory and practice.* Thousand Oaks, CA: Sage Publications, Inc.

Kastner, S., De Weerd, P., Desimone, R., & Ungerleider, L. G. (1998). Mechanisms of directed attention in the human extrastriate cortex as revealed by functional MRI. *Science, 282,* 108-111.

Kennedy, J. (2006). How the blind draw. *Scientific American, December,* 44-51.

Kinomura, S., Larsson, J., Gulyás, B., & Roland, P. E. (1996). Activation by attention of the human reticular formation and thalamic intralaminar nuclei. *Science, 271,* 512-515.

Koch, C. & Ullman, S. (1985). Shifts in selective visual attention: towards the underlying neural circuitry. *Human Neurobiology, 4*(4), 219-227.

Le, T., Pardo, J. V., & Hu, X. (1998). 4 T-fMRI study of nonspatial shifting of selective attention: cerebellar and parietal contributions. *Journal of Neurophysiology, 79*(3), 1535-1548.

Lynch, J. C., Mountcastle, V. B., Talbot, W. H., & Yin, T. C. (1977). Parietal lobe mechanisms for directed visual attention. *Journal of Neurophysiology, 40*(2), 362-389.

Lyon, R. (2005). *Attention, memory, and executive function.* Baltimore, MD: Paul H. Brookes Publishing Co.

Macneilage, P. (2009). Left and right brain. *Scientific American, July,* 60-65.

Mesulam, M. M. (1981). A cortical network for directed attention and unilateral neglect. *Annals of Neurology, 10*(4), 309-325.

Mesulam, M. M. (2000). *Principles of behavioral and cognitive neurology.* New York, NY: Oxford University Press.

Mirsky, A. F., Anthony, B. J., Duncan, C. C., Ahearn, M. B., & Kellam, S. G. (1991). Analysis of the elements of attention: a neuropsychological approach. *Neuropsychology Review, 2*(2), 109-145.

Mountcastle, V. B., Andersen, R. A., & Motter, B. C. (1981). The influence of attentive fixation upon the excitability of the light-sensitive neurons of the posterior parietal cortex. *The Journal of Neuroscience, 1*(11), 1218-1235.

Nakayama, K. & Silverman, G. H. (1986). Serial and parallel processing of visual feature conjunctions. *Nature, 330,* 264-265.

Neville, H. J. & Lawson, D. (1987). Attention to central and peripheral visual space in a movement detection task: an event-related potential and behavioral study, ii, congenitally deaf adults. *Brain Research, 405,* 268-283.

National Institute of Child Health and Human Development (1999). Child care and mother-child interaction in the first 3 years of life. *Developmental Psychology, 35,* 1399-1413.

National Institute of Child Health and Human Development Research Network (2000). The relation of child care to cognitive and language development. *Child Development, 71,* 960-980.

National Institute of Child Health and Human Development (2001). Nonmaternal care and family factors in early development: an overview of the N.I.C.H.D. study of early child care. *Applied Developmental Psychology, 22,* 457-492.

National Institute of Child Health and Human Development (2003). Do children's attention processes mediate the link between family predictors and school readiness? *Developmental Psychology, 39,* 581-593.

O'Connor, C. (2003) Part 2: abstracts of posters. *Brain and Cognition, 54,* 133-176.

Paletta, L. (2007). *Attention in cognitive systems: Theories and systems from an interdisciplinary viewpoint.* New York, NY: Springer-Verlag.

Parasuraman, R. (2000). *The attention brain.* Cambridge, MA: MIT Press.

Pardo, J. V., Fox, P. T., & Raichle, M. E. (1991). Localization of a human system for sustained attention by positron emission tomography. *Nature, 349,* 61-64.

Pearson, D. A. & Lane, D. M. (1990). Visual attention movements a developmental study. *Child Development, 61,* 1779-1795.

Pesaran, B., Pezaris, J. S., Sahani, M., Mitra, P. P., & Andersen, R. A. (2002). Temporal structure in neuronal activity during working memory in macaque parietal cortex. *Nature Neuroscience, 5*(8), 805-811.

Petersen, S. (1994). P.E.T. studies of parietal involvement in spatial attention: comparison of different task types. *Canadian Journal of Experimental Psychology, 48,* 319-338.

Pineda, A. (2009). *Mirror neuron systems.* New York, NY: Springer Verlag.

Posner, M. (1980). Attention and the detection of signals. *Journal of Experimental Psychology, 109,* 160-174.

Posner, M. (2004). *Cognitive neuroscience of attention.* New York, NY: The Guilford Press.

Posner, M. I., & Petersen, S. E. (1990). The attention system of the human brain. *Annual Review of Neuroscience, 13,* 25-42.

Posner, M. I., Walker, J. A., Friedrich, F. J., & Rafal, R. D. (1984). Effects of parietal injury on covert orienting of attention. *The Journal of Neuroscience, 4*(7), 1863-1874.

Posner, M. I., Walker, J. A., Friedrich, F. A., & Rafal, R. D. (1987). How do the parietal lobes direct covert attention? *Neuropsychologia, 25,* 135-145.

Prinzmetal, W., Presti, D. E., & Posner, M. I. (1986). Does attention affect feature integration? *Journal of Experimental Psychology, 12,* 361-369.

Richards, J. E. & Holley, F. B. (1999). Infant attention and the development of smooth pursuit tracking. *Developmental Psychology, 35,* 856-867.

Rizzolatti, G., Riggio, L., Dascola, I., & Umiltá, C. (1987). Reorienting attention across the horizontal and vertical meridians: evidence in favor of a premotor theory of attention. *Neuropsychologia, 25,* 31-40.

Rizzolatti, G. (1998). Language within our grasp. *Trends in Neurosciences, 21,* 188-194.

Robertson, I. H., Tegnér, R., Tham, K., Lo, A., & Nimmo-Smith, I. (1995) Sustained attention training for unilateral neglect: theoretical and rehabilitation implications. *Journal of Clinical Experimental Neuropsychology, 17,* 416-430.

Robinson, D., Goldberg, M. E., & Stanton, G. B. (1978). Parietal association cortex in the primate: sensory mechanisms and behavioral modulations. *Journal of Neurophysiology, 41,* 910-931.

Ruff, H. (1996). *Attention in early development.* New York, NY: Oxford University Press.

Sakata, H., Shibutani, H., & Kawano, K. (1983). Functional properties of visual tracking neurons in posterior parietal association cortex of the monkey. *Journal of Neuropsychology, 49,* 1364-1380.

Schmidt, T. (2002). The finger in flight: real-time motor control by visually masked color stimuli. *Psychological Science, 13,* 112-118.

Schneider, W. (1998). *Mechanisms of visual attention: A cognitive neuroscience perspective.* Oxfordshire, UK: Taylor & Francis, Inc.

Schoenfeld, M. A., Tempelmann, C., Martinez, A., Hopf, J. M., Sattler, C., Heinze, H. J., & Hillyard, S. A. (2003). Dynamics of feature binding during object selective attention. *Proceedings of the National Academy of Sciences, 100*(20), 11806-11811.

Selemon, L. D. & Goldman-Rakic, P. S. (1988). Common cortical and subcortical targets of the dorsolateral prefrontal and posterior parietal cortices in the rhesus monkey: evidence for a distributed neural network subserving spatially guided behavior. *The Journal of Neuroscience, 11,* 4049-4068.

Sheliga, B. (1995). Spatial attention and eye movements. *Experimental Brain Research, 105,* 261-275.

Shiu, L. (1994). Negligible effect of spatial precuing on identification of single digits. *Journal of Experimental Psychology, 20,* 1037-1054.

Sieroff, E. (1988). Cueing spatial attention during processing of words and letter strings in normals. *Cognitive Neuropsyhcology, 4,* 451-472.

Sohlberg, M. (2001). *Cognitive rehabilitation.* New York, NY: The Guilford Press.

Sohlberg, M. M. & Mateer, C.A. (1987). Effectiveness of an attention-training program. *Journal of Clinical and Experimental Neuropsychology, 9*(2), 117-130.

Steinman, B., Steinman, S. B., & Lehmkuhle, S. (1995). Visual attention mechanisms show a center-surround organization. *Vision Research, 35*(13), 1859-1869.

Steinmetz, M. (1995). Neurophysiological evidence for a role of posterior parietal cortex in redirecting visual attention. *Cerebral Cortex, 5,* 448-456.

Sturm, W., de Simone, A., Krause, B. J., Specht, K., Hesselmann, V., Radermacher, I., . . . Willmes, K. (1999). Functional anatomy of intrinsic alertness: evidence for a fronto-parietal-thalamic-brainstem network in the right hemisphere. *Neuropsychologia, 37*(7), 797-805.

Treisman, A. (1982). Perceptual grouping and attention in visual search for features and for objects. *Journal of Experimental Psychology, 8*(2), 194-214.

Treisman, A. (1990). Conjunction search revisited. *Journal of Experimental Psychology: Human Perception and Performance, 16,* 459-478.

Treisman, A. (1996). The binding problem. *Current Opinion in Neurobiology, 6,* 171-178.

Treisman, A. (1998). Feature binding, attention and object perception. *Philosophical Transactions of the Royal Society B, 353,* 1295-1306.

Treisman, A. M. & Gelade, G. (1980) A feature-integration theory of attention. *Cognitive Psychology, 12,* 97-136.

Treisman, A. & Paterson, R. (1984). Emergent features, attention and object perception. *Journal of Experimental Psychology, 10*(1), 12-31.

Tucker, M. & Ellis, R. (1998). On the relations between seen objects and components of potential actions. *Journal of Experimental Psychology: Human Perception and Performance, 24*(3), 830-846.

Vidyasagar, T. R. & Pammer, K. (1999). Impaired visual search in dyslexia relates to the role of the magnocellular pathway in attention. *NeuroReport, 10*(5), 1283-1287.

Vidyasagar, T. R. (2001). From attentional gating in macaque primary visual cortex to dyslexia in humans. *Progress in Brain Research, 134*(19), 297-312.

Wickens, C. & McCarley, J. S. (2008). *Applied attention theory.* Boca Raton, FL: CRC Press.

Wojciulik, E. & Kanwisher, N. (1999). The generality of parietal involvement in visual attention. *Neuron, 23,* 747-764.

Wolfe, J. M. (1989). Guided search: an alternative to the feature integration model for visual search. *Journal of Experimental Psychology, 15*(3), 419-433.

Wolfe, J. M. (1994). Guided search 2.0 a reused model of visual search. *Psychonomic Bulletin and Review, 1*(2), 202-238.

Yantis, S. (1992). Multielement visual tracking; attention and perception organization. *Cognitive Psychology, 24*(3), 295-340.

Zimmer, C. (2009). The brain. *Discover Magazine, July-Aug,* 24-25.

SUGGESTED READING

Craighero, L. (1998). Visuomotor priming. *Visual Cognition, 5*(1/2), 109-125.

3

Memory

Philosophers have speculated about memory for at least 2,000 years, but scientific investigation only began 100 years ago. Historical examples have shown us that memory capabilities among people differ widely. Julius Caesar's memory was so superior that he could dictate four letters to his secretaries simultaneously. Milton, who was blind, composed *Paradise Lost* in his mind, 40 lines at a time, and then recited them to a scribe. Aruro Tosacani, conductor of the NBC Symphony for 17 years, knew every note of more than 400 scores from Bach to Wagner. At 87, he momentarily forgot a passage from Lannbauser in midperformance. He left the stage that night and never returned.

Memory is a broad term used to refer to a number of different brain functions. The common feature of these functions is the re-creation of past experience by the synchronous firing of neurons that were involved in the original experience (Carter, 2009).

Memory is the result of changes in synaptic connections as the result of experience. Long-and short-term changes in synaptic effectiveness occur in different regions of the brain. Loss of memory after seizures or head injury and the susceptibility of recent learning to interference by later learning indicate that memories require time to become consolidated. The period before a memory is completely consolidated may be several years in humans, although, after head injury, usually only events that occurred in the preceding few minutes are completely forgotten. It has been suggested that brain trauma completely interrupts the recording of a memory, which takes only a short time to complete, and impairs the effectiveness of recently produced synaptic changes for several days or weeks until the damage has healed. Early theories of consolidation attributed the effect to a two-stage process in which information is first stored as a neural "reverberation" and later by structural changes. Recent evidence suggests that the initial storage involves local modification of receptor and second-messenger proteins followed some time later by the production of a new protein by an effect on gene expression. When undisturbed, the initially affected synapses retain a chemical tag that allows the new protein to find them and thus produce the more permanent change at the correct synapses (Milner, 2006). It does not take many synaptic connections to be altered to encode a memory. The brain fires an electric charge so it can rewire itself as a new memory is formed, and so it can send the new information to other cells. It is a chemical in the brain called phosphotidyl inositol, or protein kinase C (PKC), that forms short- and long-term memories.

Once a cell is alerted to the fact that it needs to format a memory, a second chemical messenger notifies PKC. PKC then connects to another protein, F1, and adds a phosphate molecule to it. The phosphate alerts F1, which changes the synaptic connections. These are temporary changes, lasting long enough to dial a phone number after looking it up in a telephone book. When permanent memory is required, PKC goes to the cell nucleus and launches a genetic process that results in the production of more F1. This increase in F1 starts to rearrange the architecture of the brain cell connections, and more permanent memories are formed.

Research has shown how synapses are altered physically to become stronger with learning. The learning changes the surfaces of synapses from flat to bumpy. The bumps form compartments that store an increased amount of

Lane, K. A. *Visual Attention in Children:*
Theories and Activities (pp. 61-74).
© 2012 SLACK Incorporated.

information. With disuse, these compartments fade, and surfaces flatten out, erasing the memories that were once there (Kotulak, 1996).

ATTENTION: THE GATEWAY FOR MEMORY

Attention is the gateway for memory and awareness. Human learning and behavior are dependent upon the ability to pay attention to critical features in the environments; retain and retrieve information; and select, display, monitor, and control cognitive strategies to learn, remember, and think. Without these abilities, we could not plan, solve problems, or use language. Likewise, without the capacity to attend, remember, and organize and structure data within our world, we would be incapable of modifying our behavior when confronted with new situations (Lyon, 2005; Styles, 2006).

Memory and attention go together. You cannot have one without the other. If there was no attention, our world would be confusing and disorganized and would appear to be a maze of unrelated parts. There would not be anything to store in memory because there would not be anything organized enough to store. If there was no memory, there would not be any top-down information to help us to decide what to attend. We would be no better than a lower life form that just relies on instincts and reflexes to guide its way through life.

Long-Term and Short-Term Memories

Long-term memory is a complex storage system with several different types of storage distributed throughout the brain. Numerous classifications of long-term memory have been proposed, including memory for faces, music, etc. Information is generally stored as visual images, verbal units, or both. Consequently, long-term storage is generally partitioned into visual and auditory or verbal memory. The retention and reconstruction of visual images are the main characteristics of visual memory. Auditory and verbal memory are more complex, with several subtypes. There are several characteristics of long-term memory that distinguish it from short-term memory (STM):

- Long-term representations change slowly and incrementally after repeated exposures to the same information, whereas STM can instantaneously represent new information.

- Long-term memory is based on neural growth, whereas STM consists of temporary electrical activation.

- Long-term memory maintains long-term, relatively stable structured representations of the world, whereas short-term memories are less structured and less distinct. These differences illustrate why it is likely that long-term memory must certainly make a contribution to STM performance. When information enters phonological STM, related phonological and semantic information is immediately and automatically activated. When the individual is required to recall the information temporarily stored in STM, long-term memory enhances recall by drawing on the activated phonological and semantic representations. This explains why memory span is greater for real words than nonwords. Long-term memory also facilitates short-term recall in another way. Each verbal item recalled must be reorganized from the stream of information in the phonological store. This re-recognition is aided by long-term memory representations. This process explains how partially delayed information can be recalled and why those with normal memory span have more difficulty recalling rhyming than nonrhyming words (Dehn, 2008).

Memory has long been described as a function of brain cells getting together and forming connections. A new study shows that single cells can remember things. Individual nerve cells in the front part of the brain can hold traces of memories by themselves for up to 1 minute and perhaps longer (LiveScience, 2009).

Studies have shown that the "pop-out" effect is an STM phenomenon. It reflects the operation of one of the most important visual integrative systems that higher primates are likely to possess—the system for directing visual attention and guiding saccadic eye movements. Studies show that visual perception is surprisingly tenuous and that we are aware only of what we are specifically interested in and attending to. These ideas are confirmed in studies using natural scenes as stimuli. These findings demonstrate that visual attention is needed to be aware of individual elements and that without such attention, we are essentially blind. We also show that "preattentive" aspects of attention actually require visual attention as well. Studies that recorded eye movements during a visuomotor task show that we seem to make an unusual number of eye movements to recently fixated portions of a scene. This constant need for "checking" suggests that, at any given moment, our STM is limited. Thus, visual attention plays a more important role in perception than previously suspected. Rather than just modulating perception, it is its vital prerequisite. Conscious perception outside the confines of attention is almost nonexistent. It is estimated that we make two to four saccadic eye movements every second of our waking hours. As such, the system makes approximately 200,000 such shifts per day. Studies have shown very different patterns of eye fixations over the same picture in response to alternative questions put to the observer regarding a scene. Thus, we have a curious combination of conscious and automatic control with the bulk of eye movements conducted without any supervision on our part (Maljkovic, 2000).

STM is 20 to 30 seconds in the absence of rehearsal (Farah, 2000). It is located in the frontal cortex behind the forehead and enables us to follow and remember such things as conversations or phone numbers. STM consists of information that is within the grasp of immediate consciousness or focus of attention and is limited to five to nine items (Baddeley, 1998). It can be disrupted by irrelevant movements. This last fact is obvious to any teacher or parent who has worked with a child with attention deficit/hyperactivity disorder (AD/HD). The main difference between short- and long-term memory when we deal with schoolwork is that short-term storage retains words in terms of their sounds, while long-term memory stores words in terms of their meanings (Logie, 1995). When you look at people who have amazing memories, you have to ask yourself, what is normal? Most researchers feel that the average person can remember up to seven chunks of information (Baddeley, 1998). They call this the magical number seven. This means that if you were to show the average adult numbers in a row, he or she can remember seven numbers. What can the average child remember? The average child of 6 can remember four to five numbers, a 7 or 8 year old can remember five numbers, and a 9 or 10 year old should remember six numbers. Does this mean if a 6-year-old can only remember three numbers that he or she is going to have school difficulty? The answer is perhaps. Learning disabled children are usually inferior in both visual and auditory sequential memory. It is important that you are aware of what kind of sequential memory is important. Just clapping your hands and having a child repeat it is not important. What is important is sequential memory for units of speech (e.g., words or vowel letters' sounds). This is a more important test than just numbers in a row for determining if a child will have difficulty in school.

WORKING MEMORY

Working memory (WM) has been defined as the use of temporarily stored information in the performance of more complex cognitive tasks. Overall, WM is viewed as a comprehensive system that unites various long- and short-term memory subsystems and functions. To summarize, WM is limited to the management, manipulation, and transformation of information drawn from either short- or long-term memory. The chief differences between STM and WM are as follows:

- STM passively holds information; WM actively processes it.

- STM capacity is domain specific (verbal and visual). WM capacity is less domain specific.

- WM has a stronger relationship with academic learning and with higher-level cognitive functions.

- STM automatically activates information stored in long-term memory; WM consciously directs retrieval of desired information from long-term memory.

- STM has no management functions; WM has some executive functions.

- STM can operate independently of long-term memory; WM operations rely heavily on long-term structures.

- STM retains information coming from the environment; WM retains products of various cognitive processes (Dehn, 2008).

SUMMARY ON WORKING MEMORY

- WM is a complex system responsible for the temporary storage and processing of information (Logie, 1995).

- WM is structurally and functionally distinct from the different forms of permanent or long-term memory. More specifically, there appears to be a basic disassociation between long- and short-term memory in both the verbal domain and the visuospatial domain.

- The contents of WM consist of the set of representations that are currently being activated by interpretative processes in long-term memory. This provides the mechanism by which semantic knowledge about objects and language can be brought to bear on uninterpreted phenomenal experiences.

- The effecting capacity of WM is constrained by (a) long-term memory and (b) the limited attentional resources that are available to activate and maintain task-relevant information and to inhibit and remove irrelevant information.

- The core of this system is a central processor that is involved in a wide variety of executive functions, including the coordination of performance in skilled tasks and the encoding of episodic (i.e., an incident in a series of events) information in long-term memory.

- Some of the storage functions of the central executive system can be discharged to auxiliary subsystems that are structurally and functionally distinct from one another by subsiding to the central executive. These include the phonological loop, the visuospatial sketchpad, and perhaps a third subsystem involved in the representation of familiar body movements (Richardson, 1996).

- It has been found that good readers have a larger WM capacity than do poor readers, regardless of the task being performed.

The adjective *working* implies that this kind of memory, in contrast to the iconic (very brief visual memory) and echoic (very brief auditory memory) sensory memory stores, encompasses more than just passive storage of information. *Working memory* can be defined as the alliance of temporary memory systems that play a crucial role in many cognitive tasks, such as reasoning, learning, and understanding (Pickering, 2006). It can be distinguished from long-term memory, which is the more or less permanent collection of facts, knowledge, and records of experiences. The WM model consists of three components: (1) a phonological loop, (2) visuospatial sketchpad, and (3) a central executive function. The phonological loop is called upon to store and manipulate speech-based information and the visuospatial sketchpad is responsible for storing and manipulating visual images. The central executive is an all-purpose attentional controller that is presumed to supervise and coordinate the work of the other two systems (Johnson, 2004).

Phonological Loop

The phonological loop is thought to contain phonological information (i.e., information according to how it sounds). It appears that if the memory span (length of a list of items that can be repeated back 50% of the time) for dissimilar words (e.g., hat, nut, log, cup) is seven items, memory span for phonologically similar words (e.g., top, pop, shop, chip, tip) may be only five items. It seems that the presentation of speech-like sounds directly interferes with the information held in the phonological loop. The more similar it is in sound, the greater the interference. This limited capacity of the phonological loop is also reflected in the dependence of memory span on the time it takes to pronounce the items to be remembered. The more time it takes to pronounce an item, the fewer items that can be remembered. In general, people can remember the amount of information that they can pronounce within 2 seconds (Johnson, 2004). This is why a child will often read a word in one paragraph but not recognize it in the next paragraph. If he or she cannot pronounce it within 2 seconds, it will not make it to long-term memory.

Several studies have indicated that short-term phonological memory capacity probably plays an important role in the acquisition of vocabulary by both normal children and children with a specific language disability. Phonological loop capacity also appears to be crucial in the case of children learning a second language (Baddeley, 1998).

The loop has been further fractionated into two subcomponents: the phonological short-term store and an articulatory subvocal rehearsal process. The store retains phonological representations of verbal information, and these representations decay with time. Decay can, however, be offset by means of the subvocal rehearsal process, which restores the fading phonological representations. Long periods between rehearsals of an item are likely to result in the phonological representation becoming indiscriminable as a result of decay and hence unrehearsable. As we mentioned before, it is more difficult to remember words or letters that sound alike than if they were more phonologically distinct (e.g., K, X, M). Also, ordered recall of memory lists is better when the elements in the list are short (e.g., sum, wit, hate) than long (e.g., university, opportunity, aluminum) in articulating duration. According to the working memory model, this word length effect is due to the extra time it takes to rehearse words that are slow to articulate, which leads to greater decay from the phonological store between successive rehearsals. Auditory phonological material is believed to gain obligatory access to the phonological store. Thus, irrelevant speech in a memory test interferes with memory performance even when the subjects are instructed to ignore the sounds. This is known as the "unattended speech effect." Visual linguistic material, on the other hand, has to be converted by means of the subvocal rehearsal process into a phonological form appropriate for representation in the phonological store. A few things concerning the phonological loop are as follows:

1. Memory span is greater for words with short rather than long articulatory durations, even if the two sets of words have the same number of syllables.

2. Children's memory spans increase in direct proportion with their increase in rate of speaking as they get older.

3. Poor phonological memory skills are closely associated with immature speech production abilities during childhood: short utterance lengths, small productive vocabularies, and low syntactic complexity of spontaneous speech.

4. Neuropsychological data indicate that the phonological loop plays a critical role in vocabulary acquisition (Gazzaniga, 2004).

Visuospatial Sketchpad

The visuospatial sketchpad (also called visuospatial working memory) is responsible for the short-term storage of visual and spatial information, such as memory for objects and their locations. It also plays a key role in the generation and manipulation of mental images. Like the phonological loop, it consists of a passive temporary store and an active rehearsal process. Decay in the temporary visuospatial store seems to be as rapid as the phonological decay, taking place within a matter of seconds. The rate of forgetting seems to be a function of stimulus complexity and how long the stimulus is viewed. Refreshment of the visual trace appears to result from eye movement manipulation of the image or some type of visual mnemonic. The sketchpad seems primarily designed to maintain spatial or patterned stimuli, which explains why it has been linked to the control and production of physical movement. It may also serve an important function during reading, as it visually encodes printed letters and words while maintaining a visuospatial frame of reference that allows the reader to back track and keep his or her place in the text. Much of short-term visuospatial storage, rehearsal, and processing seems dependent on other working memory components. Although the phonological loop is designed for sequential processing and the visuospatial sketchpad is better suited to holistic processing, most normal individuals will verbally recode much of their visuospatial input (Dehn, 2008). If a child does not appear to verbally recode his or her visuospatial input, he or she should be taught to do so. An example of this is number 2 under Summary and Attention Tips.

The sketchpad is divided into two storage subcomponents: visual and spatial. The visual is responsible for the storage of static visual information (i.e., information about objects' shapes and colors), and the spatial subcomponent is responsible for the storage of dynamic spatial information (i.e., information about motion and duration). Visual short-term storage is limited in capacity, typically to about three or four objects in a matter of seconds. Complex patterns are not retained as well as simple patterns (Dehn, 2008). Development of this area is associated with activity in the frontal and parietal cortices (Coull, Frith, Frackowiak, & Grasby, 1996; Pesaran, Pezaris, Sahani, Mitra, & Andersen, 2002).

There is evidence that differences between males and females with visuospatial abilities could emerge before puberty with males being better in this task. Research has found that this may be the result of the lesser development of the female frontal lobes. There may also be a difference in the development of the parietal lobe (Cornoldi, 2003).

Studies have shown that newborn infants have very good memory for visual configurations. Young children are typically successful in tasks and games that require memory for locations. Furthermore, they have an impressive tendency to imitate behaviors they have seen before, thus demonstrating a good memory for behaviors. Consistent with this view, some studies have suggested that location memory shows little age change. Other studies have shown that most visuospatial skills evolve with age, and children's performance increases significantly from 7 to 11 years in a series of tasks that tap visuospatial working memory, such as recalling spatial positions or solving a jigsaw puzzle. Visuospatial failures may be dramatic and do not necessarily mirror developmental delays. In fact, some good visual spatial working memory competencies seem to be highly developed in young children while others are characterized by different developmental trends (Cornoldi, 2003).

The maintenance of information in spatial working memory appears to recruit a network that includes the occipital, dorsal, parietal, and superior frontal cortices. Regarding the subcomponents of spatial working memory, it is suggested that this system might rely upon implicit eye movement programs analogous to the way that verbal rehearsal involves a component of subvocal articulation. Therefore, continuing to move your eyes over the object you need to remember helps in its memory. Also, unwanted eye movements away from the object will make it difficult to remember. It has also been shown that any motor act (not just eye movements) can disrupt remembering a spatial object. For example, directed arm movement can interfere with spatial memory (Awh, 2001).

Vision, attention, perception, and memory are all interrelated, with the key element being attention. Vision is somewhat of an illusion. We regard our visual world as "just there," not as something that is only acquired after sequential sampling and reconstruction. It appears to us that vision occurs in parallel, yet our actual contact with the world is serial as the result of eye movements. It is constructed as a result of pattern recognition matches. Thus, the actual amount of visual information that is explicitly used as part of memory and pattern recognition processes is but a tiny fraction of the information available. Visual objects are assemblies of features, associatively linked through visual experience and stored in memory. An example of the brain not processing and remembering information as a picture but as individual features is handwriting and printing.

Before recognizing handwriting is explained, some background information is needed. The brain forms the object; the object is not sent to the brain as a whole picture. Therefore, the letter we are looking at is organized in the brain, and because a letter cannot be processed by its whole shape, it must be processed by its parts. Letters are composed of lines and angles; therefore, letters must be recognized by the lines and angles from which they are made. This theory probably would not have been considered except for the work of D. H. Hubel and T. N. Wiesel in 1958. They were trying to get different cells in a cat's cortex to respond to light and were having a very difficult time until they noticed that the light did not get a response but the faint shadow cast by the edge of the glass they were sliding into the light slot of the microscope did. They found that when the shadow was swept across one small part of the retina, it caused the cells in the brain to respond. They also found that it only worked when it was moved in one direction. In other words, the brain cells did not respond to diffuse light but responded to lines made by shadows. Further research showed that cells in the brain's cortex would respond to only certain configurations, such as lines, or lines of different orientation or direction. In fact, they found that 70% to 80% of the cortex cells seem to be orientation-selective. It also seems that there are cells in the brain that respond to moving objects and those that respond to stationary objects. It, therefore, appears that parts of letters, such as lines, curves, and angles, stimulate different cells in the brain's cortex. This, however, still does not give the full story of letter recognition because the brain still has to combine these stimuli (lines, curves, etc.) to form a pattern, and the pattern has to be recognized. How does this happen? The prototype theory answers this problem.

The basic elements of this theory are memory representations called "prototypes." A prototype is characterized as a statistical average of all of the individual patterns that belong to a category. People feel a pattern belongs to a category if it is like the prototype. If it is like the prototype, then it belongs to that class of patterns (Boff, 1986). In other words, the letters "T" and "t" are recognized as the same by the brain because they both fit the prototype of "t" letters. Prototype theory takes into account the fact that people attend to certain critical features more than others when they classify patterns. Another way of saying this is that combinations of features are critical for pattern recognition. For example, in pattern recognition for the letter "b" in a prototype pattern of letters, the critical features may be the "loop" at the lower right and the straight vertical line on the left side. Therefore, when you are teaching children letters, do not just show them the letter, but also explain the letter, e.g., the letter "b" is a straight line with a rounded loop at the lower end of the line whereas a "p" is a straight line with the loop at the top of the line. It has been shown that basic level categories are quickly learned by children, whereas superordinate categories, such as the breed of a dog instead of dogs in general, require more prolonged development. Two studies with children demonstrated that young children (3 to 5 years old) have very little trouble making adult-like categorizations but are not fully developed until the early school years (5 to 8 years old). For example, even a 3 year old can sort pictures of chairs, cars, and shoes into correct piles, but the sorting of pictures of different furniture, vehicles, and clothing was performed perfectly only by children at least 8 years of age (Boff, 1986). This is yet another indication that children need time to develop the perceptual skills needed for success in school. It may also indicate that children should be exposed to categories early in childhood. It would be better to learn alphabet letters in categories such as all loop letters ("B" and "D") first then letters with straight lines like "T." It would be beneficial if, when learning the letter "B," you show the child the letter "B" next to a "T" so he or she is made aware of differences and similarities among letters. Because we learn the basic patterns of letters, we can recognize handwriting we have never seen. A printed "T" is a vertical line with a horizontal line on top. A written letter "t," even if it is poorly written, would still be a vertical line and horizontal line on top. The brain, therefore, will see it as a "T" because it is more similar to a "t" than any other letter.

Executive Function

This term is difficult to give one single definition. Most people stress that it must include planning and control. It should also include monitoring, organizing, coordinating, and adopting knowledge and strategic resources as well as self-regulation. Executive function (EF) is now seen as a special case of attention in which the initial response of the individual to an environmental event alters the probability of a subsequent response of that individual. That initial response is classified as an executive act or function when used only when it serves to directly modify the likelihood of another response by the individual. EFs are inherently self-regulating actions. They function to change the subsequent behavior of the individual. All executive acts by the individual can also be thought of as futures or goal-directed, principally because they indirectly function to change the likelihood of future consequences for the individual, consequences often quite distant in time. Thus, an executive function is so, not only because it is self-regulating, but also because it is ultimately future-directed (Lyon, 2005).

The wide range of cognitive capacities that have been ascribed to the central executive can be broadly classified into two categories. The first category is control activities. The executive has been suggested to house the control of attention and action to regulate information flow through the working memory system and to operate the retrieval of information from more permanent knowledge systems. The second category is storage and processing capabilities. The central executive is considered to be fueled by limited-capacity processing resources that can be flexibly deployed to respond to many different information processing requirements. Activities suggested to be supported by these resources include retrieval from long-term memory, maintenance rehearsal, and the storage and processing of linguistic material (Gathercole, 1994).

Executive functions are unique and only arise in humans. Other primates do not have this function. Executive functions include inhibition, self-awareness, self-regulation, imitation, symbolization, and generativity (mental stimulation for behavioral innovator) (Barkley, 2001).

Studies based on a variety of approaches have implicated the anterior cingulated cortex in numerous functions including emotion, pain, and attention (Garavan, 1998). This region is also involved primarily in effector or executive functions in controlling output whether to visceromotor, endocrine, or skeletomotor systems. The main area of involvement, however, is the frontal lobes (D'Esposito et al., 1995), which are responsible for planning, initiating, regulating, and verifying a sequence of actions. Some of the most common problems demonstrated by people with frontal and executive involvement include the following:

- Problems in "starting." Individuals may demonstrate markedly reduced initiation and spontaneity of behavior. In many cases, they may verbalize an intent to act but do not follow through.

- Problems with "stopping." Individuals may demonstrate disinhibition, impulsivity, and quick shifts in behavior and emotional tone.

- Difficulties in marking mental or behavioral shifts. Individuals may demonstrate rigid, inflexible, or preservative behavior, seemingly becoming fixed on a response set.

- Problems with attention. Individuals with frontal dysfunction are often distractible and display poor selective and divided attention.

- Problems with awareness of self and others. Individuals may display limited or no apparent understanding and appreciation with regard to the nature of their difficulties and the impact these have on everyday functioning.

The loss of executive skills can impair a person's ability to monitor his or her own performance and/or to use feedback to exert control over his or her own behavior. The "dysexecutive syndrome" refers to a cluster of deficits including attention, planning, problem solving, and behavior control, which are classically associated with lesions to the prefrontal cortex (Manly, Hawkins, Evans, Woldt, & Robertson, 2002).

An executive function is a special case of attention (Sohlberg, 2001). It is inherently self-regulatory, where attention need not be so. It does not require temporal (time) proximity among the components of the sequence; that is, it organizes these sequences across delays in time between components of the sequence, thereby providing considerable cross-temporal organization to human adoptive behavior. It is also directed at altering the probability of consequences to the individual in the future and not the moment and, therefore, seems to maximize the future positive outcome to the individual. Finally, it is always initiated by a delay in the proponent response to the environmental event.

The components of attention are typically conceived of as at least these four: initiate, sustain, inhibit, and shift. Each describes a certain general form of an "attending" response or reaction that may be taken to an environmental event. Similarly, the components of executive function may likewise comprise these same general forms (initiate, sustain, inhibit, shift) but refer to the actions the individual takes to modify the subsequent probability of one of these general forms of responses to the environment (the attending responses). Executive functions, then, can also be initiated, sustained, inhibited, and shifted as they are used to alter the general responses of the individual to the environment.

A second link between attention and executive function follows from the above and occurs at the neuropsychological or brain function system level of analysis. We know that three major functional brain systems (sensory-motor, spatial-sequential, and inhibitory-excitatory systems) are important in understanding attention. We can now see that the executive system provides a fourth functional system that is cross-temporal in nature and acts to govern these other systems in the service of future-oriented, goal-directed behavior.

Attention arises as a result of the dynamic interaction of the brainstem arousal/alertness systems with the limbic system, motivational and emotional centers, and these two regions with the sensory-motor and premotor zones of the cortex and tertiary posterior cortical areas related to spatial-sequential processing and movement. The prefrontal cortex housing the executive system links up neuroanatomically with all of these brain regions and regulates them, as needed, in the service of self-regulated, goal-directed, and future-oriented behavior. Richly connected to the posterior cortical sensory analyzers, the prefrontal executive cortex can redirect the event to these tertiary spatial-sequential systems for further parallel processing, the obvious advantage of a large brain. Seated above and apparently evolving out of the lower limbic system, the prefrontal cortex is similarly suited to receive, regulate, and even reciprocally kindle limbic motivational drive and emotional states to subserve goal-directed behavior (Lyon, 2005).

Executive function is critical for good reading comprehension. Reading words correctly is not what reading is about. By definition, *reading* is an interaction among the reader, the situation, the task, and the text that results in the construction of meaning. To assure that comprehension is occurring, the reader taps into the power of executive control, a volitional process that enables him or her to monitor and take charge of the construction of meaning while reading. Executive control is one of the most important, if not *the* most important, student aptitudes related to reading comprehension. Executive control processes for comprehending text deal with how individuals plan, direct, select, and orchestrate the various cognitive structures and processes available to them for attaining comprehension goals. Five of the often-cited executive processes include planning, prioritizing, organizing, shifting mindsets flexibility, and self-checking. A sixth executive control process is self-assessing. Executive control processes enable readers to monitor what they read for sense and to be in charge of whether or not they understand what they read (Meltzer, 2007).

Research has consistently found students with specific learning difficulties to be the most deficient in the executive processing component of working memory. Executive working memory serves a governing function, controlling and regulating memory subsystems. Executive-loaded working memory tasks provide the best discrimination between children with and without learning disabilities. For example, when compared with IQ-matched peers, students with learning disabilities have relatively more difficulty with a reverse digit span test (Dehn, 2008). In order to properly perform a reverse digit span, the executive function must be able to hold and then reorganize the digits in reverse order. This is a real test for the executive function.

The following is a list of memory components most highly related to types of academic learning:

- Reading decoding: Phonological short-term memory, verbal working memory, executive function of working memory

- Reading comprehension: Executive function of working memory, verbal working memory

- Written language: Executive working memory, verbal working memory, phonological working memory

- Mathematics: Visuospatial working memory, executive working memory (Dehn, 2008)

EXECUTIVE DYSFUNCTION

The EF domain includes attention and working memory. You cannot separate the two functions. It is on equal footing with other domains of the brain, such as language, visuospatial ability, visual object discrimination, verbal and visual memory storage, and motor coordination. EF, just as visual perception, is captured as "where" and "when" functions. We can speak of EF as encompassing "how" and "when" functions. Even more colloquially speaking to adolescents and parents, EF can be defined as "getting your act together." The index of inadequate inhibitory executive control is found in many studies of children with AD/HD and in some studies of children with learning disabilities (LDs), which usually means reading disability as well as language and processing difficulties.

As for a child with AD/HD and executive dysfunction (EDF) (you cannot focus on one without the other), there is usually an impact on basic reading skills. One 8-year-old little boy captured the EDF issue better than most professionals do: he explained that, although he could recite the rule of the silent terminal "e" and explain short and long vowels, he found that when he got involved in reading text, he "forgot to look ahead." He could recall the strategy but forgot to be strategic, the very "curious disassociation between knowing and doing" that is the core of EDF. As this child grew older, the repetitive practice effect obviated strategic approach, but he did poorly in extracting from text answers to questions posed by the teachers to assess reading comprehension.

It is the difficulty in planning (often called sequencing in LD terms) and working memory that is at the core of most LD children's difficulties. If you add poor ability to move their eyes across a line of print and often being distracted due to poor focused and sustained attention, you can easily see the problem many LD children face.

Children in our information age are flooded with stimulation from multiple media sources and are exposed to an intensity of technology-assisted multitasking that was not required by earlier generations. It seems reasonable to speculate that such experience could be reflected in the quality of neural connectivity, especially for those brain systems that are most involved in interface with environmental context. The flood of information may stimulate the development of more efficient and finely tuned executive systems, or it may result in less well-regulated execution systems. It is unfortunate that children often lack highly structured environments that are crucial in shaping behaviors (Meltzer, 2007).

WORKING MEMORY CAPACITY

At age 4, the typical child can recall an average of three digits in order. By 12 years of age, the span has doubled to six digits, and by 16, the digit span has plateaued to seven to eight digits. In most children, phonological short-term memory appears to be firmly established by 3 years of age. At 4 years of age, the typical child can remember two or three words in sequence. However, the more consequential occurrence at age 4 is the emergence of subvocal rehearsal. The traditional explanation for growth in phonological short-term memory is that age-related improvements in span depend primarily on increases in speech rote. Increases in articulation rates during childhood are assumed to enhance the effectiveness of subvocal rehearsal processes.

The capacity for visuospatial working memory doubles between ages 5 and 11, when span reaches an adult level of approximately four items. It seems that nearly all humans naturally gravitate toward recording visuospatial information into verbal code. Visuospatial recording emerges between the ages of 6 and 8 years at about the same time children learn to read.

Neuropsychological studies have documented that growth in executive working memory and in general working memory capacity is related to prefrontal cortex maturation. Whereas 9-year-old children have considerable difficulty preventing unrelated information from entering working memory, 14 year olds have much better developed inhibitory mechanism. Thus, younger children may need more executive resources to inhibit or resist potential interference from irrelevant items, leaving fewer executive resources for other tasks. Executive working memory develops until 16 to 17 years of age (Dehn, 2008).

MEMORY DEVELOPMENT

The fact that every part of the brain takes part in some form of information storage helps make sense of the way memory emerges during infancy. Implicit (unconscious) memories, the kinds of habits and conditional responses that can be stored in more precocious lower-brain areas like the spinal cord and brainstem, dawn first (Eliot, 1999). These occur without conscious awareness. In fact, most brain systems are plastic and work outside of consciousness. They can be thought of as implicit memory systems. Those aspects of the self that are learned and stored in implicit systems make up the implicit aspects of the self. We use this information all the time even though we are not aware of it. The way we characteristically walk and talk and even the way we think and feel all reflect the working of systems that function on the basis of past experience, but their operations take place outside of awareness (LeDoux, 2003) and start forming in infancy. Babies' repertoire of implicit memory skills grows broader as structures such as the basal ganglion and cerebellum rapidly mature during early infancy. Memories that depend on the cerebral cortex emerge slowly because the cortex lags well behind subcortical structures in its maturation. Cortical development may not be the only factor limiting conscious memory in babies. Important evidence suggests that the hippocampus is also responsible for the phenomenon of infantile amnesia. First, it is one of the very few brain areas in which neurons are still being formed after birth; some 20% of cells in the first hippocampal relay are added between birth and around 9 months of age. Second, several of the major input and output pathways of the hippocampus are among the slowest to myelinate of all fiber tracts in the brain. One tract in particular, the fornix, which carries information from the hippocampus to the thalamus, does not even begin myelinating until the second year after birth and continues the process into late childhood. To some degree, infantile amnesia is the same problem faced by adults with amnesia, the lack of a functional hippocampus (Eliot, 1999).

Around 9 months of age, emerging motor skills, such as crawling, play an important role in infants because they can attend to new aspects of their physical and social environment. They also have an increase in memory function at this time. This improves such abilities as retrieving representations of past experiences when minimal cues are present (Ruff, 1996). In fact, at 9 months, babies can remember an event and reproduce it 20 to 24 hours later. By 13 months, they can remember up to 1 week later. Children as young as 14 months are known to imitate actions that they have observed only on TV. By 3 years of age, when children are speaking in complete sentences, they can remember events that happened up to 1 year before. Language is not, as psychologists once believed, a prerequisite for storing conscious memories. On the contrary, it is now thought that children remember much more than they can talk about, at least until about 6 years of age, when their language skills finally catch up with their various memory abilities (Eliot, 1999).

LAYING DOWN A LONG-TERM MEMORY

- 0.2 seconds—Attention: Attention causes the neurons that register the event to fire more frequently. Such activity makes the experience more intense because the more the neuron fires, the stronger the connections. Attention is the critical element in the beginning of a memory.

- 0.25 seconds—Emotion: Intensely emotional experiences, such as the birth of a child, are more likely to be laid down in memory because the emotion increases attention.

- 0.5 seconds to 10 minutes—Working memory: Working memory is like text on a blackboard that is constantly refreshed. It begins with an experience and continues as that experience is "held in the mind" by repetition.

- 10 minutes to 2 years—Hippocampal processing: Particularly striking experiences "break out" from working memory, where they undergo further processing.

- 2 years onward—Consolidation: It takes up to 2 years for a memory to become firmly consolidated in the brain, and, even after that, it may be altered or lost. During this time, the neural firing patterns that encode an experience are played back and forth between the hippocampus and the cortex (Carter, 2009).

INFANTILE AMNESIA

Most of us do not recall anything before age 3.5. In fact, memories remain very sketchy until 5 or 6 years of age. A 75-year-old person can recognize high school classmates even if he or she has not seen them in 50 years, but a 10 year old finds it very difficult to identify preschool friends whom he or she saw just 6 years earlier. Why is this? Most feel infantile amnesia is due to an absence of certain cognitive skills such as language. We now know that infantile amnesia is the result of the fact that some circuits in the brain that are responsible for storing permanent memories take years to develop. It is, therefore, a problem of storage, not retrieval. Early experiences never make it to long-term memory because the brain's recording machinery is not yet functional. Recent evidence suggests that it is the functional immaturity of the association areas of the cortex that may be the cause of infantile amnesia (Lyon, 2005). This does not mean very young children are not capable of storing some information. For example, even 4 month olds can recognize familiar people or toys. A child in preschool can recite facts and even remember his or her second birthday; however, he or she will not remember them when he or she is an adult (Eliot, 1999).

Who has better memory: boys or girls? With young children, it is probably girls, and this can be blamed on testosterone (Eliot, 1999). Testosterone slows cellular development in certain cortical regions, including the inferior temporal cortex. It has different growth-related effects in different parts of the brain, promoting certain features of boys' mental functions at the expense of some of their memory skills. Toward the end of the first year, girls are about a month ahead in tests of short-term memory, like remembering where a toy is hidden. Girls tend to perform better on tests of verbal recall, like remembering details about recent events, a difference that emerges in the fourth year and persists into adulthood. The main reason for this is testosterone.

The human memory seems capable of maintaining a great amount of information for a very short period of time while still being capable of holding part of it in a transitory memory system for tenths of a second, even when the person does not have the possibility of refreshing it. These capacities are not specific to human beings as they can also be found in animals. Furthermore, infants aged less than 1 year also demonstrate good and quite stable visual memory abilities, remembering more than one element in a series of visual stimuli presented serially.

WORKING MEMORY ACTIVITIES

Number-Letter Location

Area of attention: Working memory

Materials: Chart 3-1

Procedure: The charts are an example of how you will set up this activity. Show the child the top chart for a few seconds, then take it away. He or she is to have a blank chart. His or her job is to draw in the blank chart where he or she saw the number or letter. In this example, it may be the number 3.

Letter Location

Area of attention: Working memory

Materials: Chart 3-2

Procedure: Show the child the entire chart of letters. Ask him or her where one of the letters is located after you take the chart away. See how long it takes him or her to fill in the entire chart of letters. The fastest he or she could do it would be in nine attempts.

Fastest Route

Area of attention: Working memory

Materials: Chart 3-3

Procedure: Show the child the chart with the "start" in one of the squares and the letter "X" in another square. Show him or her the chart for 5 seconds. He or she is then to tell you the fastest route to the "X." He or she is allowed to go diagonally. In the top example, the fastest way would be four squares. Two to the left and two left diagonal. The bottom would be three. Two diagonal and one up.

Math Problems

Area: Phonological working memory

Materials: A list of math problems—some correct and some incorrect. For example, $5 + 2 = 4$, $6 - 3 = 3$, $7 + 7 = 14$.

Procedure: Each of the math problems will be followed by a word. For example, $6 - 3 = 3$ CAT, $5 + 2 = 4$ HOUSE, $7 + 7 = 14$ MAN.

The child must look at each math problem and tell you if it is true and remember the word after it. At the end of the last problem, the child must repeat all of the words in correct order.

Maps

Area: Visuospatial sketchpad

Materials: Map of a state, blank paper

Procedure: Show the child a map and explain to him or her where the different towns are located.

1. Name a large town or city, and see how fast he or she can find it. Give him or her clues, such as downright, etc., to help him or her.

2. After he or she has become familiar with the map, have him or her make a map with his or her blank sheet of paper. You name three towns that he or she has seen on the state map, and he or she marks where they go on his or her paper in relation to each other.

Faces

Area: Visuospatial sketchpad

Materials: Faces that you have cut out of magazines. Try to have a lot of these to vary the activities.

Procedure: Show the child 10 faces. Give him or her about 30 seconds to study them. Then, put the faces away.

1. Mix some of the extra faces with the 10 that he or she looked at. He or she is to tell you which ones were in the original 10.

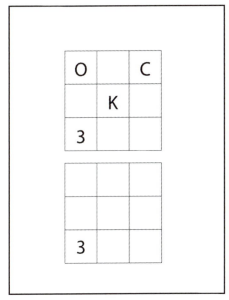

Chart 3-1. Number-letter location.

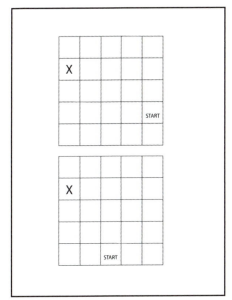

Chart 3-3. Fastest route.

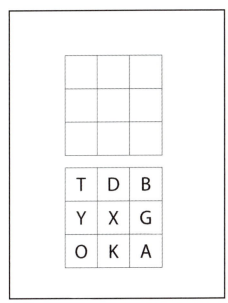

Chart 3-2. Letter location.

Delayed Response

Area: Executive function

Materials: Brockstring (a 1.5-foot string with colored beads), metronome. The child holds one end to his or her nose and the other at arm's length.

Procedure: Child is to move his or her eyes from bead to bead, starting with the nearest and going to the one at the end and then back toward the nearest bead again. At every beat of the metronome, he or she moves his or her eyes.

1. Vary this by telling him or her to wait until two or three beats of the metronome before he or she moves his or her eyes. Continue to vary this from every beat to multiple beats.

2. Tell him or her a sequence you want him or her to follow. At each beat, go from red to blue to yellow beads. Make up different sequences. Encourage him or her to vocalize to him- or herself to remember the sequence.

Pseudowords

Area: Phonological working memory

Materials: A list of pseudowords (words that sound like real words, e.g., cam, lovz, dat, lup)

Procedure: Show the child a list of pseudowords. Start with three and work up to seven. He or she is to look at the words for 1 second per word (three words = 3 seconds) and then repeat them to you. In the correct sequence, encourage him or her to vocalize the words to him- or herself to improve his or her ability to remember them. You can make this more difficult by adding multisyllable words, (e.g., socamlot).

Last Letter

Area: Phonological working memory

Materials: Paper with a list of words that the child should know: cat, boy, house, man, lady.

Procedure: Have the child read the words aloud in sequence. When he or she is done, have him or her close his or her eyes and see how many ending letters he or she can remember. Start with two words, and try to work up to five or seven words. He or she does not have to remember the letters in sequence. The above example would be t, y, e, m, y.

Reverse Alphabet

Area: Phonological working memory

Materials: A list of letters not in alphabetical order (e.g., H, C, B, O).

Procedure: Have the child look at the list of letters. He or she is to remember these and then write them in alphabetical order. Encourage him or her to continue to say the letters to himself or herself. The above example would be B, C, H, O.

Rehearsal Training

Area: Phonological working memory

Materials: A list of words

Procedure: Slowly repeat a string of words to the child. Start with two or three and work up until he or she cannot repeat them back to you. For example, you say "dog, man." He or she repeats this. Now, add a word: "dog, man, horse." He or she repeats this. Continue until the child cannot remember the list. The goal is five to seven words or more.

Rhyming Game

Area: Phonological working memory

Materials: None

Procedure: This is very good for preschool and young children. Tell the child you are going to say part of a word. He or she is to try and guess what the word is. Start with one syllable, and continue to add syllables until he or she correctly guesses the word. For example, vacation. Start with VA—then VACA—then VACATION. You can give him or her clues like, this is what you do each summer with your parents.

Objects Series

Area: Working memory
Materials:

1. A series of numbers and letters, etc.

    T   B   3   W

2. A grid with these four figures in it (Chart 3-4).

3. Another series of letters and numbers.

    4   0   3   X

4. A blank grid

Procedure: Show the child a series of figures. Now, show him or her a grid with four figures. Show him or her another series of figures. His or her job is to look at this new series and tell you which one was in the original series and where it was in the last grid that was shown to him or her. For example, show him or her:

    T   B   3   W

Now show grid #1.

Now show him or her:

    X   D   3   P

He then picks out the 3 and puts it in his grid at the correct location in his blank grid.

This exercise explores three parts of working memory.

Word Grid

Area: Working memory

Materials: Two grids: one a blank grid with six to nine squares and another with an equal amount of squares with letters (Chart 3-5).

Procedure: The child looks at the grid with the letters for 20 seconds. You then take the grid away and tell how to spell a word in his or her grid using the same letter locations as the grid he or she saw. For example, spell "dog" by putting the letters in the correct squares.

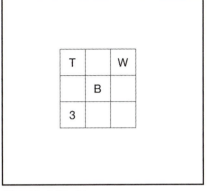

Chart 3-4. Working memory.

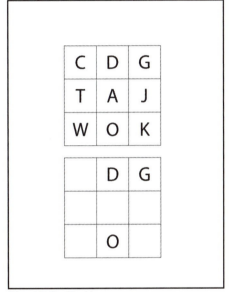

Chart 3-5. Working memory.

SUMMARY AND ATTENTION TIPS

1. To test a child's memory, having him or her repeat your hand clapping is not important. What is important is sequential memory for units of speech, e.g., words or vowel letter's sound.

2. Teach the child to use subvocal (saying it to him- or herself) to improve his or her memory. This restores the fading phonological representation. With spatial memory, he or she must scan the objects several times to improve his or her spatial memory. He or she may also learn to verbally recode the visuospatial input. For example, repeating to him- or herself such things as "the red object is below the green object."

3. You can always make a spatial memory task more difficult by having the child tap his or her fingers on the table while he or she is trying to remember the task.

4. When you teach children letters, do not just show them the letters; explain the letter. For example, the letter "p" is a straight line with a loop at the top of the line on the right side.

5. Show the child a list of words in sequence (e.g.,"boy, dog, cat). He or she is then to repeat it. Gradually increase the number of words he or she is to remember.

6. Have the child repeat a spoken sentence.

7. Have several geometric shapes or letters on paper in front of the child. Slowly show him or her parts of the shapes or letters, gradually building to the finished shape or letter. See how fast he or she can identify the correct shape or letter.

8. Chunking is a good way for a child to remember long strips of numbers. For example, instead of remembering 784962, it is easier to remember 78-49-62 or 784-962.

9. Any of the above can be made into go-no-go tests by having the child hold his or her response for a period of time.

REFERENCES

Awh, E. (2001). Overlapping mechanisms of attention and spatial working memory. *Trends by Cognitive Sciences, 5*(3), 119-126.

Baddeley, A. (1998). *Human memory: theory and practice.* Upper Saddle River, NJ: Pearson Education.

Barkley, R. A. (2001). The executive functions and self-regulation: an evolutionary neuropsychological perspective. *Neuropsychology Review, II*(1), 1-29.

Boff, K. (1986). *Handbook of perception and human performance* (vol. II). New York, NY: John Wiley and Sons.

Carter, R. (2009.) *The human brain.* New York, NY: D.K. Publishers.

Cornoldi, C. (2003). *Visuo-spatial working memory and individual differences.* London, UK: Psychology Press.

Coull, J. T., Frith, C. D., Frackowiak, R. S., & Grasby, P. M. (1996). A Fronto-parietal network for rapid visual information processing: a pet study of sustained attention and working memory. *Neuropsychologia, 34*(11), 1085-1095.

Dehn, M. (2008). *Working memory and academic learning.* New York, NY: John Wiley & Sons, Inc.

D'Esposito, M., Detre, J. A., Alsop, D. C., Shin, R. K., Atlas, S., & Grossman, M. (1995). The neural basis of the central executive system of working memory nature. *Nature, 378*(16), 279-281.

Eliot, L. (1999). *What's going on in there?* New York, NY: Bantam Books.

Farah, M. J. (2000). *The cognitive neuroscience of vision.* Malden, MA: Blackwell Publishers, Inc., U.S.A.

Garavan, H. (1998). Serial attention within working memory. *Memory and Cognition, 26*(2), 263-276.

Gathercole, S. (1994). Neuropsychology and working memory: a review. *Neuropsychology, 8*(4), 494-505.

Gazzaniga, M. (2004). *The cognitive neurosciences iii.* Cambridge, MA: The MIT Press.

Johnson, A. (2004). *Attention theory and practice.* Thousand Oaks, CA: SAGE Publications.

Kotulak, R. (1996). *Inside the brain: Revolutionary discoveries of how the mind works.* Kansas City, MO: Andrews McMeel Publishing.

LeDoux, J. (2003). *Synaptic self: How our brains become who we are.* New York, NY: Penguin Group (USA), Inc.

Logie, R. (1995). *Visuo-spatial working memory.* Oxfordshire, UK: Taylor & Francis, Inc.

Lyon, R. (2005). *Attention, memory, and executive function.* Baltimore, MD: Paul H. Brookes Publishing Co.

Maljkovic, V. (2000). Priming of popout: iii: a short-term implicit memory system beneficial for rapid selection. *Visual Cognition, 7*(5), 571-595.

Manly, T., Hawkins, K., Evans, J., Woldt, K., & Robertson, I. H. (2002). Rehabilitation of executive function: facilitation of effective goal managements on complex tasks using periodic auditory alerts. *Neuropsychologia, 40,* 271-281.

Meltzer, L. (2007). *Executive function in education.* New York, NY: The Guilford Press.

Milner, D.A. (2006). *Visual brain in action.* New York, NY: Oxford University Press.

Pesaran, B., Pezaris, J. S., Sahani, M., Mitra, P. P, & Andersen, R. A. (2002). Temporal structure in neuronal activity during working memory in macaque parietal cortex. *Nature Neuroscience, 5*(8), 805-810.

Pickering, S. J. (2006). *Working memory and education.* Philadelphia, PA: Elsevier.

Richardson, J. (1996). *Working memory and human cognition.* New York, NY: Oxford University Press.

Ruff, H. (1996). *Attention in early development.* New York, NY: Oxford University Press.

Sohlberg, M. (2001). *Cognitive rehabilitation.* New York, NY: The Guilford Press.

LiveScience Staff. (2009). Single cell can hold a memory. *Brain in the News, 16*(2), 7.

Styles, E. (2006). *The psychology of attention.* London, UK: Psychology Press.

SUGGESTED READING

Garavan, H., Ross, T. J., Murphy, K., Roche, R. A., & Stein, E. A. (2002). Dissociable executive functions in the dynamic control of behavior: inhibition, error detection, and correction. *Neuroimage, 17,* 1820-1829.

Olesen, P.J., Nagy, Z., Westerberg, H., & Klingberg, T. (2003). Combined analysis of DTI and fMRI data reveals a joint maturation of white and grey matter in a fronto-parietal network. *Cognitive Brain Science, 18*(1), 48-52.

Parachin, V. (1997). A good memory means success: seven ways to sharpen memory. *Supervision, 10,* 9-11.

Posner, M. (2004). *Cognitive neuroscience of attention.* New York, NY: The Guilford Press.

Rugg, M. (2010). How are memories saved? where does the recording take place and how? *Scientific American Mind, January/February,* 74.

Stix, G. (2009). Turbocharging the brain. *Scientific American, Oct,* 46-49.

4

Attention Deficit/ Hyperactivity Disorder

It is estimated that during the past 10,000 years, humans have evolved as much as 100 times faster than at any other time since the split of the earliest hominid from the ancestors of modern chimpanzees. In most parts of the world, babies no longer die in large numbers. People with genetic damage that was once fatal now live and have children. Some scientists speculate that more inheritable traits could be accumulating in the human species and that these traits are anything but good for us. For example, behavior disorders such as Tourette's syndrome and attention deficit hyperactivity disorder (AD/HD) may be encoded in a few genes in which case their heritability could be very high. David Comings, a specialist in these two diseases, has argued that these conditions are more common than they used to be and that evolution might be the reason: women with these syndromes are less likely to attend college and thus tend to have more children than those who do. However, other researchers have brought forward serious concerns about Comings' methodology. It is not clear whether the incidence of Tourette's syndrome and AD/HD is in fact increasing at all (Ward, 2009).

AD/HD is one of the many labels for one of the most prevalent and, undoubtedly, the most controversial conditions in child psychiatry. AD/HD is conservatively estimated to occur in 3.0% to 7.5% of school-aged children, but more permissive criteria yield estimates up to 17%, and up to 20% of boys in some school systems receive psychostimulants for the treatment of AD/HD. Despite the absence of controlled studies in preschool-aged children and concern about potential long-term adverse effects, stimulant medications are increasingly being administered to children as young as 2 years of age (Castellanos & Tannock, 2002).

Longitudinal epidemiological studies demonstrate that AD/HD is no more common today than in the past. The apparent statistical rise in the number of cases may be explained by increased public awareness and improved diagnosis. Researchers using state-of-the-art imaging techniques have found differences in several brain regions of AD/HD and non-AD/HD children of similar ages. On average, both the frontal lobe and the cerebellum are smaller in AD/HD brains, as are the parietal and temporal lobes. AD/HD seems to be the result of abnormal information processing in these brain regions, which are responsible for emotions and control over impulses and movements. Experts now believe that neural information processing—the foundation of experience and behavior—may break down in children with AD/HD, especially when many competing demands suddenly flood the brain. In this circumstance or when faced with tasks requiring speed, thoroughness, or endurance, the performance of AD/HD brains decreases dramatically compared with the brains of other children. A lack of stimulation, on the other hand, quickly leads to boredom.

The attention deficit is particularly evident whenever children are asked to control their behavior—stopping an impulsive action or maintaining a high level of performance in a given task (Rotenberger, 2007). Most argue that AD/HD involves a central deficiency in response inhibition (Barkley, 2006). A deficit in the inhibition of behavior will produce an adverse impact on executive functioning, self-regulation, and the cross-temporal organization of behavior toward the future. Behavior inhibition is critical to the development, privatization, and proficient performance of the four executive functions. The four executive functions

Lane, K. A. *Visual Attention in Children: Theories and Activities* (pp. 75-84). © 2012 SLACK Incorporated.

are nonverbal working memory, internalization of speech (verbal working memory), the self-regulation of affect/ motivation/arousal, and reconstitution (planning and generativity). These executive functions can shift behavior from control by the immediate environment to control by internally represented forms of information through their influence over motor control (Barkley, 1997).

The uniquely human executive function affected by AD/ HD affects the following functions:

- The senses of time, hindsight, and forethought
- Self-awareness
- The internalization of language and its governance over behavior (Berk & Potts, 1991)
- The separation of effect from content in responding to events or objectivity
- The regulation of effective and motivational states in subservience to goal-directed behavior
- Reconstitution, or the dissembling of events and messages from others, the progressive distribution of their components to parallel brain systems for processing of their particulars and their reconstruction into novel messages or responses (Lyon, 2005)

Hyperactivity has been a hallmark of the diagnosis of AD/HD. These children have been found to be more active, restless, and fidgety than same-aged peers; however, their greatest difficulties are with sustaining attention to tasks or with vigilance. The problem is often defined as a pattern of rapid, inaccurate responding to tasks. It may also be described as poor sustained inhibition of responding, poor delay in gratification, or impaired adherence to commands to regulate or inhibit behavior in social contexts (Incorvaia, 1999).

Studies of children with AD/HD have shown that critical points of their brains develop more slowly than other children's brains. The lag can be as much as 3 years and can involve several brain areas that include the frontal lobe and the cerebellum, parietal, and temporal lobes (Rotenberger, 2007). One research team used scans to measure the cortex thickness at 40,000 points in the brains of 223 children with AD/HD and 223 others who were developing in a typical way. The scans were repeated two, three, or four times at 3-year intervals. In both groups, the sensory processing and motor control areas at the back and top of the brain peaked in thickness earlier in childhood, while the frontal cortex areas responsible for higher-order executive control functions peaked later, during the teen years. Delayed in children with AD/HD was development of the higher-order functions and areas that coordinate those with the motor areas. The only area of the brain that matured faster in the children with AD/HD was the motor cortex, a finding that the researchers said might account for the restlessness and fidgety symptoms common among those with this disorder (Schmid, 2007).

WHAT AREAS OF ATTENTION ARE AFFECTED BY ATTENTION DEFICIT HYPERACTIVITY DISORDER?

Selective attention appears to be the area of attention that is most affected. Selective attention is the process of selecting what is relevant to current behavior from our environment while ignoring that which is not. The extent to which an individual can ignore irrelevant information may be dependent on a number of factors, including age, state of arousal, visual processing abilities, the nature of the stimuli, and the presence of any attentional difficulties. Developmental studies of selective attention have consistently shown that children between ages 2 and 12 years improve considerably in their ability to attend selectively.

Studies have shown that all children were slower responding in the presence of distractors. Children with AD/HD did not respond differently on trials with meaningful and irrelevant distractors, whereas children without AD/HD were significantly faster (lower distractor difference scores) in the irrelevant distractor condition compared to the meaningful distractor condition (Brodeur & Pond, 2001).

AD/HD can also affect children in other areas besides the motor area and can affect their later school years. In contrast to earlier reports claiming that hyperactive children "outgrow" their symptoms, more recent studies suggest that at adolescence, these children still have serious educational, emotional, and social problems despite some improvement in their symptoms. It was found that when compared to normal children, these children have failed more grades and had received significantly poorer report card marks on nearly all academic subjects. These studies found that hyperactive adolescents also showed signs of emotional immaturity, lack of ambition, feelings of hopelessness, and markedly low self-esteem as well as some social difficulties. The study showed that 25% had a history of antisocial behavior, 30% were reported by their mothers to have no steady friends, 25% showed acting out behaviors, and 10% had been court referrals. Academic underachievement, low self-esteem, and antisocial behavior would appear to be common characteristics of children with AD/ HD at adolescence (Hoy, Weiss, Minde, & Cohen, 1978).

One of the symptoms of hyperactive boys when compared to normal boys was a deficient motor inhibition/ control system. This was shown as difficulty in making discrete, isolated (as opposed to massive global) movements. For example, the flexion of a finger requires that an individual be able to activate the called-for flexions and to inhibit the reflex-associated contraction of the other finger flexors. These associated (overflow) movements appear to be the stigmata of deficient motor inhibition/control and are the central symptoms of AD/HD (Denckla & Rudel, 1978).

Optometrists have noticed for years the poor motor control of AD/HD children concerning saccadic fixations. We know that executive and motor control systems develop in parallel, suggesting shared neural circuitry including frontostriated systems and the cerebellum. The model of frontal lobe structure and function describe at least five parallel frontal-subcortical circuits. The most posterior are related to motor and oculomotor functions (originating in skeletomotor and oculomotor regions of the cortex). The more anterior are thought to be crucial in control of higher-order behavior (e.g., cognitive, "executive," and socio-emotional control). Children with AD/HD often present with motor dysfunction, including inefficient motor speed and coordination, excessive overflow movements, slowed processing speed, and variability of motor response, which has also been linked to anomalous function of the frontal-subcortical circuits.

These children often demonstrate deficits in oculomotor response inhibition, including increased errors on three different paradigms:

1. Antisaccades (AS)—In this test, two penlights are held in front of the child. You are to turn one of them on, and the child is to make a quick saccadic eye movement to the opposite light (the one not on).

2. Memory-guided saccades (MES)—This test has the child remember the location of the light that was flashed, and he or she has to move his or her eyes quickly to the remembered location.

3. Go-no-go (GNG)—In this case, the child is instructed to look at the center white square and to keep his or her eyes on the square until told to move them. He or she is to make a quick saccadic eye movement to the target that flashed red. If it flashed green, he or she is to ignore it and not move his or her eyes.

These test results show that children with AD/HD have more difficulty with these tests compared to normal children. One interesting finding was that girls had a great deal of difficulty in visually guided saccades (VGS). In fact, they had more difficulty than the boys, so this can be a good test to see if a girl may fit AD/HD. In this test, the child was told, "When the target light comes on, immediately, with your eyes only (not moving the head), look at the target light. When it goes off, look back to the center target" (Mahone, Mostofsky, Lasker, Zee, & Denckla, 2009).

Another oculomotor area that is easily evaluated and is a good test for AD/HD is smooth pursuits. This test must be done monocularly (one eye). Have the child cover one eye, and as you slowly move a pencil in a horizontal direction, he or she is to keep his or her eye on the pencil without moving his or her head. This test is almost pure attention, and you will notice very poor pursuit skills in children with AD/HD. You may also notice numerous losses in fixation and often large midline flicks.

RIGHT SIDE INVOLVEMENT

We have discussed in an earlier chapter the role of the right hemisphere in attention. Now, neuropsychological studies suggest that the core deficit in AD/HD is a failure to inhibit or delay motor responses while sensory detection or early information processing is intact. Phenomenological and neuropsychological studies have implicated prefrontal dysfunction in AD/HD. In light of findings of partial left visual field "neglect" (loss of attention to targets on the left side), deficits in delayed response tasks, and poor gating of irrelevant stimulus, studies have proposed a right-sided dysfunction of frontal-striatal circuitry for AD/HD (Carter, Krener, Chaderjian, Northcutt, & Wolfe, 1995; Casey et al., 1997; Castellanos et al., 1996).

DOPAMINE THEORY

AD/HD is as real as Down syndrome and schizophrenia. There appears to be striking differences in the brain's motivational machinery in people with AD/HD symptoms. Brain scans of adults with AD/HD show a flaw in the way they process dopamine, which, among other things, alerts people to new information and helps them anticipate pleasure and rewards. It seems that children and adults with AD/HD may have a net deficit in dopamine. People with AD/HD also have difficulty with a lack of motivation as well as a deficit of attention. They cannot generate the same degree of enthusiasm as other people for activities they do not automatically find appealing. This is why children can do something they like for hours but cannot pay attention in class (Ellison, 2009). This syndrome could also be called "an interest deficit." Imaging has shown that in people with AD/HD, the dopamine receptors and transporters are significantly less abundant in midbrain structures composing the so-called reward pathway, which is involved in associating stimuli with pleasurable expectations (Ellison, 2009).

Attention is controlled by both anterior and posterior brain systems. It is neither the property of a single brain area nor of the entire brain. Attentional effects are mediated through enhancement of attended or suppression of unattended items depending on the task or brain area studied. The origins of amplification effects are found in specialized cortical areas of the frontal and parietal lobes. There is a role in the parietal lobe (particularly the right) in orienting of attention. On the other hand, "executive control" is maintained by frontal systems, including the anterior cingulate and the prefrontal areas. These areas are involved in inhibition and working memory. There is also a vigilance network whose task is the maintenance of sustained state of alertness and is related to noradrenergic activity to the right frontal lobe. The role of dopaminergic systems in working memory and inhibitory processes is of central importance in AD/HD, but noradrengeric transmitters are also involved in orientation to novel stimuli and may also be involved in working memory (Levy & Swanson, 2001). Therefore, the anterior attention system depends on the neurotransmitter dopamine (prefrontal cortex, anterior cingulate, basal ganglion corpus striatum), and the posterior attention system (parietal lobe and thalamus) depends on norepinephrine (Rotenberger, 2007).

ETIOLOGY

Studies indicate that 80% of AD/HD cases can be traced to genetic factors (Durston et al., 2004). Although the etiology for AD/HD is likely multifactorial, several family studies have indicated that genetic inheritance may play a role. For example, the concordance rate of AD/HD in monozygotic twins is about 80% compared to about 30% for same-sex dyzygotic twins. One such candidate gene is the dopamine D4 receptor gene (DRD4). This gene, encoding one of five known protein receptors that mediate the post-synaptic actions of dopamine (DA), displays a very high degree of variability in the human population. This gene was chosen because (1) DA transmission is thought to play a critical role in AD/HD, (2) the distribution of the DRD4 mRNA in the brain suggests more of a role in cognition and emotional functions compared with the motor actions traditionally associated with the classical D4 receptors, and (3) the gene displays a high degree of variability that has been shown to be functionally significant. In addition, two studies have shown an association between DRD4 and novelty seeking, a well-defined and psychological trait characterized by exploratory behavior excitability and impulsiveness (La Hoste et al., 1996; Swanson, Flodman et al., 2000; Swanson, Posner, et al., 2001).

Studies have linked the neural network for alerting to connected brain regions centered in the right frontal lobe, for orienting to connected brain regions centered in the posterior parietal, and for executive control to connected brain regions centered in the anterior cingulate gyrus and including the basal ganglia. The association of dopamine genes with AD/HD suggests that the two attentional networks that include brain regions rich in dopamine receptors (the alerting network and executive control network) may be involved in the attention deficit that defines this disorder (Swanson et al., 2001).

Environmental influences may also play a role in AD/HD. For example, alcohol and nicotine consumption by a mother during pregnancy tends to increase the risk of AD/HD in offspring, much the same way it contributes to extreme prematurity, low birth weight, and food allergies. On the other hand, it is also true that mothers with a genetic predisposition to AD/HD have a propensity to smoke and drink during pregnancy. They tend to make basic child-rearing errors, too, such as failing to establish clear rules and effective limits. A chaotic household can strengthen biological AD/HD tendencies to a vicious cycle. Other psychosocial factors, including a nonsupportive school environment, psychological problems arising between parents, and poor parent-child attachment can also transform a latent tendency into a full-blown disorder (Rotenberger, 2007).

FETAL ALCOHOL SPECTRUM

Some people can trace the recognition of fetal alcohol syndrome (FAS) all the way back to the Bible, when an angel tells Samson, "Future mother, behold…thou shalt conceive and bear a son" and instructs her to "drink no wine nor strong drink." Physicians and researchers now recognize a whole range of conditions, known as fetal alcohol spectrum disorder, that can occur in children who are exposed to alcohol in utero. The effects may include physical, mental, behavioral, and learning disabilities with possible lifelong implications. The most severe condition on the spectrum is FAS. Three criteria are necessary for the diagnosis of FAS: abnormalities of the central nervous system, characteristic facial features, and poor growth.

The brain problems associated with FAS are numerous. A child with FAS may be hyperactive and impulsive and so would meet the criteria of AD/HD, but the damage that alcohol causes to the developing brain results in a constellation of mental and behavioral characteristics that go well beyond what is seen in AD/HD. Some children have generalized cognitive impairment or mental retardation. Others are not mentally retarded but still have significant learning disabilities and other developmental issues, including motor delays, problems with social skills, memory deficits, language problems, and difficulties with the complex set of mental skills—including planning, flexibility, and decision making—that are known as the "executive function."

A child with FAS has characteristic facial features that you need to be aware of. Eyes appear small, there is a thin upper lip and a longer-than-average distance from the nose to the upper lip, and often the philtrum (the vertical groove below the nose) is flattened, with a near absence of the ridges that result from the fusion of embryonic elements of the face in this area. The child could also be small for his or her age, and his or her head may seem small relative to the rest of the body (Cohen, 2010).

HOW COMMON IS ATTENTION DEFICIT HYPERACTIVITY DISORDER?

Reported prevalence varies from 1% to 2% among school-aged children (Barbaresi, 2002). Most studies put it between 7% and 16%. The prevalence of treatment with stimulant medication is 86.5% for definite AD/HD, 40.0% for probable AD/HD, and 6.6% for questionable AD/HD. Most people believe it is about 7.5% of the school population (McMullan, 2007). One study put this total at 4.4 million children between 4 and 17 years of age.

ATTENTION DEFICIT DISORDER VERSUS ATTENTION DEFICIT HYPERACTIVITY DISORDER

Behavioral disorders resembling AD/HD have been described for almost 100 years. During the past 100 years, numerous diagnostic labels have been given to this constellation of behavior, including hyperkineses, minimal brain dysfunction, and attention deficit disorder (with or without hyperactivity). Currently, the disorder is termed *attention deficit/hyperactivity disorder*, a name that places greater emphasis on the hyperactive and impulsive features of the disorder (Incorvaia, 1999).

The changing names given to attention disorders and the different behaviors that have been highlighted are reflected in concomitant changes in diagnostic criteria. For example, in the third edition of the *Diagnostic and Statistical Manual of Mental Disorders (DSM-III)* (American Psychiatric Association, 1980), two subtypes of attention deficit disorder were identified: attention deficit disorder with hyperactivity (ADD+H) and attention deficit disorder without hyperactivity (ADD–H). The three primary symptoms of inattention, impulsivity, and hyperactivity still characterized ADD+H. *ADD–H* was defined as significant problems with sustained attention alone. The diagnostic criteria were revised again for *DSM-III-R* (American Psychiatric Association, 1987). This definition included inclusionary and exclusionary criteria, recognized the situational variability of behaviors associated with AD/HD, and acknowledged the need for documenting that symptoms exceeded developmental expectations. At the time, however, there was little empirical support for two distinct subtypes. As a result, ADD–H was no longer listed as a subtype. Instead,

the label of *undifferentiated attention deficit disorder* was used to characterize those children whose primary difficulty was inattention and in whom signs of hyperactivity and impulsivity were not present. *AD/HD* was defined as difficulties with inattention, hyperactivity, and impulsivity that exceeded developmental expectations.

The *DSM-IV* (American Psychiatric Association, 1994) represents still another change in diagnostic classification. This change reflects the increasing empirical evidence that attention deficits and hyperactivity-impulsivity are two distinct dimensions, differing in level of impairment, the presence of comorbid features, social and cognitive development, and developmental course.

The symptoms of inattention, impulsivity, and hyperactivity are still present in the new diagnostic criteria. However, they may occur separately or concurrently, resulting in the following four subtypes:

1. AD/HD, predominantly inattentive type
2. AD/HD, predominantly hyperactive-impulsive type
3. AD/HD, combined type
4. AD/HD, not otherwise specified (for disorders with prominent symptoms of attention deficit or hyperactivity-impulsivity that do not meet criteria for any of the first three subtypes) (Incorvaia, 1999).

Who Is Qualified to Diagnose Attention Deficit Hyperactivity Disorder?

Table 4-1 for the National Institute of Mental Health tests the types of doctors who are qualified to diagnose and supervise treatment for AD/HD, although not all may have specific training in the disorder.

TELEVISION AND ATTENTION DEFICIT HYPERACTIVITY DISORDER

The lead author of a study on young children's TV viewing said unrealistically fast-paced visual images typical of most TV programming may alter normal brain development. The study has found that TV might overstimulate and permanently "rewire" the developing brain (Tanner, 2004). In fact, French TV has been banned from marketing shows for kids younger than 3 to shield them from developmental risks. The French feel that TV viewing hurts the development of children under 3 years old and poses a certain number of risks, encouraging passivity, slow language acquisition, overexcitedness, trouble with sleep and concentration, and dependence on screens (Olliver, 2009).

TABLE 4-1. DIAGNOSING AND TREATING ATTENTION DEFICIT/HYPERACTIVITY DISORDER			
SPECIALTY	CAN DIAGNOSE AD/HD?	CAN PRESCRIBE MEDICATION IF NEEDED?	PROVIDES COUNSELING OR TRAINING?
Psychiatrists	Yes	Yes	Yes
Psychologists	Yes	No	Yes
Pediatricians or family physicians	Yes	Yes	Sometimes
Neurologists	Yes	Yes	No

From www.Mayoclinic.com

One study found that for every hour of TV watched a day, two groups of children aged 1 and 3 faced a 10% increased risk of having attention problems at 7. The findings bolster previous research showing that TV can shorten attention spans and supports the American Academy of Pediatrics that children under 2 should not watch TV. About 36% of 1 year olds watch no TV, while 37% watch 1 to 2 hours daily and have a 10% to 20% increased risk of attention problems. Fourteen percent watch 3 to 4 hours daily and have a 30% to 40% increased risk compared to children who do not watch TV. Researchers feel that the unrealistically fast-paced visual images typical of most TV programming may alter normal brain development (Tanner, 2004).

Television, music videos, and video games, all of which use TV techniques, unfold at a much faster pace than real life, and they are getting faster, causing people to develop an increased appetite for high-speed transitions in those media. It is the form of the TV medium—cuts, edits, zooms, pans, and sudden noises—that alters the brain by activating what Pavlov called the "orienting response," which occurs whenever we sense a sudden change in the world around us, especially a sudden movement. The response is physiological; the heart rate decreases for 4 to 6 seconds. Television triggers this response at a far more rapid rate than we experience it in life, which is why we cannot keep our eyes off the TV screen. Because typical music video action sequences and commercials trigger orienting responses at a rate of one per second, watching them puts us into continuous orienting response with no recovery (Doidge, 2007).

In one experiment, an electrode was posted to the scalp of a woman while she first looked at a magazine and then watched TV commercials as she was reading the magazine. Her brain registered active alertness, but switching to TV viewing "instantly produced a preponderance of slow (alpha) waves, which are classically associated with lack of mental activity." Researchers say that, as viewing time of young children increased, "this prolonged idleness" of the prefrontal cortex could have serious consequences.

Child-development experts often mention the issue of "transfer," that is, how much can we expect experiences with one type of input—such as video games—to build up abilities that can be used elsewhere, such as reading? Many people feel that anything improving children's visual-spatial skills (e.g., playing fast-paced video games) should also improve their reading speed, or even their geometry abilities, which are known to call heavily on visual spatial reasoning. Unfortunately, however, the brain often seems to have difficulty applying skills it has learned in one specific area to other kinds of problems. When teachers ask how the learning will transfer, they are referring to the fact that teaching a child how to outline a story in English class does not necessarily mean he or she will automatically apply the same skills to his or her history textbooks—unless someone specifically shows him or her how and he or she practices the same outlining with history. It seems safe to say that much of children's experiences with video games will have little, if any, transfer value to traditional school tasks (Healy, 1990).

Before we leave this subject, I am including more information on video games. We know that some video games put less emphasis on violence and destruction and focus more on complex goals and strategies. These intricate virtual environments have a significant impact on a young person's brain in the frontal lobe—the region that requires further development during adolescence for abstract thinking and planning skills to take hold. However, Professor Ryuta Kawashima at the University Tohoku in Japan found that when children play video games, their brains do not use frontal lobe circuits but rather use a limited brain region that controls vision and movement. This is in sharp contrast to what they found when kids performed simple, mundane math exercises. When the study volunteers did single-digit addition calculations, their brains recruited neurons from a much wider brain area, involving the frontal lobes, regions that control learning, memory emotion, and even impulse control (Small, 2008). I have also noticed in my experience with children with AD/HD that even though they are very good at video games, their visual tracking and visual motor skills are still very poor; therefore, there does not seem to be a lot of transfer concerning these skills that are critical for success in school.

DIAGNOSING ATTENTION DEFICIT HYPERACTIVITY DISORDER

Behavioral Ratings Questionnaire

Two ways that a child can be diagnosed with AD/HD are the questionnaire and evaluating his or her responses on a computer that measures the child's response times, attention, and impulsivity.

The following criteria for AD/HD are reproduced from the American Psychiatric Association's *DSM-IV*:

A. Either (1) or (2):

1. Six (or more) of the following symptoms of inattention have persisted for at least 6 months to a degree that is nonadaptive and inconsistent with developmental level:

   Inattention

   a. Often fails to give close attention to details or makes careless mistakes in schoolwork, work, or other activities

   b. Often has difficulty sustaining attention in tasks or play activities

   c. Often does not seem to listen when spoken to directly

   d. Often does not follow through on instructions and fails to finish schoolwork, chores, duties in the workplace (not due to oppositional behavior or failure to understand directions)

   e. Often has difficulty organizing tasks and activities

   f. Often avoids, dislikes, or is reluctant to engage in tasks that require sustained mental effort (such as schoolwork or homework)

   g. Often loses things necessary for tasks or activities (e.g., toys, school assignments, pencils).

   h. Is often easily distracted by external stimuli

   i. Is often forgetful in daily activities

2. Six (or more) of the following symptoms of hyperactivity-impulsivity have persisted for at least 6 months to a degree that is nonadaptive and inconsistent with developmental level.

   a. Often fidgets with hands or feet or squirms in seat

   b. Often leaves seat in classroom or in other situations in which remaining seated is expected

   c. Often runs about or climbs excessively when it is inappropriate

   d. Often has difficulty playing or engaging in leisure activities quietly

   e. Is often "on the go" or often acts as if driven by a motor

   f. Often talks excessively

   g. Often blurts out answers before questions have been completed

   h. Often interrupts or intrudes on others (e.g., butts into conversation or games)

B. Some hyperactive-impulsive or inattentive symptoms that caused impairment were present before age 7 years.

C. Some impairment from the symptoms is present in two or more settings (e.g., at school [or work] and at home).

D. There must be clear evidence of clinically significant impairment in social, academic, or occupational functioning.

E. The symptoms do not occur exclusively during the course of a pervasive developmental disorder, schizophrenia, or other psychiatric disorders and are not better accounted for by another mental disorder (e.g., mood disorder, anxiety disorder, dissociative disorder, or a personality disorder).

Reprinted with permission from the Diagnostic and Statistical Manual of Mental Disorders, Fourth Edition, Text Revision, *(Copyright ©2000). American Psychiatric Association.*

Test of Variables of Attention

It is generally agreed that no single procedure, observation, or behavioral characteristic is sufficient to support a diagnosis of AD/HD. For example, it has repeatedly been demonstrated that correlations between teacher and parent ratings of hyperactivity are, at best, modest and frequently low or even absent. Similarly, it is well known that there may be little correspondence between a child's behavior in a psychologist's clinic or medical office and behavior at home or school (Forbes, 1998). The Test of Variables of Attention (TOVA) is a continuous performance test that a child completes on a computer. He or she is given a very boring task to perform for 23 minutes, and then the computer will analyze his or her responses compared to his or her age level to children who have already been clinically diagnosed as AD/HD. This test has been shown to correctly identify 80% of a sample of AD/HD children and 72% of those without AD/HD. What makes the test extremely useful is that it can be run before and after medication to see if the medication is correctly helping the AD/HD.

Is the best treatment a combination of drugs and behavior training? The answer to this question is probably yes.

A comprehension examination conducted in 2000 by the National Institute of Mental Health rated the effectiveness of medical and behavioral treatments of AD/HD. Conducted over 2 years, the Multimodal Treatment Study of Children with AD/HD included 579 AD/HD children at six different university medical centers. The principal investigators divided the test subjects, all of whom were between the ages of 7 and 9, into four groups that had different treatment plans. The results strongly suggest that a combination of drug and behavioral therapies leads to the highest success (Rotenberger, 2007). Nonpharmacologic treatment for AD/HD would include counseling, cognitive behavioral therapy, support groups, parent training, educator/teacher training, herbal remedies, biofeedback, dietary intervention, and chiropractic manipulation.

The results show the success of either behavioral therapy, drug therapy, or a combination of both:

- Routine daily treatment with prescribed medication normalized behavior in 25% of children treated

- Intensive behavioral therapy without medication ended with 34% of patients exhibiting no further remarkable symptoms

- Carefully tailored medical treatment with accompanying counseling for the child and parents helped 56% of the children.

- A combination of medication and behavioral therapy resulted in a success rate of 68% (Rotenberger, 2007).

TREATING ATTENTION DEFICIT HYPERACTIVITY DISORDER

Attention-focusing drugs have been around for years. Amphetamines, nicknamed "go pills," were discovered in the late 19th century. By the 1940s, these central nervous system stimulants were widely used to treat asthma and had become popular as "pep" and diet pills. They were embraced by members of the armed forces, especially pilots, who had to remain attentive to myriad tasks despite constant danger and fatigue. Rife with serious side effects, including hallucinations, anorexia, and heart problems, dextroamphetamine (trade name Dexedrine—better known as speed) is rarely used today by civilians. But the amphetamine mix Adderall and the amphetamine-related drugs (Ritalin, Methylin, Concerta, among others) are commonly prescribed today. Exactly how these drugs work remains unknown, but stimulants like Ritalin and modafinal could influence the neurotransmitters dopamine and norepinephrine, which are essential for attention and memory skills. Both drugs inhibit re-uptake or re-absorption of these neurotransmitters by neurons, thus prolonging their action. Modafinal also indirectly alters the action of glutamate, the main neurotransmitter used by neurons in the brain. The center action of these drugs is the prefrontal cortex, the part of the brain that is responsible for executive function (Baker, 2009).

An estimated 9% of boys and 4% of girls in the United States are taking stimulant medications as part of their therapy for AD/HD. The majority of patients take Ritalin or Concerta, whereas most of the rest are prescribed an amphetamine such as Adderall.

During the past 15 years, doctors have been prescribing stimulants to a rapidly rising number of patients. In addition, patients are no longer just taking medications for a few years during grade school but are encouraged to stay on them into adulthood. As a result, prescriptions for Ritalin and Adderall rose by almost 21% a year between 2000 and 2005 according to a 2007 study.

Can these drugs cause harm over the long run? Recently, a few studies (mostly with animals) hint that stimulants could alter the structure and function of the brain in ways that may depress mood, boost anxiety, and lead to cognitive deficits. Human studies already indicate that medication can adversely affect growth in children. In 2007, a study involving 579 children compared growth rates of unmedicated 7- to 10-years-olds over 3 years with those of children who took stimulants. The drug-treated children showed a decrease in growth rate, gaining on average 2 cm less in height (an inch is 2.54 cm) and 2.7 kg less in weight. The children on medications never caught up to their counterparts. With animals, studies have shown amphetamine-induced brain damage due to lower levels of dopamine and fewer dopamine transporters on nerve endings in the striatum. Also, one possible consequence of a loss of dopamine and its associated molecules is Parkinson's disease. A study in humans published in 2006 hints at a link between Parkinson's and a prolonged exposure to amphetamines in any form (Higgins, 2009). It needs to be stressed that in human studies so far, it is only the growth rate that has been a proven consequence of these drugs. Nevertheless, in light of the emerging evidence, many doctors and researchers are recommending a more cautious approach to the medical use of stimulants.

An article in *USA Today* in 2009 stated that stimulants used to treat AD/HD could increase the risk of sudden death in children who have no underlying heart conditions. Since 2006, such drugs have carried warnings about an increased risk of sudden death in children known to have serious heart abnormalities, but this is the first time a study has linked stimulants to healthy children. Scientists compared stimulant use in 564 young people who suffered sudden unexplained death with that of 564 killed in car accidents. Of those who died suddenly for no apparent reason, 10 (1.8%) had been taking Ritalin. Only two (0.4%)

who died in car accidents had been taking stimulants (Rubin, 2009). This indicates a better chance of dying from taking Ritalin than in a car accident.

In addition to stimulant drugs, nicotine has been shown to improve attention and information-processing speed in normal adults after administration of either tobacco smoke or nicotine skin patches in cigarette smokers and low-dose nicotine skin patches in nonsmokers. Nicotine-induced attentional improvement raises the possibility that nicotine treatment may be useful for treatment of attentional disorders. The critical mechanism for the action of nicotine in attention is unclear. Nicotine potentiates the release of dopamine and norepinephrine as well as other transmitters, such as serotonin and acetylcholine. The net increase in catecholaminergic stimulation resembles the action of Ritalin and Dexedrine (Levin, Conners, Silva, Canu, & March, 2001).

Electroencephalogram Neurofeedback

For the 20% to 25% of children who do not respond well to medication, there may be a combination of reasons: (1) more serious side effects including gastrointestinal disturbances, (2) increased tic disorders when tics are present (a possible problem with Ritalin), (3) seizure disorders, (4) headaches, (5) urinary problems, or (6) changes in affect unacceptable to the person or family (Schwartz, 1995). For people who do not respond well to medication, neurofeedback is often successful. Often, the neurofeedback is administered in conjunction with medication. There are many children with AD/HD whose hyperactivity would be so pervasive that they would be unmanageable for a neurofeedback therapeutic situation.

Neurofeedback, a form of electroencephalogram (EEG) biofeedback, has developed very rapidly and was first used for AD/HD problems in the 1970s. In the past 20 years, there has been a burgeoning of interest in this area. Ten years ago, there were more than 800 groups using neurofeedback to treat attention problems. With neurofeedback, unlike medication, there is often long-term carryover (Evans, 1999).

The results of neurofeedback have often been impressive. A study in California showed an increase of 10 Wechsler Intelligence Scale for Children-Revised (WISC-R) points and a significant decrease in inattentiveness. Another study found changes of more than 10 points in verbal and performance IQ. Some individuals showed more than a 20-point change (Schwartz, 1995).

The procedure for neurofeedback involves the child coming in for an intake (baseline) evaluation to determine

---

SUMMARY AND ATTENTION TIPS

1. Go-no-go activities should be part of every therapy program. AD/HD children have difficulty controlling their behavior. For example, make the child delay a response or do the opposite of what you ask, such as go right and he or she turns left.

2. Have the child anticipate an outcome. For example, have five playing cards on a table (face up), and ask him or her to draw what they would look like after he or she knocks them off of the table and they land on the floor (Incorvaia, 1999).

3. Teach the child to separate gross and fine motor skills. Have the child learn to flex one finger at a time without moving the other finger.

4. Antisaccadics—Two penlights are held in front of the child. You are to turn one of them on, and the child must make a quick saccadic movement to the other one.

5. The child looks straight ahead, and you flash a light in his or her peripheral vision. The child must remember where the light was flashed and make a saccadic eye movement to that location.

6. Go-no-go—The child looks at a target, such as a white square. He or she is not to take his or her eyes off of the square until you tell him or her. He or she then makes a quick saccadic eye movement to the target you have shown him or her.

---

the percentage of theta and beta activity to determine the correct protocols to use in treatment. Theta (commonly defined as 4 to 8 Hz) is usually associated in inattentiveness, while beta (commonly 12 to 16 Hz) is normally associated with focused concentration. Electrodes are placed on the scalp at the correct location to determine the theta/beta ratio. If the theta/beta ratio is highly in favor of theta, this means that the child is more often in an inattentive mode instead of an attentive (beta) mode. The training then starts to change this ratio by decreasing theta and increasing beta.

REFERENCES

American Psychiatric Association. (1980). Diagnostic and statistical manual of mental disorders, 3rd ed. Washington, DC: Author.

American Psychiatric Association. (1987). *Diagnostic and statistical manual of mental disorders, 3rd ed*, Revised. Washington, DC: Author.

American Psychiatric Association. (1994). *Diagnostic and statistical manual of mental disorders, 4th ed.* Washington, DC: Author.

Baker, S. (2009). Building a better brain. *Discover Magazine, April,* 56-59.

Barbaresi, W. (2002). How common is ADHD? *Archives of Pediatrics & Adolescent Medicine, 156,* 217-224.

Barkley, R. A. (1997). Behavioral inhibition, sustained attention, and executive functions: constructing a unifying theory of ADHD. *Psychological Bulletin, 121*(1), 65-94.

Barkley, R. A. (2006). *Attention-deficit hyperactivity disorder.* New York, NY: The Guilford Press.

Berk, L. & Potts, M. K. (1991). Development and functional significance of private speech among attention deficit hyperactivity disorder and normal boys. *Journal of Abnormal Child Psychology, 9*(3), 357-375.

Brodeur, D. A. & Pond, M. (2001). The development of selective attention in children with attention deficit hyperactivity disorder. *Journal of Abnormal Child Psychology, 29*(3), 229-239.

Carter, C. S., Krener, P., Chaderjian, M., Northcutt, C., & Wolfe, V. (1995). Asymmetrical visual-spatial attentional performance in ADHD: evidence for a right hemispheric deficit. *Biological Psychiatry, 37*(11), 789-797.

Casey, B. J., Castellanos, F. X., Giedd, J. N., Marsh, W. L., Hamburger, S. D., Schubert, A. B., . . . Rapoport, J. L. (1997). Implication of right frontostriatal circuitry in response inhibition and attention deficit/hyperactivity disorder. *Journal of the American Academy of Child and Adolescent Psychiatry, 36*(3), 374-383.

Castellanos, F. X., Giedd, J. N., Marsh, W. L., Hamburger, S. D., Vaituzis, A. C., Dickstein, D. P., . . . Rapoport, J. L. (1996). Quantitative brain magnetic resonance imaging in attention deficit hyperactivity disorder. *Archives of General Psychiatry, 53*(7), 607-616.

Castellanos, F. X. & Tannock, R. (2002). Neuroscience of attention-deficit/hyperactivity disorder: the search for endophenotypes. *Nature Reviews, 3*(8), 617-628.

Cohen, M. (2010). Vital signs. *Discover Magazine, March,* 30-31.

Denckla, M. B. & Rudel, R. G. (1978). Anomalies of motor development in hyperactive boys. *Annals of Neurology, 3*(3), 231-233.

Doidge, N. (2007). *The brain that changes itself.* New York, NY: Penguin Group (USA), Inc.

Durston, S., Hulshoff Pol, H. E., Schnack, H. G., Buitelaar, J. K., Steenhuis, M. P., Minderaa, R. B., . . . van Engeland, H. (2004). Magnetic resonance imaging of boy with attention deficit/hyperactivity disorder and their unaffected siblings. *Journal of the American Academy of Child and Adolescent Psychiatry, 43*(3), 332-340.

Ellison, K. (2009). Brain scans, link ADHD to biological flaw tied to motivation. *Brain in the News, Oct,* 6.

Evans, J. (1999). *Introduction to quantitative EEG and neurofeedback.* Philadelphia, PA: Elsevier.

Forbes, G. B. (1998). Clinical utility of the test of variables of attention (TOVA) in the diagnosis of attention deficit/hyperactivity disorder. *Journal of Clinical Psychology, 54*(4), 461-476.

Healy, J. (1990). *Endangered minds.* New York, NY: Simon & Schuster.

Higgins, E. (2009). Do ADHD drugs take a toll on the brain? *Scientific American Mind, July/August,* 38-43.

Hoy, E., Weiss, G., Minde, K., & Cohen, N. (1978). The hyperactive child at adolescence: cognitive, emotional, and social functioning. *Journal of Abnormal Psychology, 6*(3), 311-324.

Incorvaia, J. (1999). *Understanding, diagnosing, and treating AD/HD in children and adolescents.* Lanham, MD: Jason Aronson, Inc.

La Hoste, G., Swanson, J. M., Wigal, S. B., Glabe, C., Wigal, T., King, N., & Kennedy, J. L. (1996). Dopamine d4 receptor gene polymorphism is associated with attention deficit hyperactivity disorder. *Molecular Psychiatry, 1*(2), 121-124.

Levin, E. D., Conners, C. K., Silva, D., Canu, W., & March, J. (2001). Effects of chronic nicotine and methylphenidate in adults with attention deficit/hyperactivity disorder. *Experimental and Clinical Psychopharmacology, 9*(1), 83-90.

Levy, F. & Swanson, J. M. (2001). Timing, space and ADHD: the dopamine theory revisited. *Australian and New Zealand Journal of Psychiatry, 35*(4), 504-511.

Lyon, R. (2005). *Attention, memory, and executive function.* Baltimore, MD: Paul H. Brookes Publishing Co.

Mahone, E. M., Mostofsky, S. H., Lasker, A. G., Zee, D., & Denckla, M. B. (2009). Oculomotor anomalies in attention-deficit/hyperactivity disorder: evidence for deficits in response preparation and inhibition. *Journal of the American Academy of Child and Adolescent Psychiatry, 48*(7), 749-756.

McMullan, D. (2007). Inside your child's brain. *D Magazine, April,* 66-70.

Olliver, C. (2009). *French TV banned from marketing shows for kids younger than 3.* Associated Press.

Rotenberger, A. (2007). Informing the ADHD debate. *Scientific American, September,* 36-39.

Rubin, R. (2009). Sudden death in kids, ADHD drugs linked. *USA Today.* Tuesday, June 16, 2009.

Schmid, R. (2007). ADHD kid's brains develop more slowly. *Brain in the News, December,* 1-2.

Schwartz, M. (1995). *Biofeedback: a practitioner's guide.* New York, NY: The Guilford Press.

Small, G. (2008). *iBrain: Surviving the technological alteration of the modern mind.* New York, NY: Collins Living Publishers.

Swanson, J., Flodman, P., Kennedy, J., Spence, M. A., Moyzis, R., Schuck, S., . . . Posner, M. (2000). Dopamine genes and ADHD. *Neuroscience and Biobehavioral Reviews, 24*(1), 21-25.

Swanson, J., Posner, M., Fusella, J., Wasdell, M., Sommer, T., & Fan, J. (2001). Genes and attention deficit hyperactivity disorder. *Current Psychiatry Reports, 3*(2), 92-100.

Tanner, L. (2004). Children's TV habits may lead to attention problems. *Ft. Worth Star Telegram,* April 5.

Ward, P. (2009). What will become of homo sapiens? *Scientific American, January,* 68-73.

SUGGESTED READING

Berry, C.A. Shaywitz, S. E., & Shaywitz, B. A. (1985). Girls with attention deficit disorder: a silent minority? A report on behavioral and cognitive characteristics. *Pediatrics, 76*(5), 801-809.

Nealy, J. (1990). *Endangered minds.* New York, NY: Simon & Schuster.

Swanson, J., Oosterlaan, J., Murias, M., Schuck, S., Flodman, P., Spence, M. A., . . . Posner, M. I. (2000). Attention deficit/hyperactivity disorder children with a 7-repeat allele of the dopamine receptor d4 gene have extreme behavior but normal performance on critical neuropsychological tests of attention. *Proceedings of the National Academy of Sciences, 97*(9), 4754-4759.

5

Autism

"At his second birthday party, we found our son, Jake, lying face down in the driveway, his cheek pressed to the ground. He did not look at us or talk to us. It was as if we—his own mother and father—were not there.

"Two weeks later, Jake was diagnosed with autism.

"In the first seventeen months of his life, Jake hit every developmental milestone—he walked, and he talked. He was within the age appropriate weight and height percentile. By all accounts, he was a typical child, and then, over a 6-month period, Franklin and I watched as our once active and talkative toddler gradually developed into a lethargic and silent little boy. It was as if, one by one, all of the circuit breakers in his brain were clicking off" (Exkom, 2006, p. 85).

The autism spectrum disorders (ASDs) are a group of developmental disabilities that are characterized by significant impairments in social interaction and communication as well as repetitive stereotyped behaviors. Individuals who have ASD often are affected by their ability to attend, learn, and process sensory stimuli. The term *spectrum* refers to the tremendous variation in how the condition is manifested. For instance, cognitively, those with ASD may range from gifted to severely challenged, from talkative to completely nonverbal, and from performing independently to needing constant one-on-one attention. Symptoms of ASD begin before the age of 3 and exist throughout an individual's life. ASD occurs in all racial, ethnic, and socioeconomic groups and is four times more common in boys than girls.

Three areas are evaluated for behaviors consistent with a diagnosis of ASD:

1. Social interaction—Decreased eye contact, very little facial expression, an inability to develop peer relationships, and a lack of social or emotional reciprocities.

2. Communication—Marked delay in the development of spoken language, being unable to carry on a conversation, and very limited abilities to make-believe or show imaginative play.

3. Repetitive, stereotyped behavior patterns—Inflexibility to changes in routine, repetitive motor mannerisms such as lining up objects, and marked preoccupation with the parts of an object rather than its use as a whole object (Coulter, 2009).

Current research suggests there may be multiple factors involved in the pathways leading to ASD. There is a great deal of research supporting genetic influences. Genetic factors and prenatal development processes are likely to predispose a child to autism or create vulnerabilities to prenatal and postnatal challenges that have the same effect (Greenspan, 2004).

Autism is an etiologically heterogeneous disorder. Nevertheless, it is now widely accepted that most causes arise because of a complex genetic predisposition. Since autism was first described in 1943, hypotheses about its etiology have ranged from the psychological to the biological. During the 1970s and 1980s, however, twin and family studies provided unequivocal evidence for a genetic component to autism (Moldin, 2006).

Lane, K. A. *Visual Attention in Children: Theories and Activities* (pp. 85-100).

HISTORY OF AUTISM

More than 50 years ago, Leo Karmer presented case studies of children who displayed unusual development of communication skills and a disturbance of affective contact. These children were also noted to have odd behaviors, unusual sensory interests, and an "insistence on sameness." Karmer used the term *autistic* to describe these children, borrowing from Blueler in 1911 who used the label to describe the social withdrawal observed in schizophrenia. Particularly striking in these children was the contrast between the ability to develop effective relationships and the child's intelligent relations to objects. Karmer recognized that deficits in social interactions and communications can occur in individuals who may otherwise be considered intelligent based on their ability to function in nonsocial tasks. The differentiation of social competing skills and intelligence is key in making the diagnosis of autism (Huebner, 2001).

We now know that genes play a large part in the autism spectrum. Latent class analysis of twin and family data has suggested that as few as three to four predisposing genes may be implicated, although as many as 15 loci have been proposed to be involved (Risch et al., 1999). In the case of a multilocus model, no single variant is necessary or sufficient per se, and multiple predisposing variants in one or more genes have to be inherited to develop the phenotype. Other factors such as gender and environmental influences may also influence the severity of phenotype expressions.

The identification of chromosomal abnormalities in autism has helped to reinforce the view that genetic influences are important in the development of this disorder. Numerous reports in the literature have documented chromosomal aberrations associated with autism (Gillberg, 1998). Abnormalities of chromosome 15 and structural and numerical abnormalities of the gender chromosomes are most frequently reported. The most prevalent chromosome 15 abnormalities are supernumerary isodicentric chromosome 15 and internally derived interstitial duplications of the 15q11-q13 region, particularly in individuals with mental retardation and seizures. The concordance of the linkage findings of chromosome 7 has recently made this region the focus of several gene studies (Moldin, 2006).

What is probably happening is that genes and the environment interact, in either a fetus or a young child, changing cellular function all over the body, which then affects tissue and metabolism in many vulnerable organs. It is the interaction of this collection of troubles that lead to altered sensory processing and impaired coordination in the brain. A brain that causes these kinds of problems produces the abnormal behaviors that we call autism (Neimark, 2009).

EARLY SIGNS

Many children with autism have a history of food and airborne allergies, 20 to 30 ear infections, eczema, or chronic diarrhea (Neimark, 2009). However, most parents notice that something is not right with their children when the children are 2 or 3 years old. In some cases, parents pick up signs even earlier, when their children are in infancy, according to the National Institute of Mental Health (NIMH). Some possible early indicators of ASD include the following:

- Does not babble, point, or make meaningful gestures by 1 year of age
- Does not speak one word by 16 months
- Does not combine two words by 2 years of age
- Does not respond to his or her name
- Loses language or social skills
- Avoids eye contact
- Does not seem to know how to play with toys
- Excessively lines up toys or other objects
- Is attached to one particular toy or object
- Does not smile
- At times seems to be hearing impaired (Exkom, 2006).

At least 30% to 50% of parents recall abnormalities dating back to the first year, including extremes in temperament and behavior ranging from alarming passivity to marked irritability, poor eye contact, and lack of response to the parents' voices or attempts to play and interact. Core symptoms of speech delay and stereotyped behavior are often evident in the second year. There is absence of social smiling, lack of facial expression, lack of pointing/showing, and abnormal muscle tone, posture, and movement patterns. Early abnormalities in attention, behavioral reactivity, emotion regulation, and activity level may compromise both the quality and quantity of early social interaction and thus the prerequisite experiential input for developing neural systems critical to later social-communicative competencies.

There seems to be prolonged latency to disengage visual attention—a tendency to fixate on particular objects in the environment and delayed expressive and receptive language. There is also preoccupation with parts of an object, such as the wheels on a toy, and unusual sensory responses, such as smelling toys (LeCouteur et al., 1989).

All of this taken together suggests a striking clinical picture of the child with autism during the first year of life.

Children with autism are observed at 6 months to be somewhat passive, with relatively few initiations and less responsiveness to efforts to engage their attention. These children vocalize less than other infants at 12 months of age. An assessment of behavioral features finds that eye contact is poor and there are marked abnormalities in visual attention, including poor visual tracking (Zwaigenbaum et al., 2005).

The cerebral cortex and its affiliated white matter make up about 80% of normal overall brain volumes, so cerebral overgrowth is clearly likely to be a contribution to abnormal increases in brain and head size. As with overall brain volume, there is evidence of overgrowth during the earliest years of life in autism. Independent studies have examined cerebral volume in children in the important time period before 5 years of age (Courchesne, Saitoh et al., 1994). These studies found that significant enlargement was already present in young children. Clearly, at some time prior to these early years, the cerebrum has undergone an abnormal schedule of growth. The greatest degree of enlargement in 2 and 3 year olds was found in the frontal lobe (15% parenchymal enlargement) followed by the temporal and parietal lobes (14% and 9% parenchymal enlargement, respectively). It is not surprising to see that the areas of more extreme abnormality are also the cerebral areas bearing the greatest proportion of higher-order multimodal cortex. The most noticeable deficits in autism are related to higher-order cognitive functions. These areas, particularly the frontal lobe, are normally the slowest to develop ontogenetically.

The hurried development of the autistic brain may mean that, at a point when experience-driven plasticity becomes biologically essential for prototypical development of higher-order areas, lower-level primary or secondary sensory areas may not have fully matured. This would mean that the input (experience) provided by these lower-level areas may be noisy or information poor. With inadequate input, normal experience-driven construction of association areas will be derailed (Moldin, 2006).

STATISTICS

It has been noted that the frequency of individuals demonstrating at least one of the disorders on the spectrum was 3.4/1,000 for children 3 to 10 years of age with the Centers for Disease Control (CDC) now estimating that 2 to 6/1,000 (from 1 in 500 to 1 in 150) children have the disorder. Boys have a three to four times greater risk of having the disorder than girls. Although this ratio is lower than that found for intellectual disability (9.7 per 1,000), it is higher than the prevalence of cerebral palsy (2 to 8 per 1,000), deafness (1.1 per 1,000 children), and severe visual impairment (0.9 per 1,000 children) (Maino, 2009).

Other studies estimate that the rate of autism is from 2 to 4 per 1,000. A study by the CDC showed that the rate was 1 per 250 for autism and approximately 1 per 150 for ASD. In comparison to these current estimates, the rates 10 or 15 years ago were considerably lower. Although they tended to vary a great deal by the study conducted, the most widely cited rate then was 1 per 2,000 to 2,500 for autism. Although some believe these increasing rates are due to better identification and diagnosis, many investigators believe there is an alarming increase in autism (Greenspan, 2004).

DIAGNOSTIC ASSESSMENT

The following are taken from the fourth edition of *Diagnostic and Statistical Manual of Mental Disorders (DSM-IV)*—Autistic Disorder 299.00:

A. A total of six (or more) items from (1), (2), and (3), with at least two from (1) and one each from (2) and (3).

1. Qualitative impairment in social interactions as manifested by at least two of the following:

   a. Marked impairment in the use of multiple nonverbal behaviors, such as eye-to-eye gaze, facial expression, body posture, and gestures to regulate social interaction

   b. Failure to develop peer relationships appropriate to developmental level

   c. A lack of spontaneous seeking to share enjoyment, interests, or achievements with other people (e.g., by a lack of showing, bringing, or pointing out objects of interest)

   d. Lack of social or emotional reciprocity

2. Qualitative impairments in communication as manifested by at least one of the following:

   a. Delay in or total lack of the development of spoken language (not accompanied by an attempt to compensate through alternative modes of communication, such as gesture or mime)

   b. In individuals with adequate speech, marked impairment in the ability to initiate or sustain a conversation with others

   c. Stereotyped and repetitive use of language or idiosyncratic language

   d. Lack of varied, spontaneous make-believe play or social initiative play appropriate to developmental level

3. Restricted, repetitive, and stereotyped patterns of behavior interests and activities, as manifested by at least one of the following:

   a. Encompassing preoccupation with one or more stereotyped and restricted patterns of interest that is abnormal either in intensity or focus

b. Apparently inflexible adherence to specific nonfunctional routines or rituals

c. Stereotyped and repetitive motor mannerisms (e.g., hand or finger flapping or twisting) or complex whole-body movements

d. Persistent preoccupation with parts of objects

B. Delays or abnormal functioning in at least one of the following areas with onset prior to age 3 years.

1. Social interaction
2. Language as used in social communication or symbolic imaginative play

C. The disturbance is no better accounted for by Rett syndrome or childhood disintegrative disorder.

Reprinted with permission from the Diagnostic and Statistical Manual of Mental Disorders, Fourth Edition, Text Revision, *(Copyright ©2000). American Psychiatric Association.*

SENSORY PROCESSING DISORDERS

Sensory integration is a growing area of practice in occupational therapy. The term *sensory integration dysfunction* was founded in the publication *Sensory Integration and Learning Disorders* by A. Jean Ayres in 1972. Later scholars have clarified the many uses of the term *sensory integration*. Sensory integration theory refers to constructs that discuss how the brain processes sensation and resulting motor, behavior, emotional, and attention responses. Sensory integration assessment is the process of evaluating people for problems in processing sensation. Sensory integration treatment is a method of intervention.

Since Ayres first proposed the theory of sensory integration, many theorists, researchers, and clinicians have further developed the theory. What has evolved is the term *sensory processing disorder* (SPD). It has been suggested that this term be used only if the sensory processing difficulties impair daily routines or roles. There are three categories of SPD. Each of these is further refined into patterns and subtypes.

Pattern 1: Sensory Modulation Disorder

Sensory modulation is the capacity to regulate and organize the degree, intensity, and maturity of responses to sensory input in a graded and adaptive manner so that an optimal range of performance and adaptation to challenges can be maintained. Research with attention deficit/hyperactivity disorder (AD/HD) children has revealed two subgroups within AD/HD: one group with normal sensory processing functions and one with sensory modulation disorder (SMD). Identifying a subgroup within AD/HD who have sensory dysfunction may inform more effective treatment options (Mangeot et al., 2001).

Sensory modulation occurs as the central nervous system regulates the neural messages about sensory stimuli. SMD results when a person has difficulty responding to sensory input with behavior that is graded relative to the degree, nature, or intensity of the sensory information. Responses are inconsistent with the demands of the situation, and inflexibility adapting to sensory challenges encountered in day-to-day life is observed. Three subtypes of SMD exist.

Sensory Modulation Disorder Subtype 1: Sensory Over-Responsivity

People with sensory over-responsivity (SOR) respond to sensation faster, with more intensity, or for a longer duration than those with typical sensory responsivity.

SOR prevents people from making effective functional responses. Difficulties are particularly evident in new situations and during transitions. The atypical responses are not willful; they are automatic, unconscious, physiologic reactions to sensation. Emotional responses include irritability, moodiness, inconsolability, or poor socialization. People with SOR are often rigid and controlling.

Sensory Modulation Disorder Subtype 2: Sensory Under-Responsivity

People with sensory under-responsivity (SUR) disregard or do not respond to sensory stimuli in their environments. They appear not to detect incoming sensory information. Behavior of people with SUR is often described as withdrawn, difficult to engage, inattentive, or self-absorbed. Commonly, SUR is not detected in infancy or toddlerhood.

Sensory Modulation Disorder Subtype 3: Sensory Seeking/Craving

People with sensory seeking/craving (SS) desire an unusual amount or type of sensory input and seem to have different capacities in each modality (e.g., a visual or auditory discrimination disorder but good discriminations in all other modalities). He or she may require extra time to process the salient aspects of sensory stimuli, leading to "show" performance. Low self-confidence, attention-seeking behavior, and temper tantrums may result.

Pattern 2: Sensory Discrimination Disorder

People with sensory discrimination disorder (SDD) have difficulty interpreting qualities of sensory stimuli and are unable to perceive similarities and differences among stimuli. They can perceive that stimuli are present and can regulate their response to stimuli but cannot tell precisely what or where the stimulus is. SDD can be observed in any sensory modality. A person with SDD may have different capacities in each modality (e.g., a visual or auditory discrimination disorder but good discrimination in all other modalities).

Pattern 3: Sensory-Based Motor Disorder

People with sensory-based motor disorder (SBMD) have poor postural or volitional movement as a result of sensory problems. There are two subtypes of SBMD.

Sensory-Based Motor Disorder Subtype 1: Postural Disorder

Postural disorder (PD) is a difficulty stabilizing the body during movement or at rest to meet the demands of the environment of a given motor task. PD is characterized by inappropriate muscle tension, hypotonic or hypertonic muscle tone, inadequate control of movement, or inadequate muscle contraction to achieve movement against resistance. Poor balance between flexion and extension of body parts, poor stability, poor righting and equilibrium reactions, poor weight shifting and trunk rotation, and poor oculomotor control may also be noted.

Sensory-Based Motor Disorder Subtype 2: Dyspraxia

Dyspraxia is an impaired ability to conceive of, plan, sequence, or execute novel actions. People appear awkward and poorly coordinated in gross, fine, or oral-motor areas. People with dyspraxia seem unsure of where their body is in space and have trouble judging their distances from objects, people, or both. They may seem accident prone, frequently breaking toys or objects because of difficulty grading force during movements. They are often inactive, preferring sedentary activities, such as watching TV, playing video games, or reading books, which can result in a tendency toward obesity (Miller, Anzalone, Lane, Cermak, & Osten, 2007).

Children with autism commonly have difficulty with various sensory processing skills, such as orienting responses, filtering information, habituation, and interpreting sensory events in the environment. They may over-react or under-react to sensory events or may fluctuate in their responses over time. Many children with autism have difficulties with motor planning and initiation or regulation of movement.

Two types of sensory processing disorders have been defined for children with autism. The first is the registration of, or orientation to, sensory input. Children with this type of sensory processing problem may react normally to sensory stimuli one minute, and the next minute, they may over-react or under-react to the same stimuli. This inconsistent responding is attributed to inconsistent registration due to a high threshold for sensory input.

The second sensory processing disorder involves the control or modulation of a stimulus once it is registered by the child's nervous system. Children with poor modulation may be able to exert control of behavior at certain times but not at others. They may be overly reactive to sensations, thereby exhibiting sensory defensiveness.

An extensive chart review of 200 children with autism showed that 95% exhibited sensory modulation difficulties. In a survey of occupational therapists, it was reported that they frequently observed difficulty in sensory modulation, tactile and vestibular function, and body awareness among children with autism (Huebner, 2001).

ASPERGER'S SYNDROME AND HIGH-FUNCTIONING AUTISM

The following are examples of high-functioning autism (Asperger's syndrome):

1. Joseph had "always seemed like a brilliant child. He began talking before his first birthday, much earlier than his older sister and brother. He expressed himself in an adult way and was always very polite... He showed a very early interest in letters and by 18 months could recite the whole alphabet. He taught himself to read before his third birthday. Joseph wasn't much interested in typical toys like balls and bicycles, preferring instead what his proud parents considered 'grown-up' pursuits like geography and science. Starting at age 2, he spent many hours lying on the living room floor looking at maps in the family's world atlas. By age 5, he could name anywhere in the world from a description of its geographical location (What is the northernmost coastal city in Brazil?)" Just as his parents suspected, Joseph is brilliant. He also has Asperger's syndrome.

2. Nine-year-old Seth was playing video games in the family room while his mother hurried about the house cleaning up for the guests who would soon arrive. As she climbed a stepladder in the living room to change a light bulb, she lost her balance and fell backward. While she lay on the floor gasping for breath, Seth walked by on his way to the kitchen for a snack, stepped over her and said, "Hi, Mom." Seth has high-functioning autism.

3. Clint turns 30 soon. He graduated from college with a degree in engineering, lives in an apartment in a nice section of town, recently bought a used car, and enjoys going to the movies. He is troubled, however, by his difficulty finding and keeping a job. Time and again, supervisors get frustrated by his slow work pace and difficulty getting along with coworkers. Clint gets stuck on details and finds it difficult to

set goals that eventually lead to completion of projects. After finishing a seasonal job cleaning hotel rooms at a ski resort, he tells prospective employers that he was "let go" without realizing that this term means "fired" to most people. Unable to find work for months, he visits a vocational counselor, who suggests that he have a psychological evaluation. It reveals that Clint has high-functioning autism, which was never diagnosed (Ozonoff, 2002).

The following is taken from the *DSM IV* Diagnostic Criteria: Asperger's disorder (299.80)

A. Qualitative impairment in social interaction, as manifested by at least two of the following:

1. Marked impairment in the use of multiple nonverbal behaviors such as eye-to-eye gaze, facial expression, body postures, and gestures to regulate social interaction

2. Failure to develop peer relationships appropriate to developmental level

3. A lack of spontaneous seeking to share enjoyment interests or achievements with other people (e.g., by a lack of showing, bringing, or pointing out objects of interest)

4. Lack of social or emotional reciprocity

B. Restricted repetitive and stereotyped patterns of behavior interest and activities as manifested by at least one of the following:

1. Encompassing preoccupation with one or more stereotyped and restricted patterns of interest that is abnormal either in intensity or focus

2. Apparently inflexible adherence to specific non-functional routines or rituals

3. Stereotyped and repetitive motor mannerisms (e.g., hand or finger flapping or twisting or complex whole-body movements)

C. The disturbance causes clinically significant impairment in social, occupational, or other important areas of functioning.

D. There is no clinically significant general delay in language (e.g., single words by age 2 years, communication phrases used by 3 years).

E. There is no clinically significant delay in cognitive development or in the development of age-appropriate self-help skills, adaptive behavior (other than in social interactions).

F. Criteria are not met for another specific pervasive developmental disorder or schizophrenia.

The prevalence of Asperger's syndrome using the *DSM IV* or International Classification of Diseases (ICD) criteria varies in each study with reported rates of between 0.3 per 10,000 children to 8.4 per 10,000 children (Baird et al., 2000). The expected rate varies in research studies between 1 in 330,000 and 1 in 12,000 (Attwood, 2007).

ETIOLOGY OF AUTISM

Vaccines

A paper by Gerber and Offet noted that on February 28, 1998, Andre Wakefield, a British gastroenterologist, and his colleagues published in the *Lancet* a paper that described eight children whose first symptoms of autism appeared within 1 month of receiving a measles, mumps, rubella (MMR) vaccine. All of these children had gastrointestinal symptoms and signs as well as lymphoid nodular hyperplasia. Wakefield postulated that the MMR vaccine caused intestinal inflammation that led to a translocation of usually nonpermeable peptides to the bloodstream and the brain. These then went on to affect the child's development. However, there were several problems that undermined his unwarranted conclusions. These problems included a self-referred subject cohort, a lack of control subjects, no determination of causation versus coincidental occurrence, and a poor study design (not a double-blind methodology, incomplete data collection in an unsystematic fashion) (Maino, 2009). *Lancet,* in March 2010, retracted the study tying vaccines to autism (Wang, 2010).

Everyone is not in agreement that vaccines are not somehow related to ASD. After years of insisting there is no evidence to link vaccines with the onset of ASD, the U. S. government has quietly conceded a vaccine-autism case in the Court of Federal Claims.

The claim, one of 4,900 autism cases currently pending in Federal "Vaccine Court," was conceded by U. S. Assistant Attorney General Peter Keisler and other Justice Department officials, on behalf of the Department of Health and Human Services, the "defendant" in all Vaccine Court cases.

The child's claim against the government—that mercury-containing vaccines were the cause of her autism—was supposed to be one of three "test cases" for the thimerosal-autism theory currently under consideration by a three-member panel of Special Masters, the presiding justices in Federal Claims Court.

Keisler wrote that the medical personnel at the Division of Vaccine Injury Compensation (DVIC) had reviewed the case and "concluded that compensation is appropriate."

The doctors conceded that the child was healthy and developing normally until her 18-month well-baby visit, when she received vaccinations against nine different diseases all at once (two contained thimerosal).

Days later, the girl began spiraling downward with illnesses and setbacks that, within months, presented as symptoms of autism, including no response to verbal direction, loss of language skills, no eye contact, loss of "relatedness," insomnia, incessant screaming, arching, and "watching the florescent lights repeatedly during examination."

Seven months after vaccination, the patient was diagnosed by Dr. Andrew Zimmerman, a leading neurologist at the Kennedy Krieger Children's Hospital Neurology clinic, with "regressive encephalopathy (brain disease) with features consistent with autistic spectrum disorder, following normal development." The girl also met the *DSM-IV* official criteria for autism.

In its written concession, the government said the child had a pre-existing mitochondrial disorder that was "aggravated" by her shots and that ultimately resulted in an ASD diagnosis. Mitochondria are the little powerhouses within cells that convert food into electrical energy, partly through a complex process called oxidative phosphorylation. If this process is impaired, mitochondrial disorder will ensue (Kirkby, 2011).

The Wakefield study was the "starting pistol" to the vaccine controversy. Research has shown that as many as 2.1% of U.S. children were not immunized with the MMR vaccine in 2000, up from 0.77% of children in 1995.

While Wakefield has been outspoken about his concern about the measles vaccine, he has continuously pushed the view that the vaccine caused autism, said Greg Poland, Professor of Medicine and Infectious Diseases at the Mayo Clinic and Director of the Vaccine Research Group in Rochester, Minn. With the retraction, the hypothesis that Wakefield has put forward has been debunked (McKhann, 2009; Wang, 2010).

AREAS OF THE BRAIN AND AUTISM

The Brain Component

Research shows that there is a disruption of circuitry in the brains of children with ASD. Some parts are overconnected; some are underconnected. Studies on brain circuitry have found that people with ASDs process information in different parts of their brains from those in typical people. For example, they recall letters of the alphabet in the part of the brain that normally processes shapes.

There are early developmental cues that point to brain abnormalities—smaller head size at birth followed by a period of excessive head growth between 6 months and 2 years of age, where chronic inflammation occurs in the areas of excessive growth. The frontal lobes, where nerve cells are responsible for higher-order processing like decision making and social reasoning, undergo the greatest increase, even though they are normally the last brain region to develop. Children with ASD may have problems in these cognitive areas because even though their frontal lobes are enlarged, their nerve cells are actually much smaller than normal.

The underconnectivity theory may help explain why some people with ASD have typical or even superior skills in some areas, while lacking skills in other areas. Dr. Marcel Just, Director of Carnegie Mellon's Center for Cognitive

Brain Imaging uses a sports analogy to explain this concept. In the brain of a typical person, the team members work together to coordinate their efforts, whereas in the brain of someone with ASD, they do not. This may account for the difficulties in complex thinking, social skills, and overall behavior (Exkom, 2006).

The Amygdala and Autism

This brain region has been implicated in several component processes of social behavior, including social motivation, evaluation of social significance, and generation of emotion in social situations.

The behavioral manifestation of amygdala pathology in autism is not yet understood. It is possible that pathology of the amygdala may alter the ability to correctly regulate fear and anxiety responses. Indeed, anxiety appears to be a common, though understated, feature of autism.

There is substantial evidence that individuals with autism are impaired in their ability to process social information from faces (Grelotti, Gauthier, & Schultz, 2002). Autism subjects show abnormal visual scan paths during eye tracking studies when viewing faces, typically spending little time on core social features such as the eyes. It is unclear whether these findings represent active avoidance of the eye region, potentially involving the amygdala, or that failure to look at the eyes represents a more global lack of social interest or motivation. An emerging hypothesis is that the amygdala may play a role in mediating or directing visual attention to the eyes (Grelotti, Gauthier, & Schultz, 2002). Although inattention to faces, particularly the eyes, is one of the earliest and most consistent symptoms of autism, little is known regarding the underlying causes of this abnormal pattern of social attention. One possibility is that people with autism simply lack social motivation and thus lack interest in attending to the face. An alternative view is that individuals with autism perceive social interactions as threatening and, therefore, avoid the interaction as a means of alleviating anxiety (Moldin, 2006).

Investigations that have measured point of regard during face perception indicate that normal adults direct most of their attention to core features of the face (i.e., eyes, nose, mouth) and spend very little time on nonfeatures. In fact, participants donated the vast majority of their fixations to the eyes, nose, and mouth with nearly 70% of those fixations directed to the eyes. The autistic individuals seem to rely more on individual parts of the face for identification (e.g., the lower face and mouth area) than the overall configuration. It seems autistic individuals adopt segmental perceptual strategies that are more characteristic of those of normal individuals during nonface object perception (Pelphrey et al., 2002). Autistic people inspect our faces as an object and not an emotional face.

In another experiment, it was investigated whether the fixation behavior for faces that were presented either upright or upside down differed between normal and autistic children. It was observed that the autistic children spent the same amount of time looking at upright faces as upside-down faces, whereas the normal children spent less time looking at the upside-down faces. The fact that autistic children are less sensitive to the orientation of a face is an indication that autistic individuals indeed rely less on holistic modes of processing (Van Der Geest, Kemner, Verbaten, & van Engeland, 2002).

Frontal Cortex

Studies show a delayed postnatal maturation of the frontal lobes in children with primary autism. At 3 to 4 years, the autistic children had a regional cerebral blood flow (CBF) pattern characterized by clean-cut frontal hypoperfusion, similar to the pattern reported for normal children about 2 years younger. In spite of these clear early differences, the same autistic children, 3 years later, had frontal CBF at normal values. In autistic children, delayed CBF maturation of the frontal lobe is highly consistent with several key abnormalities in cognitive development. For example, autistic children have been shown to perform poorly on executive tasks, which are closely linked to the frontal lobes (Ozonoff, Pennington, & Rogers, 1991). In addition, the prefrontal cortex is probably necessary for the formation of second-order cognitive representations of the world, which are dramatically impaired in autistic children. This results in an inability to predict and explain the behavior of other human beings in terms of their mental states, which is considered by some to be the central cognitive dysfunction in autism.

These findings suggest abnormal cortical connectivity and/or activation in autism. Because the late phase of cortical maturation is thought to reflect synapse selection and elimination, in part depending on neural activity and occurring during critical periods, it is conceivable that postnatal shaping of neural connections is altered in many brain structures of autistic children because of lack of normal frontal input between ages 2 and 4. To summarize, delayed frontal maturation is consistent with recent theories suggesting incomplete development of the distributed neural network for complex information processing (Zilbobius et al., 1995).

Cerebellum

One of the most consistent neuropathological findings in autism has been a reduction in the number of Purkinje cells in the cerebellum on the average of a 30% decrease. Surprisingly, studies of children under age 5 with autism report a significant enlargement of the cerebellum. An enlargement of about 7% was found in 3 and 4 year olds and in 2 and 3 year olds (Courchesne, Saitoh et al., 1994). This effect disappeared, however, in older children, in which the volume of the cerebellar gray matter, in par-

ticular, was significantly smaller than normal. Contrary to previous thought, this suggests that Purkinje cell loss in the cerebellum may occur later in life, perhaps in late childhood (Moldin, 2006).

Limbic System

Limbic structures, specifically the amygdala and hippocampus, have been studied by MRI studies. These provide information that indicates that there is an important effect of age in the development and maturation of this region, just as there is in the cerebrum. It appears that the amygdala is abnormally enlarged in both early (2 to 4 years or 3 to 5 years) and late (7.5 to 12.5 years) childhood. But in adolescence and adulthood, the volume is either normal or smaller than normal, suggesting an early overgrowth followed by either an arrest of growth or an atrophy of tissue in later years, much as we saw in the cerebrum (Schumann et al., 2004).

Brainstem

Assuming that brain system dysfunction may be involved in autism, to what extent can abnormal brainstem mechanism account for autistic behavior? The autistic disturbances of social relation, language and communication, and reaction to objects represent a profound disruption of adoptive integrative and motivated behavior. There are deficits in communicative skills, ability to apply experience to present transactions and future planning, a sense of self in relation to others, and the capacity to make decisions and choices. Social awareness and motivation seem to be dominated by disordered perceptual processes, which depend on compensation by abnormal motor activity, and autistic children "rely more on perceptual activity than on perceptual analysis" and may use their abnormal motility to make sense out of sensation. These latter disturbances of the modulation of sensory input and motor output are likely to involve the brain stem (Ornitz, Atwell, Kaplan, & Westlake, 1985).

DNA and Autism

A specific structural variation on chromosome 16 dramatically increases the risk of autism.

Autism is known to have a strong genetic influence with up to 90% of cases thought to have a genetic component. However, because the disorder is linked to a combination of genetic variations, each playing a minor role, identifying specific genetic triggers has been difficult. In a study, scientists used microarrays to scour DNA of more than 2,000 individuals with autism. They found that deletion or duplication of approximately 500 of the same DNA letters on chromosome 16 was strongly linked to autism (Singer, 2008).

Mirror Neurons

Evidence from electroencephalogram, functional magnetic resonance imaging (fMRI), and transcranial magnetic stimulation (TMS) studies suggest there is a dysfunction of the mirror neuron system in children and adults with autism. The mirror neuron theory of autism simply proposes that dysfunction of the execution/observation matching system does not allow for the internal representation of others' observed behavior, expressions, movements, and emotions. This prevents the individual with autism from having an immediate, direct experience of the other through this internal representation. Social deficits, including deficits in imitation, empathy, and theory of mind, therefore, cascade from this lack of immediate, experimental understanding of others in a social world. A disruption of the connections between the mirror neuron circuit and brain regions related to the inhibition of imitative acts could also account for another aspect of autism symptomatology—echolalia and repetitive behaviors (Pineda, 2009).

Faulty attentional circuitry could impact the input to the mirror neuron system in autism. Research has shown that individuals with autism even as young as 8 months old demonstrate reduced attention to social information. This decreased social attention could result in subsequent dysfunction of differential activation of the mirror neuron system. The cerebellum and the amygdala, as well as other brain regions such as the fusiform gyrus and ventromedial prefrontal cortex, have been implicated in autism, and understanding the interconnections between those brain regions and the mirror neuron systems will be necessary to understand the nature of the neural basis in autism.

The outstanding questions concerning the input to the mirror neuron system are the next step in better understanding the differential activity of this system in individuals with autism. The most parsimonious explanation is that disruptions to multiple circuits acting in concert result in the pattern of social impairments seen in autism (Pineda, 2009).

Motor

As much as people with Asperger's syndrome have a different way of thinking, they can also have a different way of moving. When walking or running, the child's coordination can be immature, and adults with Asperger's syndrome may have a strange, sometimes idiosyncratic gait that lacks fluency and efficiency. On careful observation, there can be a lack of synchrony in the movement of the arms and legs, especially when the person is running. Parents often report that the child was delayed by a month or two in learning to walk and needed considerable guidance in learning activities that required manual dexterity, such as tying shoelaces, dressing, and using eating utensils. Teachers may notice problems with fine motor skills, such as the ability to write

and use scissors. Activities that require coordination and balance can also be affected, such as learning to ride a bicycle, skate, or use a scooter. Children with Asperger's syndrome can have difficulty knowing where their bodies are in space, which may often cause them to trip, bump into objects, and spill drinks. The overall appearance can be of someone who is clumsy (Attwood, 2007).

Abnormal postures, such as toe walking, bizarre posturing of trunk and extremities, arching of the back, hyperextension of the neck, and so forth, have been consistently noted in children with autism. The findings from one study suggest that postural abnormalities in children with autism appear to be the most consistent with abnormalities arising at the level of the mesocortex or cerebellum rather than the vestibular system per se (Kohen-Raz, Volkmar, & Cohen, 1992).

ATTENTION/PERCEPTION/ VISION

These three areas are combined into one section because, after reviewing many studies, it is difficult to separate them, nor should they be separated.

The ability to attend selectively to meaningful stimuli while ignoring irrelevant ones is essential to cognitive functioning. Impaired selective attention results in increased distraction and diminished cognitive functioning because responses to irrelevant stimuli interfere with the processing of targeted information (Lane, 1982). It is widely reported that autistic children appear to ignore relevant stimuli in favor of apparently meaningless stimuli in their environment. But we should remember that the decision about which stimuli are relevant and which are meaningless depends on the common stack of experiences and knowledge. Autistic people might attend to what they think is important, but usually it turns out to be different from what nonautistic people think is important and is described as idiosyncratic focus of attention (Bogdashina, 2003).

Without selective interest, experience is an utter chaos (James, 1890). Anecdotally, this chaos is often observed in ASD, in which individuals appear to fixate inappropriately on seemingly irrelevant information in the environment.

Theories of early selection (in attention) assert that perception requires selective attention in order to proceed; therefore, selection occurs after only basic physical properties of stimuli have been processed. Conversely, the argument for late selection studies is that selection takes place only after stimuli have been perceived fully in an automatic, parallel fashion. Lance put forward a proposal that seems to resolve the dispute. She suggested that the focus of selection is dependent on the perceptual load (amount of potentially task-relevant information) of the task in question. When the perceptual load of a task is low and does not exceed perceptual capacity, distractors are processed. However, when the perceptual load is high, irrelevant distractors are not processed. It should be noted that perceptual load is not synonymous with task difficulty.

The perceptual load effect has been investigated within subsets of the population. Children and the elderly demonstrate early selection at lower set sizes than young adults, which suggests that children and the elderly have reduced perceptual capacity. This means that a crowded scene makes it difficult for selective attention in these groups. However, with ASD, it is the opposite. Individuals with ASD appear to have an inefficient, overly broad attentional lens that fails to contract appropriately when attending stimuli. It seems that individuals with ASD would require a higher level of perceptual load to eliminate distractor processing, according to the load theory. Such a finding would indicate increased perceptual capacity in individuals with ASD (Figure 5-1).

Figure 5-1A shows a high perceptual load, while Figure 5-1B shows a low perceptual load. If the target is X, children with ASD who have a high perceptual load would be less distracted by the other letters in A. The L would be very distracting in B to the ASD children compared to A. This is the opposite as to what we usually think. With normal children, they would be more distracted and have a difficult time selecting their attention to the X in A compared to B (Remington, Swettenham, Campbell, & Coleman, 2009).

Children with autism have a very narrow focus of attention. This is because in order to avoid sensory information overload, autistic people acquire voluntary and involuntary strategies and compensations such as monoprocessing when they focus their attention to one single channel or so-called "tunnel perception," when they concentrate on details instead of a whole. Autistic individuals often compare this attentional pattern with having a mind like a flashlight, a laser pointer, or a laser beam that highlights only a single dot (an area of high focus that they can see very clearly) while everything around it is gray or fuzzy. This is a form of attention tunneling (Bogdashina, 2003). An extreme example of such highly focused attention is the autistic child watching a spinning top who cannot be distracted from his or her preoccupation. This inattention appears similar to that observed in patients with acquired lesions in the posterior cortex who also fail to respond to sensory information outside their attentional focus (Townsend, 1994).

Consistent with behavioral similarities of autistic and lesion patients is evidence that a subgroup of patients with autism have damage to the posterior cortex. The most commonly reported structured pathology in autism is abnormality of the neocerebellum, but now both neuroradiological examination and quantitative estimates from MRI images have formed bilateral abnormally increased sulci width in the parietal cortex of a large group (43%)

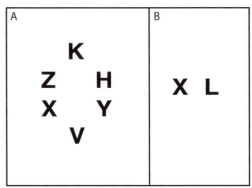

Figure 5-1. (A) High and (B) low perceptual loads.

of autistic adults. This parietal damage appears to result in diminished ability to process stimulation outside an attended location (i.e., spotlight attention). Such inattention may reflect a narrowed distribution of attentional resources that produces abnormally strong enhancement of sensory stimulation at the selected focus and/or abnormally weak enhancement in surrounding locations (Townsend, 1994). This could lead to difficulty disengaging attention and also could cause the autistic individual to have poor attention to his or her left side. Training that would include peripheral training especially to his or her left side would be very important to autistic patients.

Shifting of attention is another large difficulty with autistic patients. Studies have shown that (a) the cerebellum might play a role in the coordination of attention in a fashion analogous to the role it plays in motor control and that (b) in autism, cerebellum maldevelopment is a consistent feature that renders the child unable to adjust his or her mental focus of attention to follow the rapidly changing verbal, gestural, postural, tactile, and facial cues that signal changes in a stream of social information. Cerebellar pathology has now been verified by 16 quantitative magnetic resonance (MR) and autopsy reports from nine independent research groups involving 240 autistic cases. These results indicate that, like patients with acquired cerebellar damage, patients with autism are severely impaired in their ability to coordinate accurate and rapid voluntary shifts of attention between sensory modalities (Courchesne, Townsend et al., 1994).

A training procedure could be to train the autistic patient to increase his or her speed in shifting between sensory modalities (e.g., visual and auditory).

Hypersensitivity is a major concern for autistic children. For example, a child frequently covering his or her ears (even if you do not hear any disturbing sounds) may mean his or her hearing is hypersensitive, and it is your job to find out which sounds disturb him or her. If a child licks his or her fingers in front of his or her eyes, the child may have problems with hypersensitive or hyposensitive vision (Bogdashina, 2003).

Photosensitivity has long been noted to be a symptom associated with autism. Up to 50% of those who have autism may have severe sensitivity to fluorescent lighting. Researchers found that repetitive behaviors for ASD children increased when they were in a room illuminated by fluorescent light versus when they were in a room with equal intensity incandescent light (Colman, Frankel, Ritvo, Freeman, 1976). Individuals with autism may be hypersensitive to the flicker of the fluorescent lighting with some reports suggesting they can see a 60-cycle flicker. Accounts of hypersensitivity include descriptions of increased light sensitivity and harshness to colors.

Studies of color perception in children with ASD have demonstrated differences in color memory, discrimination abilities between colors, and detection of color when presented on achromatic (free from color) background. Individuals with autism have been noted to only eat white foods or to never play with toys of a certain color. Optometrists have had some success with varying color overlays to increase reading speed, and tinted lenses have helped some individuals (Coulter, 2009).

Visual hypersensitivity may also provide superior visual search skills in children with autism, possibly by heightened feature discrimination or failure to inhibit reception of some information.

Hyposensitivity to visual information can also occur as individuals with ASD struggle to regulate their level of alertness, body position, touch, and auditory stimuli.

The following is a list of environmental offenders that may be difficult for hypersensitive individuals:

- Clothing on others
  - Synthetic fibers
  - Intricate patterns
  - Metallic look
  - Reflecting accessories (e.g., sequins, watches)
  - Noise makers (e.g., bangle jangle bracelets)
- Lighting
  - Fluorescent lights
  - Halogen lights
  - Strobe lights
  - Flickering sunlight (e.g., through leaves or blinds)
  - Severe contrast
  - Lighted mirrors
  - Reflective materials
  - Certain colors (e.g., yellow-orange)
  - Color contrasts (e.g., black/red)
  - White paper (glossy magazines)
  - LCD signboards
    - Automobile lights at night or in the rain
    - Automobile lights in white-tiled tunnels (Lemer, 2008)

Hand Flapping and Finger Flicking

The voluntary, repetitious movements of the fingers and hands often within the line of the subject's vision is another symptom closely linked to ASD. The behaviors of hand flapping or finger flicking near the face have been explained as compensations for poor visuospatial skills and also for attention/focus in order to deal with overstimulation. These individuals lack the visuospatial abilities to know where their body parts are or where their bodies are in relationship to other objects. As a result, individuals with ASD compensate by seeking additional sensory input to tell them where they are in space (Coulter, 2009).

TUNNEL VISION

Studies have shown that autistic children responded to multiple cues when these cues were positioned closely together (Rincover & Ducharme, 1987). This is a form of tunnel vision, which may be a critical deficit in autistic children, accounting for many of the behavioral deficiencies of autism, including delays in speech and social behavior and the failure for autistic children to acquire new behaviors or observational learning. It has been shown that, as the distance between stimulus features increases, children with autism show evidence of selectively responding to only a small part of the stimulus array. This results in individuals with autism being able to respond quicker to central rather than lateralized stimuli (Wainwright & Bryson, 1996). The mechanism of tunnel vision hinders the child's auditory abilities to peripherally select and respond to chosen stimuli, thus creating overselectivity (Searfoss, 2000).

POOR EYE CONTACT (GAZE AVERSION)

Gaze aversion is a visual behavior noted in autism in which the individual looks away or avoids eye contact. Although gaze aversion occurs in nonaffected developing babies when they are overstimulated or tired, gaze aversion is more severe and persists longer in individuals with ASD (Coulter, 2009).

Typical newborns will turn their heads in the direction of their mother's voices, and, as they develop, their eyes will be drawn to their mother's faces. Later on, faces in general will continue to hold a special fascination for them. Typical children perceive a face as a whole. Our brains are not wired to register features discretely—eyes, nose, mouth, chin, forehead—then piece them together as if they were objects. When tested, typical children perceive faces more quickly than objects, whereas children with ASD see faces feature-by-feature without compiling them into a whole.

Eye control can be particularly difficult for children with ASD because faces are rarely static: our eyebrows rise when we show surprise, our eyes look up or to the side when we are thinking, and the corners of our mouths curl up or down to connote happiness or disappointment. For children with ASD who view faces as components rather than as a whole, looking at a face may be overwhelming.

Neuroscientists now believe that a specific part of our brain is responsible for recognizing faces—a small patch of the cerebral cortex that is activated when people look at pictures of faces but not objects. They refer to this part of the brain as the fusiform face (FFA). A study using fMRI was conducted at the Yale Child Center. When typical subjects were shown pictures of faces, there was a high level of activity in the FFA. When subjects with ASD were shown pictures of faces, there was little activity in the FFA, but the researchers did note a high activation level in the nearby brain regions—the ones used for recognizing objects (Exkom, 2006).

Mind Blindness

Mind blindness can be tied to lack of eye contact. By avoiding looking at people's faces, particularly the eyes, children with ASD are missing out on being able to read affect or emotional states. Because our words do not necessarily convey our true emotional states, the expression, "I can see it in your face" is a perfect example of how much we rely on intuition and nonverbal cues to identify another person's mood. To the person with ASD, someone's facial expression may give absolutely nothing away because he or she cannot read it. Because many children with ASD experience mind blindness, they may unconsciously alienate others through their behavior. This can be especially difficult at home or school. Family members or peers may feel ignored or dismissed (Exkom, 2006).

JOINT ATTENTION

A deficit of joint attention (JA) is one of the defining criteria of autism in most diagnostic instruments as well as in measures developed for the screening for autism in infancy (Moldin, 2006). JA refers to the parent and child coordinating their attention so that they are looking at the same object or sharing in an activity. JA between a parent and a typically developing baby becomes evident when the baby is around 8 months old. At this time, babies check with their mothers to make sure it is okay for them to touch something, such as a new toy or a wall outlet. Babies will look at their mothers' faces to gauge their expressions. A smile means okay, whereas a furrowed brow means "stay away." At 10 months, JA is usually seen in children as they begin to point to things in their environment. But, typical babies are not simply interested in the objects they are pointing to. They are interested in their parents' responses to those objects, and they do not necessarily want the objects they are pointing to: they may just want to share the experience of looking at the object with their parents.

One of the first warning signs of a lack of JA in children with ASD appears in infancy when children do not look for their parents' facial reactions and do not have the ability to physically point out things in their environments. Children with ASD who can point use pointing to get something they want rather than sharing the experience with someone else.

As children with ASD get older, the lack of JA can be evident in those who have more fully developed speech and language skills. These individuals often have trouble carrying on two-way communications because they do not have an awareness of the other person's intentions or mental state. Many people with ASD will dominate the conversation, engaging in one-way communication and expressing little interest in the other person (Exkom, 2006).

In a series of experiments by Dr. Ami Klin of Yale University School of Medicine, she found that toddlers with autism paid more attention to human motions when they were accompanied by synchronous sounds. In contrast, typical toddlers paid more attention to the normal biological range of human motion. The finding may help explore the observation that children with autism tend to watch the mouths of other people—where sound and motion are synchronized. The researchers hypothesized that toddlers with autism would predictably pay preferential attention to points with synchronous motion and sound (Smith, 2009).

EYE MOVEMENTS AND AUTISM

There have been numerous studies on eye movements and autism; however, several points seem to prevail.

- It has been reported that individuals with autism look at others less frequently or show deviant use of reciprocal gaze. Although it is usually thought that the deviant behavior is a consequence of a social deficit, it may be possible that it is caused by abnormalities in visual attention. It is generally accepted that eye movements and visual attention processes are closely related. They may be directly connected or share common brain resources. Indeed, indications of abnormal visual attention in individuals with autism have been found in several reaction-time studies (Courchesne, Saitoh et al., 1994). There have been reports of deficits in high-functioning individuals with autism in neuropsychologic tests that required shifts of visual attention. These studies showed that autistic children had difficulties establishing a new focus of attention, suggesting deficits in the disengagement of attention. Kemner, Verbaten, Cuperus, Camfferman, and van Engeland, (1998) showed that autistic children made more saccadic eye movements in a passive visual task than did control children. It was proposed that a weaker attentional engagement could be related to this abnormally high saccadic frequency in autistic children. It has also been shown that the parietal lobe is a likely candidate as the source of attentional disturbances in autistic individuals. It seems that it is not deficits in attentional disengagement in children with autism, but probably that they have a lower level of attentional engagement (Van Der Geest et al., 2002).

- One of the clearest findings in children with autism is the abnormal high saccadic frequency between stimulus presentations. It is possible that the abnormal saccadic activity has been present in autistic children from birth on. One indication is the clinical observation that young autistic children do not show appropriate-looking behavior, which might be the result of interruption of saccades and/or might reflect the general indifferentiation with respect to stimulus presence. It has been known for a while that children with autism make more saccadic eye movements in between visual stimulus presentations (Kemner, Verbaten, Cuperus, Camfferman, & van Engeland, 2004).

- The pursuit system in autistic individuals may be abnormal, especially after midadolescence. Visual pursuit requires rapid, temporally precise integration of activity within several brain areas in order to visually track moving targets though space. The relevant brain circuitry includes the extrastriate areas of the visual cortex devoted to the processing of visual motion information, cortical eye fields, and cerebellum that are involved in translating sensory information to motor commands and the striatum and brainstem, which are involved in initiating motor

commands. It appears that pursuit deficits in autism are related to problems of praxis rather than deficits in visual attention (unlike saccadics, which were related to attention). The association between the pursuit deficits and impairment in praxis suggests that the observed pursuit deficits result from a more general problem in visual sensorimotor transformation rather than a highly selective disturbance in the sensory analysis of visual motion information or pursuit control. Further, these findings suggest that impairment in sensorimotor integration is not specific to types of visual information (visual motion versus visual spatial) or types of motor output (eye versus hand movements). These studies indicate that individuals with autism, because they have prolonged manual response latencies to stationary visual cues presented in the right hemisphere, may have a problem using visual information from the right visual hemifield to produce accurate motor responses (Takarae, Minshew, Luna, Krisky, & Sweeney, 2004).

PRISMS AND AUTISM

The prisms most often used by optometrists when treating an autistic individual are called yoked prisms because the bases of these prisms are in the same direction. Therefore, instead of helping eyes that have a binocular (an alignment) problem, they bend or deviate the perceived image in one direction—either up, down, right, or left. When these prisms are worn by a child, his or her visual image of the world will shift in the opposite direction of the base of the prism. So, a base-down pair of prisms will shift his or her perceived image up. What happens next is that the brain gets a mismatch between the visual system and the motor system. The image was shifted up, but the body still feels that it is straight ahead. In effect, the brain has to address a mismatch between visual and motor to create balance and a coherent body schema. The body experiences a shift in motor orientation not because the eye muscles change in alignment but because the brain is trying to match the motor and visual information with the vestibular process—the kinesthetic and proprioception processes. This is a reorganization of the senses (Lemer, 2008). It has been found that yoked prisms stimulate spatial awareness, redirect vision focus, increase visual attention, and facilitate change. All of these are critical to help the autistic child. Optometrists who are familiar with yoked prisms spend time with the child and try different prisms to see which ones will benefit the child the most. They will try different prisms and have the child do different activities to identify the proper prism to prescribe. They will not just automatically write out the same prism prescription for each child. When you refer a child to an optometrist for possible yoked prisms, find out first if the optometrist is going to do a proper work-up on the child or just automatically prescribe prism glasses.

SUMMARY AND ATTENTION TIPS

1. Autistic children do better when the visual space is crowded (high perceptual load), which is different from other children. It is better to have numerous distractors in front of the child than just one or two distractors.

2. Autistic children have difficulty paying attention to events on their left side. Stand slightly to their right when you want their attention.

3. Do a lot of peripheral training, especially toward their left side.

4. Autistic children respond faster to central rather than lateralized stimuli.

5. Train shifting of attention activities. Go for speed in shifting attentions—both visual and auditory.

6. Half of autistic children may have sensitivity to fluorescent lighting. Use incandescent lighting.

7. Colored overlays (light blue) may help some autistic children with reading.

8. The following is a list of environmental offenders to hypersensitive children:

   Clothing on others

      Synthetic fibers

      Intricate patterns

      Metallic look

      Reflecting accessories (e.g., sequins, watches)

      Noise makers (e.g., bangle jangle bracelets)

(continued)

SUMMARY AND ATTENTION TIPS (CONTINUED)

8. (continued)

   Lighting

      Fluorescent lights

      Halogen lights

      Strobe lights

      Flickering sunlight (e.g., through leaves or blinds)

      Severe contrast

      Lighted mirrors

      Reflective mirrors

      Certain colors (e.g., black/red)

      White paper (glossy magazines)

      LCD signboards

      Automobile lights at night or in the rain

      Automobile lights in white-tiled tunnels

9. Do pursuit activities. Remember, start one eye at a time if he or she will let you cover one of his or her eyes.

10. They may have a great deal of difficulty looking at visual cues on their left side.

11. When you send a child to an optometrist who prescribes prism glasses, make sure he or she does a full work-up on the child before prescribing the glasses.

12. Hyper-reactivity due to vision:

   Blinks excessively

   Covers eyes

   Picks up specks of dust

   Poor eye contact

   Poor focus

   Lack of awareness

   Fascinated by reflections

   Flicks fingers by eyes

(Lemer, 2008)

REFERENCES

Attwood, T. (2007). *The complete guide to Asperger's syndrome.* London, UK: Jessica Kingsley Publishers.

Ayres, J. A. (1972). Sensory integration and learning disorders. *Western Psychological Services.*

Baird, G., Charman, T., Baron-Cohen, S., Cox, A., Swettenham, J., Wheelwright, S., & Drew, A. (2000). A screening instrument for autism at 18 months of age: a 6 year follow-up study. *Journal of the American Academy of Child and Adolescent Psychiatry, 39*(6), 694-762.

Bogdashina, O. (2003). *Sensory perceptual issues in autism and Asperger syndrome.* London, UK: Jessica Kingsley Publishers.

Colman, R. S., Frankel, F., Ritvo, E., Freeman, B. J. (1976). The effects of fluorescent and incandescent illumination upon repetitive behaviors in autistic children. *Journal of Autism and Developmental Disorders, 6*(2), 157-162.

Coulter, R. (2009). Understanding the visual symptoms of individuals with autism spectrum disorder (ASD). *Optometry & Vision Development, 40*(3), 164-175.

Courchesne, E., Saitoh, O., Yeung-Courchesne, R., Press, G. A., Lincoln, A. J., Haas, R. H., & Schreibman, L. (1994). Abnormality of cerebellar vermian lobules vi and vii in patients with infantile autism: identification of hypoplastic and hyperplastic subgroups with MR imaging. *American Journal of Roentgenology, 162*(1), 123-130.

Courchesne, E., Townsend, J., Akshoomoff, N. A., Saitoh, O., Yeung-Courchesne, R., Lincoln, A. J., . . . Lau, L. (1994). Impairment in shifting attention in autistic and cerebellar patients. *Behavioral Neuroscience, 108*(5), 848-865.

Exkom, K. (2006). *The autism sourcebook.* New York, NY: Harper-Collins Publisher.

Gillberg, C. (1998). Chromosomal disorders and autism. *Journal of Autism and Developmental Disorders, 28*(5), 415-425.

Greenspan, S. I. (2004). *The first idea.* New York, NY: Da Capo Press.

Grelotti, D. J., Gauthier, I., & Schultz, R. T. (2002). Social interest and the development of cortical face specialization: what autism teaches us about face processing. *Developmental Psychobiology, 40*(3), 213-225.

Huebner, R. (2001). *Autism: a sensorimotor approach to management.* Austin, TX: Pro-Ed.

James, W. (1890) *The principles of psychology.* New York, NY: Dover.

Kemner, C., Verbaten, M. N., Cuperus, J. M., Camfferman, G., & van Engeland, H. (1998). Abnormal saccadic eye movements in autistic children. *Journal of Autism and Developmental Disorders, 28*(1), 61-67

Kemner, C., van der Geest, J. N., Verbaten, M. N., & van Engeland, H. (2004). In search of neurophysiological markers of pervasive developmental disorders: smooth pursuit eye movements. *Journal of Neural Transmission, 111*(112), 1617-1626.

Kirkby, D. (2011). *Government concedes vaccine-autism case in federal court. Now what?* Internet, Jan, 2011.

Kohen-Raz, R., Volkmar, F. R., & Cohen, D. J. (1992). Postural control in children with autism. *Journal of Autism and Developmental Disorders, 22*(3), 419-431.

Lane, D. (1982). The development of selective attention. *Merrill-Palmer Quarterly, 28,* 317-337.

LeCouteur, R., Rutter, M., Lord, C., Rios, P., Robertson, S., Holdgrafer, M., & McLennan, J. (1989). Autism a diagnosis interview: a standardized investigator-based instrument. *Journal of Autism and Developmental Disorders, 19*(3), 363-387.

Lemer, P. (2008). *Envisioning a bright future: Interventions that work for children and adults with autism spectrum disorders.* Santa Ana, CA: Optometric Extension Program Foundation.

Maino, D. (2009). The etiology of autism. *Optometry & Vision Development, 40*(3), 150-156.

Mangeot, S., Miller, L. J., McIntosh, D. N., McGrath-Clarke, J., Simon, J., Hagerman, R. J., & Goldson, E. (2001). Sensory modulation dysfunction in children with attention-deficit-hyperactivity disorder. *Developmental Medicine & Child Neurology, 43*(6), 399-406.

McKhann, G. (2009). A decade of research shows no link between vaccines and autism. *Brain in the News, March,* 3.

Miller, L. J., Anzalone, M. E., Lane, S. J., Cermak, S. A., & Osten, E. T. (2007). Concept of evolution in sensory integration: a proposed nosology for diagnosis. *The American Journal of Occupational Therapy, 61*(2), 135-140.

Moldin, S. (2006). *Understanding autism.* Oxfordshire, UK: Taylor & Francis, Inc.

Neimark, J. (2009). Solving the mystery: an affliction. *Discover Magazine, Summer,* 73-77.

Ornitz, E. M., Atwell, C. W., Kaplan, A.R., & Westlake, J. R. (1985). Brain-stem dysfunction in autism. Results of vestibular stimulation. *Archives of General Psychiatry, 42,* 1018-1025.

Ozonoff, S., Pennington, B. F., & Rogers, S. J. (1991). Executive function deficits in high functioning autistic children: relationship to theory of mind. *Journal of Child Psychology and Psychiatry, 32*(7), 1081-1105.

Ozonoff, S. (2002). *A parent's guide to Asperger syndrome & high functioning autism.* New York, NY: The Guilford Press.

Pelphrey, K. A., Sasson, N. J., Reznick, J. S., Paul, G., Goldman, B. D., & Piven, J. (2002). Visual scanning of faces in autism. *Journal of Autism and Developmental Disorders, 32*(4), 249-260.

Pineda, J. (2009). *Mirror neuron systems.* New York, NY: Springer-Verlag.

Remington, A., Swettenham, J., Campbell, R., & Coleman, M. (2009). Selective attention and perceptual load in autism spectrum disorder. *Association of Psychological Science, 20*(11), 1388-1392.

Rincover, A. & Ducharme, J. M. (1987). Variables influencing stimulus overselectivity and "tunnel vision" in developmentally delayed children. *American Journal of Mental Deficiency, 91*(4), 422-430.

Risch, N., Spiker, D., Lotspeich, L., Nouri, N., Hinds, D., Hallmayer, J., . . Myers, R. M. (1999) A genomic screen for autism: evidence for a multilocus etiology. *American Journal of Human Genetics, 65*(2), 493-507.

Schumann, C. M., Hamstra, J., Goodlin-Jones, B. L., Lotspeich, L. J., Kwon, H., Buonocore, M. H., . . . Amaral, D. G. (2004). The amygdala is enlarged in children but not adolescents with autism: hippocampus is enlarged at all ages. *The Journal of Neuroscience, 24*(28), 6392-6401.

Searfoss, J. (2000). Tunnel vision: a loss of visual sensitivity in school age children. *Journal of Optometric Vision Development, 31,* 117-130.

Singer, E. (2008). DNA deletion linked to autism. *Brain in the News, Feb,* 1-2.

Smith, M. (2009, March). Combined sound and motion draw autistic children. *Nature.* Retrieved from http://www.medpagetoday.com/Pediatrics/Autism/13472.

Takarae, Y., Minshew, N. J., Luna, B., Krisky, C. M., & Sweeney, J. A. (2004). Pursuit eye movement deficits in autism. *Brain, 127*(Pt. 12), 2584-2594.

Townsend, J. (1994). Parietal damage and narrow "spotlight" spatial attention. *Journal of Cognitive Neuroscience, 6*(3), 226-232.

Van Der Geest, J. N., Kemner, C., Verbaten, M. N., & van Engeland, H. (2002). Gaze behavior of children with pervasive developmental disorder toward human faces: a fixator study. *Journal of Child Psychology and Psychiatry, 43*(5), 669-678.

Wainwright, J. & Bryson, S. E. (1996). Visual-spatial orienting in autism. *Journal of Autism and Developmental Disorders, 26*(4), 423-438.

Wang, S. (2010). Lancet retraction study tying vaccine to autism. *Brain in the News, March,* 1-2.

Zilbobius, M., Garreau, B., Samson, Y., Remy, P., Barthélémy, C., Syrota, A., & Lelord, G. (1995). Delayed maturation of the frontal cortex in childhood autism. *American Journal of Psychiatry, 152*(2), 248-252.

Zwaigenbaum, L., Bryson, S., Rogers, T., Roberts, W., Brian, J., & Szatmari, P. (2005). Behavioral manifestations of autism in the first year of life. *International Journal of Developmental Neuroscience, 23,* 143-152.

SUGGESTED READING

Courchesne, E., Karns, C. M., Davis, H. R., Ziccardi, R., Carper, R. A., Tigue, Z. D., . . . Courchesne, R. Y. (2001). Unusual brain growth patterns in early life in patients with autistic disorder: an MRI study. *Neurology, 57*(2), 245-254.

Lavie, N. (1995). Perceptual load as a necessary condition for selective attention. *Journal of Experimental Psychology, Human Perception and Performance, 21*(3), 451-468.

Reading Disability

I am starting this chapter discussing three children who were all recently dismissed from my vision therapy clinic. These children are typical of the hundreds of children I have worked with for the past 30 years. My vision therapy practice is not much different from many other optometrists' vision therapy practices. I do, however, stress oculomotor activities with the vast majority of my therapy exercises dealing with the oculomotor system. Along with oculomotor, we also work on convergence and accommodation. The three areas of oculomotor, convergence, and accommodation have a lot of interaction with the right parietal lobe, which is largely involved with the magnocellular pathway, visuospatial skills, and most importantly, visual attention. Because reading is mostly a visual task, by improving the visual skills and visual attention that are critical for reading efficiency, we can greatly improve a child's overall reading speed. As I will mention later, a truly dyslexic child is uncommon. The majority of children you work with are not dyslexic but have a learning disability made worse by very poor visual attention causing very poor oculomotor abilities. By improving visual attention and oculomotor skills, the child's reading efficiency can be greatly increased. This is accomplished by decreasing the amount of time a child has to re-read (regressions), caused by losing his or her place or skipping letters or words. You decrease the re-reading; you increase the reading speed. If you make reading easier for the child, he or she will read more, which will make his or her decoding speed faster because of practice.

The three children are Breanna, Greer, and MacGregor. All were in our vision therapy program for 6 months on a twice-weekly basis and were dismissed after their second re-evaluation in February 2010.

Breanna is a 9-year-old fourth grader who complained of print blurring and did not like to read. Her initial evaluation showed a reading speed of 115 words per minute with 60% comprehension. Her last evaluation showed that her reading speed increased to 300 words per minute with 90% comprehension. Breanna now enjoys reading.

Greer is a 10-year-old, female, fourth grade student who complained of reading difficulties and had to use her finger to keep her place. She also complained of skipping words during reading. In addition to this, she had poor visual motor skills and scored at age level 7.9 in this area. Her initial reading speed was 162 words per minute. Her reading speed at her final evaluation was 210 words per minute, and her visual motor improved to age level 10.7.

MacGregor is a first grader who is 6 years old. He hated to read and would avoid it. His initial reading speed was 56 words per minute with a visual memory score in the lower 25th percentile for his age level. His last evaluation showed a reading speed of 87 words per minute, and his visual memory improved to the 75th percentile for his age level.

None of these children received any additional help in reading during the 6 months in our program. These results are not uncommon, and there are children in your practice who you could help by incorporating oculomotor activities. The type of child you need to be aware of is the child who has poor visuomotor skills and is struggling with reading. He or she is probably in your program to improve his or her fine motor skills. The child also probably has poor

Lane, K. A. *Visual Attention in Children: Theories and Activities* (pp. 101-108).

gross motor and balance abilities. Add oculomotor and the attention activities in this book to his or her program, and you will make reading easier.

DIAGNOSTIC AND STATISTICAL MANUAL-IV DEFINITION OF READING DISORDER

A. Reading achievement as measured by individually administered standardized tests of reading accuracy or comprehension is substantially below that expected given the person's chronological age, measured intelligence, and age-appropriate education.

B. The disturbance in criteria A significantly interferes with academic achievement or activities of daily living that require reading skills.

C. If a sensory deficit is present, the reading difficulties are in excess of these usually associated with it.

The term *dyslexia* is often used in the public school system to classify children who are behind in reading. By a child having this diagnosis, the school systems can offer additional help and modifications.

The question is, are all of these children dyslexic? For a child to be dyslexic, he or she would need to be in the lower 5% of the reading population. True dyslexia is rare. In all of the years I have worked with children, I have only seen fewer than 10 who were truly dyslexic. These children have extreme reading difficulties. For example, a dyslexic child, in my opinion, would still be slow at letter recognition in first grade. These children also are very slow at color naming. What you will most likely see in your practice is a child with a learning disability. This is about 20% of the school population, and these children fit the diagnosis given above for reading disorders but they are not in the lower 5% of the population. Occupational therapists will see a lot of learning disabled children because most of them have very poor fine motor and gross motor skills. The most telling symptoms are poor visuomotor skills with very poor spatial skills. In the case history, there is also a good possibility that one of the parents had difficulty in school, and there may also be some delay in speech or motor development.

The book *The Cognitive Neurosciences III* has an interesting lead sentence to one of its paragraphs on developmental dyslexia. "It is quite remarkable that even after the more obvious causes of failure are excluded, about 5% of school children still have great difficulty learning to read" (Gazzaniga, 2004, p. 818). The real question should be: with as complex a neurological process that reading is, why are there not more children who are having difficulty learning to read? This is a quote from 1962 Nobel Prize winner John

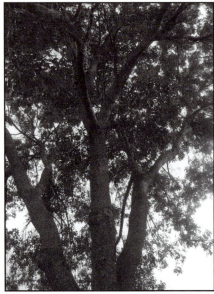

Figure 6-1. Angles and curves made by tree branches.

Steinbeck: "Some people there are who, being grown, forget the horrible task of learning to read. It is perhaps the greatest single effort that the human undertakes, and he must do it as a child."

As I mentioned before, it is a wonder that more children do not have dyslexia considering the complexity of the reading processes. British neuropsychologist Andrew Ellis declared that whatever dyslexia turns out to be, "it is not a reading disorder" (Wolf, 2007, p. 168). Ellis was referring to the fact that, in terms of human evolution, the brain was never meant to read; as we have seen, there are neither genes nor biological structures specific only to reading. Instead, in order to read, each brain must learn to make new circuits by connecting older regions. It was originally designed and genetically programmed for other things, such as recognizing objects. Dyslexia cannot be anything so simple as a flaw in the brain's "reading center," for no such thing exists. In fact, because all alphabets use similar lines, angles, and curves to form their letters, it is a good bet that the early humans who started alphabets developed letters out of visual angles, lines, and curves that they were used to seeing all day (Figure 6-1).

If they used something else, we would never have learned to read. To find the causes of dyslexia, we must look to older structures of the brain and their multiple levels of processes, structures, neurons, and genes, all of which have to come together in rapid synchrony to form the reading circuit (Wolf, 2007).

It is really amazing what we expect of our children. Because there are not reading genes, each new brain has to start from scratch to learn to read. Despite the fact that it took our ancestors about 2,000 years to develop an alphabetic code, children are regularly expected to crack this code in about 2,000 days (that is, by 6 or 7 years of age). Something this difficult needs all the attention a child can generate.

It is obvious that evolution did not plan on language—thus, the long time period between the vocal tract and speaking. It is also obvious that it did not plan on reading. If it was not planned, how did language and finally reading find brain areas to use? New brain areas were not developed. It appears that the brain used pre-existing areas and then expanded on them. The areas that it picked and the reason they were picked, I feel, holds the key to understanding reading difficulties. The brain chose the left hemisphere for language and speech because this is the hemisphere that was involved in processing rapid sequential motor skills (such as hand movements). The brain did not have to start a new section—it picked an existing section that fit its needs. Three brain areas are involved in language: the supplementary motor cortex and Broca's area in the frontal lobe and Wernicke's area around the fissure of Sylvius where the temporal lobe joins the parietal lobe (Diamond, 1999).

START OF READING

When written symbols used to convey words started 5,000 years ago, the brain was caught in the same dilemma that it was when spoken language started. What part of the brain could it use? Language was dealing not only in auditory processing but, for the first time, visual as well. It needed to use an area that performed similar functions. Again, the left hemisphere was chosen. It used cerebral regions that it had used for performing similar functions, such as object recognition. We are able to learn to read because the primate visual system evolved to do a different job that was sufficiently similar to allow it to be "recycled" into a reading machine. The area of the brain that is used lies on the left side of the brain within a strip of cortex that takes part in our object-recognition pathway (De Haene, 2003). It is interested only in visual form, not meaning. The activation of this visual word form region increases progressively with expertise in reading. This region seems to be activated in an all-or-nothing manner in which, just as an object would be recognized as a whole object, the whole group of letters in a word is perceived at once, meaning longer words do not take longer to read than shorter words. In adults with dyslexia, who never attain ease in recognizing the visual form of words, the region's activity never achieves the usual adult levels. This reduced response is most likely the result of difficulties in reading rather than the cause. This region of the brain is capable of analyzing the series of letters that make up words and then supplying other cortical regions with some sort of representation of their identity and order. What is extremely important to understand is that this region is not interested in which visual field the word may be located. It responds the same way to words presented

on the left or right visual fields. Words presented to our left are analyzed initially by the right side of the brain and words on the right by the left side of the brain. The visual word form area, which is on the left side, must collect visual signals from both hemispheres, and all of this happens in less than one-fifth of a second (De Haene, 2003). It seems clear that this region of the brain that recognizes words was originally developed to recognize visual shapes. Our visual system automatically recognizes objects as the same regardless of whether they have been rotated or face in a different direction. This makes it easy for us to recognize an object from any angle, but is a disadvantage for reading (De Haene, 2003). The fact that our brain was thrown into a situation where it had to adapt to a new situation whether that was language or reading and had to use pre-existing areas that were used for similar but not the same things may be part of the reason why some children have difficulty learning to read.

VISUAL ATTENTION AND READING

The exact relationship between attention deficit/hyperactivity disorder (AD/HD) and other forms of learning disabilities (LDs) is unclear, but experts estimate a 50% to 90% overlap between the two categories. Many feel that the reason for the LD category growing so large is because of the dramatic increase in the number of children with attention disorders (Healy, 1999).

To demonstrate the importance of attention in word recognition, the following is taken from *Proust and the Squid* by Maryanne Wolf under the section called "Every word has 500 milliseconds (msec) of fame" (Wolf, 2007, p. 145):

First 0 to 100 msec: All reading begins with attention—in fact, several kinds of attention. When expert readers look at a word (like "been"), the first three cognitive operations are (1) to disengage from whatever else we are doing; (2) to move our attention to the new focus (pulling ourselves to the text); and (3) to spotlight the new letter and word. This is the orienting network of attention and imagery research showing that each of these three operations involve different regions of the brain.

To disengage attention involves areas in the back of the parietal lobe; to move our attention involves parts of the midbrain responsible for eye movements called the superior colliculi; and to spotlight something involves part of our internal switchboard called the thalamus, which coordinates information from all five layers of the brain.

Between 50 and 150 msec: Many visual and orthographic representational processes happen between 50 and 150 msec; then, sometime between 150 and 200 msec, the executive and attentional systems of the frontal lobes activate. This is when our executive system influences the next eye movements. The executive system determines whether there is enough information about letters and word forms to move forward to a new saccade at 250 msec or whether a regression backward is needed to get more information.

Between 100 to 200 msec: This is the time the brain connects letters to sounds and orthography to phonology. The current research on phonological processes shows great anatomical activity for these processes between 150 to 200 msec in multiple cortical areas including frontal, temporal, and some parietal areas.

Between 200 to 500 msec: Research finds bursts of electrical activity between 200 and 600 msec. Often, we see an incongruous word search such as "mermaid" peaking at 400 msec. Research gives us two bits of information for this time period. First, it indicates that the retrieval of semantic information first comes in around 200 msec for typical readers. Second, it indicates that we continue to add information, particularly around 400 msec, if there is a semantic mismatch with our predictions.

This shows how complex word recognition is for the normal reader with good attention. You can only imagine how different it is for a child who has poor attention to read.

Studies have shown that children scoring at least 1 year below grade level in reading ability differ significantly both from children who are good readers and from adults in performance in a visual attention task. Good readers and adults are able to allocate attention across different points in visual space without making eye movements. Unlike good readers and adults, poor readers do not use location—information provided by parafoveally presented cues to report which of these letters is also appearing parafoveally. This suggests an attentional deficit of some kind in poor readers (Brannan & Williams, 1987). Studies have shown that poor readers were generally slower than normal readers in shifting attention automatically in response to peripheral visual cues. It seems reasonable to state that the deficit of the automatic orienting mechanism could be due to (1) a selective impairment of the ability to process peripheral visual onset stimuli and/or (2) a reduced speed in the elementary operation of moving attention. A deficit of automatic orienting of attention could hamper the exact planning of ocular movements (saccadics), which are critical for fast decoding during reading and which are known to be altered in children with dyslexia (Facoetti & Molteni, 2001).

Many studies have shown that people with dyslexia are slower and less accurate in visual search tasks requiring selection of a target (Casco, Tressoldi, & Dellantonio, 1998). Research has shown that subjects with LDs (reading disabilities [RDs]) made more errors than the control group on a selective attention task (Facoetti & Molteni, 2001). This was again shown in 2003 (Facoetti, Lorusso, Paganoni, Umiltà, & Mascetti) and showed a general attentional deficit to visual stimuli in dyslexia (Heiervang & Hugdahl,

2003). It is easy to demonstrate how we keep ahead of any words that we identify as we read. Ask a friend to turn out the light while you read aloud, so that you are suddenly deprived of visual information, and you will find that your voice is able to continue "reading" another four or five words. Your eyes were a second or more—perhaps three or four eye movements—ahead of the point your voice had reached when the lights went out. This phenomenon is known as the *eye-voice span*, a term that is rather misleading because it might suggest that we need more than a second to organize in speech the sounds of the particular word that we are looking at. But this is incorrect. We do not need a second to identify a word. The difference in time is not so much a reflection of how far thought lags behind the eye as of how far thought is ahead of the voice. We use our eyes to scout ahead so that we can make decisions about meaning and, thus, about individual words in advance. Indeed, the eye-voice span exists only when we can make sense of what we read. If we read nonsense ("dog lazy the over jumps fox quick") rather than something that makes more sense ("the quick fox jumps over the lazy dog"), then the eye and voice tend to converge on the same point, and the eye-voice span disappears (Smith, 1994). You can see from this that if a child had to read each word individually or had to continually read due to poor oculomotor and attention, the reading process would be extremely slow.

Apart from learning the meaning of words, the very mechanics of reading are arduous to master. There is a hurdle that needs to be overcome as a child learns to read. Normal serial search is a random process without memory. It is not a systematic procedure that keeps track of the locations that have been searched. However, in the case of reading, the shifting of attention cannot proceed in the same fashion but has to be conducted sequentially across the characters and spaces in each line. It has been suggested that it is the need for this kind of training that makes learning to read difficult. When we read, the eyes are moved from one fixation point to another by saccades, each fixation point lasting approximately 250 msec and the saccades themselves lasting about 25 msec. During each fixation period, most readers take in about seven or eight letters. It is proposed that the attentional spotlight shifts focus of attention from one letter to another during the fixation period, thus allowing only one or two letters to be processed at any one time (Vidyasagar, 2004).

What this research says is if visuospatial attention can be improved, then the process of reading is made less difficult. The eye movement patterns of dyslexic children and adults have a characteristic pattern of numerous re-readings and long pauses at each fixation.

Figure 6-2 shows a child who was diagnosed as being dyslexic and was in the fourth grade. The top row shows her eye movements on 10/13/09. The bottom row shows her eye movement 3 months later on 01/29/10. You can see how

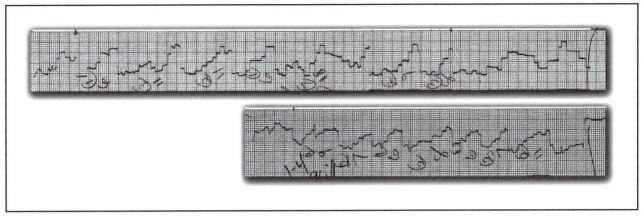

Figure 6-2. Eye Trac analysis before and after vision therapy.

much faster she read in January (both same comprehension of 90%) after visual training activities. Her reading speed increased from 157 words per minute to 214 words per minute. This was mainly the result of decreasing her re-reading from 40% to 28%. It was also noted that her decoding speed also decreased. This child made such a drastic improvement that a college student is now writing her thesis on this case.

Occupational therapists and Optometrists can greatly help dyslexic children by including spatial attention training in their sensory integration (SI) and visual therapy (VT) programs. This is accomplished by training the child to process visual spatial information in a sequential left to right duration. This is something that must be learned, and it needs to be part of every SI and VT program, especially if the child is being referred to you for fine motor training.

Dyslexia has in the past been thought to be caused by deficits in phonological decoding (Shaywitz, 1998). In the past few years, research on developmental dyslexia has shown a renewed interest in the visual aspects of dyslexia. For example, it has been shown that reading difficulties are more evident when an individual is asked to read words embedded in text than single words (Lovegrove, 1990).

Optometrists have always known that oculomotor deficits contribute to reading disabilities. They may not be the only causes, but they are part of the problem. As we have discussed earlier, convergence issues are also common with RD children. Attention, however, is still the key element. It has been shown that poor readers have difficulty concentrating on the fixated area and in suppressing the information from the peripheral areas. This appears to interfere both with a sequential left-to-right scanning strategy characteristic of slow phonological decoding and with a quick visual word recognition in a direct way (Lorusso et al., 2004).

Both the frontal eye fields and the parietal cortex are involved in the process of directing visual attention. The posterior parietal cortex and midtemporal (MT) also project to the frontal eye fields, and this may further influence attention. Both the frontal eye fields and the superior

colliculus send information to the brainstem, which in turn issues the motor command to the muscles of the eye. These anatomical connections illustrate the multilevel involvement of eye movement control, providing numerous areas that are required to participate accurately and possibly under the control of attention. Damage at any of these points may result in reading deficits. A key participator involved in this multilevel processing of eye movement control is the right parietal cortex. Other studies have demonstrated that RD children also perform visual tasks worse on their left side compared to the right (Eden, Stein, Wood, & Wood, 1994).

We know that RD children have reduced attention spans. This interferes with ocular motor processing as attention moves from word to word and from fovea to parafovea to fovea. In normal readers, when the location of fixation and attention coincide, visual tasks are performed more efficiently because the direction of gaze and the direction of attention are identical in space. This skill is called voluntary attention and is clinically trainable. Remember, oculomotor readiness depends on the shift in visual attention that precedes executing refixation. This attention drives saccades (Solan, Hansen, Shelley-Tremblay, & Ficarra, 2003).

I can tell you from experience that there are individuals who will tell you that eye exercises have no effect on a child's reading. While oculomotor training does not teach a child to read, you will make reading easier for the child. During the past decade, there are now new theories on vision and reading. One of the newer theories is the magnocellular theory on vision and reading disabilities.

MAGNOCELLULAR THEORY

Earlier in this book, I mentioned the two visual pathways from the retina to the brain. These two parallel pathways are responsible for 85% of cortical projections in the visual system (Chase, Ashourzadeh, Kelly, Monfette, & Kinsey, 2003). These pathways are sensitive to different visuospatial and temporal (time) characteristics. The parvocellular

(P) pathway is the visual pathway for object recognition and central vision of fine detail, while the magnocellular (M) pathway, which projects to the parietal lobe, is more concerned with peripheral vision and spatial organization. The M pathway has for some time been considered as a possible cause for reading problems (Borsting et al., 1996; Burr, Morrone, & Ross, 1994; Cornelissen, Hansen, Hutton, Evangelinou, & Stein, 1996; Demb, Boynton, & Heeger, 1998; Heiervang & Hugdahl, 2003; Pammer, 2006; Stein & Walsh, 1997; Vidyasagar & Pammer, 1999). Livingstone, Rosen, Drislene, and Galaburba (1991) were the first to report abnormalities in the M layer of the lateral geniculate nucleus (LGN) in dyslexic children. This study and others have suggested that dyslexic M impairment can be found throughout the visual system. Therefore, what is it about the M pathway that could be causing some cases of developmental dyslexia? One early theory was prepared by Breitmeyer (1980), who proposed a reading model in which the M channel has an indirect role in text recognition. In his model, text is only processed in the P channel. Because the duration of P channel responses can outlast the saccadic fixation, the function of the M channel is to inhibit activity of the P channel (Chase et al., 2003) as the eye moves to the next fixation stop. In other words, when the eyes move from one fixation point during reading to another point in the sentence, the visual information being processed by the point just fixated is shut off. If it was not shut off, then you would have visual information from previous fixations running into each other. This would be like a series of after images running into each other, and this would cause word recognition problems. Since then, several studies have shown that it is the M channel and not the P channel that is suppressed during a saccade (Facoetti et al., 2003; Skottun, 2000). Therefore, what is it about the M pathway that could cause reading problems? It appears that the M pathway controls spatial attention, which is critical in reading because reading is a process that requires precise knowledge about letter location due to the spatial nature of the eyes' movements used in visual scanning the text in a left-to-right direction. It has been known that children who have poor performance in visual search (especially when the letters are close together) show reduced reading speed and accuracy when compared to children with higher performances (Facoetti et al., 2003). It has also been shown that children with specific LDs were especially impaired in tests of focused visual attention, and poor readers did not appear to make use of peripheral cues of rapidly orienting their visual attention (Brannan & Williams, 1987). Research shows that transient visual attention is dominated by M inputs and that the M cell pathway plays a specific role in primary visual attention. This is why visual attention therapy alone has significantly impacted reading comprehension (Solan et al., 2003).

Therefore, it seems that the M deficit causes problems in focusing spatial attention. An important physiological component in learning to read may be training the attentional spotlight to move sequentially over the words in a line. Normal visual search is random and does not keep track of the locations that have been inspected. This has been a useful strategy in our evolution because it avoids the computational load of keeping detailed track of the search history and also keeps the visual system sensitive to changes in the scene that could occur during the search (Vidyasagar & Pammer, 1999).

Reading requires visual search in an unnatural way that has not been done before in our evolution. It requires spatial attention for position information (Pammer, 2005), proper feature conjunctions, and, therefore, word recognition. Therefore, visual training that stresses visual search, especially in left-right scanning patterns, is really training visual attention and improving the function of the M pathway, which is critical for reading.

SUMMARY AND ATTENTION TIPS

1. Reading disabled children perform visual tasks worse on their left side compared to their right. Have the reading material slightly to their right side.

2. How to start an oculomotor program:

   a. Always start in free space and with smooth pursuit training. Start one eye at a time with such activities as having the child follow a pencil.

   b. Do a lot of Marsden ball activities as the child lies directly under the ball. Slowly swing the ball in a horizontal direction.

   c. When the child has developed good pursuit movements with each eye, do both eyes together.

   d. You can start saccadic fixation training after the child has shown some success in pursuit training.

   e. Start one eye at a time and have him or her fixate between two objects, such as pencils or alphabet pencils (pencils with the alphabet on the side). When possible, use a metronome to add sound to the task.

   f. Now, have him or her fixate between several targets, such as pins on a yardstick.

(continued)

SUMMARY AND ATTENTION TIPS (CONTINUED)

2. Continued

g. When he or she can perform several targets equally in each eye, have him or her do it binocularly.

h. In addition to saccadic training, use workbooks so that he or she can continue training at home. The workbooks we use are the following:

  i. Visual Scanning—This trains the child to quickly scan and locate a number or letter in a page of print.

  ii. Spelling Tracking—Trains the proper left-to-right visual scanning needed during reading and helps develop sequencing abilities.

  iii. Visual Tracing—Trains eye-hand coordination and the concept of "left" and "right."

  iv. Number Tracking—Trains the rapid eye movement needed for good reading skills and increases reading speed and efficiency.

  v. Visual Motor—Helps to develop visual motor skills in young children.

  vi. Recognition of Reversals—Trains a child in the proper orientation of letters and numbers and helps to eliminate reversals in printing and reading.

  vii. Visual Memory—Helps to develop visual concentration and sequential memory.

i. Use the oculomotor activities in *Developing Ocular Motor and Vision Perception* by Kenneth A. Lane, published by SLACK Incorporated, 1995.

j. The Wayne saccadic fixator. This is a very good training activity to improve peripheral vision and eye-hand speed. The child stands in front of the saccadic fixator and must touch the lights as they come on in a desired sequence.

(continued)

SUMMARY AND ATTENTION TIPS (CONTINUED)

k. Peg board rotator (Figure 6-3)—The child stands in front of the rotator and has to add pegs into the rotator as it is turning.

l. Eye port (Figure 6-4)—This can be used for saccadics as the child has to move his or her eyes to keep up with the lights that flash in sequence.

m. Activities such as the Brock string and visual motor control bat with a hanging ball are all good activities to train oculomotor skills.

n. Guided reader (Figure 6-5)—This may be one of the best eye-tracking activities we have ever used. This program uses a moving window to force the child to read faster without being able to re-read.

REFERENCES

Borsting, E., Ridder, W. H. 3rd, Dudeck, K., Kelley, C., Matsui, L., & Motoyama, J. (1996). The presence of a magnocellular defect depends on the type of dyslexia. *Vision Research, 36*(7), 1047-1053.

Brannan, J. & Williams, M. C. (1987). Allocation of visual attention in good and poor readers. *Perception & Psychophysics, 41*(1), 23-28.

Breitmeyer, B. C. (1980). Unmasking visual masking: a look at the "why" behind the veil of the "how." *Psychology Review, 87,* 52-69.

Burr, D. C., Morrone, M. C., & Ross, J. (1994). Selective suppression of the magnocellular visual pathway during saccadic eye movements. *Nature, 371,* 511-513.

Casco, C., Tressoldi, P. E., & Dellantonio, A. (1998). Visual selective attention and reading efficiency are related in children. *Cortex, 34,* 531-546.

Chase, C., Ashourzadeh, A., Kelly, C., Monfette, S., & Kinsey, K. (2003). Can the magnocellular pathway read? evidence from studies of color. *Vision Research, 43*(10), 1211-1222.

Cornelissen, P. L., Hansen, P. C., Hutton, J. L., Evangelinou, V., & Stein, J. F. (1996). Magnocellular visual function and children's single word reading. *Vision Research, 38*(3), 471-482.

De Haene, S. (2003). Natural born readers. *New Scientist, 179*(2402), 30.

Demb, J. B., Boynton, G. M., & Heeger, D. J. (1998). Functional magnetic resonance imaging of early visual pathways in dyslexia. *The Journal of Neuroscience, 18*(17), 6939-6951.

Diamond, J. (1999). *Guns, germs and steel: The fates of human societies.* New York, NY: WW Norton and Company.

Eden, G., Stein, J. F., Wood, H. M., & Wood, F. B. (1994). Differences in eye movements and reading problems in dyslexic and normal children. *Vision Research, 34*(10), 1345-1358.

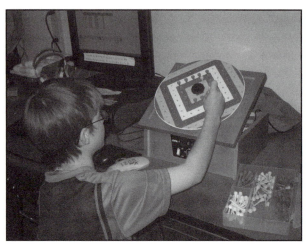

Figure 6-3. Peg board rotator.

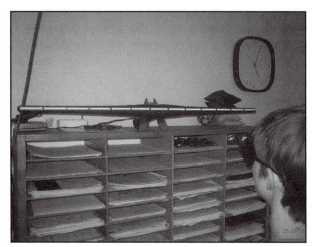

Figure 6-4. Eye port.

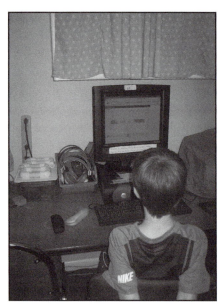

Figure 6-5. Guided reader.

Facoetti, A. & Molteni, M. (2001). The gradient of visual attention in developmental dyslexia neuropsychologia. *Neuropsychologia, 39,* 352-357.

Facoetti, A., Lorusso, M. L., Paganoni, P., Umiltà, C., Mascetti, G. G. (2003). The role of visuospatial attention in developmental dyslexia: evidence from a rehabilitation study. *Cognitive Brain Research, 15,* 154-164.

Gazzaniga, M. (2004). *The cognitive neurosciences iii.* Cambridge, MA: MIT Press.

Healy, J. (1999). *Endangered minds.* New York, NY: Simon & Schuster.

Heiervang, E. & Hugdahl, K. (2003). Impaired visual attention in children with dyslexia. *Journal of Learning Disabilities, 36*(1), 68-73.

Livingstone, M., Rosen, G. D., Drislane, F. W., & Galaburda, A. M. (1991). Physiological and anatomical evidence for a magnocellular defect in developmental dyslexia. *Proceeds of the National Academy of Science, 88,* 7943-7947.

Lovegrove, W. (1990). The effect of text presentation on reading in dyslexic and normal readers. *Perception, 19*(A), 46.

Lorusso, M., Facoetti, A., Pesenti, S., Cattaneo, C., Molteni, M., & Geiger, G. (2004). Wider recognition in peripheral vision common to different subtypes of dyslexia. *Vision Research, 4,* 2413-2424.

Pammer, K. (2005). Integration of the visual and auditory networks in dyslexia: a theoretical perspective. *Journal of Research in Reading, 28*(3), 320-331.

Pammer, K. (2006). Attentional shifting and the role of the dorsal pathway in visual word recognition. *Neuropsychologia, 44,* 2926-2936.

Shaywitz, S. (1998). Dyslexia. *The New England Journal of Medicine, 338*(5), 307-312.

Skottun, B. C. (2000). The magnocellular deficit theory of dyslexia: the evidence from contrast sensitivity. *Vision Research, 40,* 111-127.

Smith, F. (1994). *Understanding reading* (5th ed.). Mahweh, NJ: Erlbaum.

Solan, H., Hansen, P. C., Shelley-Tremblay, J., & Ficarra, A. (2003). Coherent motion threshold measurements for M-cell deficit differ for above- and below-average readers. *Optometry, 74*(11), 727-734.

Stein, J. & Walsh V. (1997). To see but not to read; the magnocellular theory of dyslexia. *Trends in Neurosciences, 20*(4), 147-152.

Vidyasagar, T. R. & Pammer K. (1999). Impaired visual search in dyslexia relates to the role of magnocellular pathway in attention. *NeuroReport, 10,* 1283-1287.

Vidyasagar, T. R. (2004). Neural underpinnings of dyslexia as a disorder of visuo-spatial attention. *Clinical and Experimental Optometry, 85*(1), 4-10.

Wolf, M. (2007). *Proust and the squid: The story and science of the reading brain.* New York, NY: HarperCollins Publishers.

SUGGESTED READING

Facoetti, A., Paganoni, P., & Lorusso, M. L. (2000). The spatial distribution of visual attention in developmental dyslexia. *Experimental Brain Research, 132*(4), 531-538.

Facoetti, A. Paganoni, P., Turatto, M., Marzola, V., & Mascetti, G. G. (2000). Visual spatial attention in developmental dyslexia. *Cortex, 36*(1), 109-123.

Plasticity

7

If a child's brain and, in some cases, an adult's brain cannot be modified, then training programs would be useless. The good news is that, especially in the case of children, experience can modify synapses in the brain. It is widely hypothesized that these changes are critically involved in fine-tuning sensory and motor systems, as well as cognitive processes, such as learning and memory. This chapter deals with the subject of plasticity and stresses that, because the brain can be modified, attention can also be trained.

There is clear evidence that learning and experience cause physical changes in the adult brain. Modification of synaptic activity through dendritic branching and, to a lesser extent, axonal sprouting is an ongoing process present in all children and adults on a continuous basis. A neuron that has lost input from a damaged neuron can develop new dendrites or dendritic spines to receive information from another neuron in the same circuit or even from another, more distant circuit. This synaptic plasticity is apparent in both recovery processes and normal learning. Importantly, it is directly related to and indeed dependent on experience. Without inputs that drive the system, these new connections do not form (Sohlberg, 2001).

It has been hypothesized that strengthening of synaptic connections occurs when pre- and postsynaptic neurons are activated at the same time. This simultaneous activation can occur when each of them is connected to another circuit, which when activated causes simultaneous activations in the disconnected neurons. This principle has been summed up as "cells that fire together, wire together." Current work suggests that plasticity indeed appears to be a property of the synapse, as this is where reorganization and changes in neural connectivity take place (Sohlberg, 1989).

The following is an example of the amazing plasticity of the human brain. A 10-year-old girl born with half of a brain has both fields of vision in one eye. The girl's underdeveloped brain was discovered when, aged 3, she underwent a magentic resonance imaging (MRI) scan after suffering seizures of brief involuntary twitching on her left side. Apart from the seizures, which were successfully treated, and a slight weakness in her left side, the girl had a normal developmental and medical history, attending regular school and taking part in activities such as roller skating. The right hemisphere in the girl's brain failed to develop in the womb. As you know, normally, the left and right visual fields are processed and mapped by opposite sides of the brain; however, the scans on the girl showed that retinal fibers that should go to the right hemisphere of the brain were diverted to the left (*Daily Mail*, 2009).

CHILDHOOD AND ADULT PLASTICITY

By the time a child is 1 year old, a huge number of synaptic contacts are present in the cerebral cortex. Most of these appear to be as yet unspecified for function. At this point, external input (experience) is necessary for inclusion of some of these synapses into functioning circuits, while others remain inactive and eventually disappear. Whether any given function will develop or not and how it will develop depends to a large extent on the type and timing of environmental input. For example, in language areas of the cerebral cortex, the brain of the 1 and 2 year old has nearly

109

Lane, K. A. *Visual Attention in Children: Theories and Activities* (pp. 109-118).
© 2012 SLACK Incorporated.

reached the maximum number of synaptic contacts and is ready to begin processing language. Lack of exposure to any language during infancy and childhood appears to permanently impair language development (Huttenlocher, 2002).

Young children have more plastic brains than adolescents and adults because the immature brain has 50% more neurons and synaptic connections. When a child reaches adolescence, a massive "pruning back" operation begins in the brain, and synaptic connections and neurons that have not been used extensively suddenly die off (Doidge, 2007). To give you an idea of the growth of a child's brain, consider the fact that at birth the average newborn brain weighs a mere 330 g. This is one-fourth of an adult brain weight. By the time the child is 2 years old, its weight will triple, and by age 7, it is 1,250 g and is at 90% of adult weight (Healy, 1999).

There are some negative aspects of plasticity. The best example is vision. Studies have shown that during the first 8 weeks or so of life, development of the visual cortex progresses normally or nearly so in the absence of exposure to formed visual images. There seems to be a "grace period" of at least 8 weeks postnatally during which visual deprivation is tolerated without permanent impairment. This is because, in humans, the period of rapid synaptogenes does not begin until about 2 months of age. Reversal of amblyopia is possible up to a critical age of 6.7 years. After that age, amblyopia is permanent. I need to add that, at 6 or 7, the child may never have 20/20 vision again, but amblyopic children at this age can have their vision improved and often to at least 20/40.

There is increasing evidence that changes in the early differentiated visual cortex may be of functional significance. A study in 1993 showed auditory responses found in the visual cortex of the early blind. Several studies have also found evidence of somatosensory processing in the visual cortex of subjects with early blindness. Also, PET responses have shown activation of the visual cortex during Braille reading in blind subjects. This form of plasticity, using a different sensory cortex, appears to be common. It may underlie the special skills acquired by people with impairment of sensory input in one modality, such as Braille reading and improved ability to navigate in space in the congenitally blind (Huttenlocher, 2002).

A young mind is like a computer with some basic programs built in and plenty of room left on its hard drive for additional information. As more and more data enter the computer's memory, it develops shortcuts to access that information. These shortcuts represent new neural pathways being laid down. Young children who have learned their times tables by heart no longer use the more cumbersome neural pathway of figuring out the math problem by counting their fingers or multiplying on paper. This plasticity allows an immature brain to learn new skills readily and much more efficiently than the trimmed down adult brain. One of the best examples is the young brain's ability to learn language. Young children are more receptive to the sounds of a new language and are much quicker to learn words and phrases. Scientists have found that the keen ability of normal infants to distinguish foreign language sounds begins declining by 12 months of age (Small, 2008). In fact, an infant's ability to discriminate foreign speech sounds begins to wane as early as 6 months of age. By this age, English-learning babies have already lost some of their ability, still present at 4 months, to discriminate certain German or Swedish vowels. Foreign vowels are the first sort of phoneme (minimal unit of speech sound) to go. Then, by 10 or 12 months, out goes the ability to discriminate foreign consonants, like r/s and l/s for Japanese babies. Such losses go hand in hand with a baby's growing sensitivity to his or her native language. Every time he or she hears a particular phoneme—each piece of each word spoke within earshot—that experience broadens his or her perceptual category for that sound, at the expense of neighboring sounds (i.e., those with similar physical properties) not a part of his or her native language. So, even though babies are born with the ability to discriminate among all the world's speech sounds, most of these tiny categories eventually become subsumed by the few phoneme categories needed to interpret their native language (English, for example, has just 40 phonemes in all). As each category broadens, moreover, the boundaries between them grow sharper. The end result is that babies can more rapidly identify each speech sound they hear (no matter how sloppy the pronunciation) as one of the few types that everyone around them seems to be using.

Phoneme perception is thus another example of "use it or lose it" in the developing brain. Our experience of speech sounds gets warped by experience—in this case, very early exposure to a single native language. This very early shaping phoneme perception has important implications for foreign language learning. Obviously, the better you can hear the sounds of a foreign language, the easier time you will have learning it. Even though babies begin to lose this ability very early on, their brains remain flexible enough during the early critical period for them to be able to recover foreign phoneme perception should they suddenly find themselves immersed in a new language. Adults, in contrast, literally tune out when they hear a foreign language spoken: our left hemispheres are not even activated when we listen to speech in an unfamiliar language. Although we can, with intensive effort, learn to distinguish some of the more difficult foreign speech sounds, we can never do it as easily, naturally, and completely as children, nor can we come anywhere near matching children's ability to pronounce foreign phonemes properly. This is why adults speak newly acquired languages with an obvious accent (Eliot, 1999).

Language learning in the young child is a herculean task. An early "word spurt" has been described between the ages of 14 and 22 months in most children, although word acquisition appears to be more gradual in some. During the early word spurt, the child may learn up to an average of three new words a day, mainly object words. Vocabulary growth is even more rapid later in childhood. Between grades 1 and 3, there is an average increase in estimated vocabulary of about 9,000 words or about 12 new words per day. This amounts to about one new word every 90 waking minutes.

In the case of language learning in the child, the brain regions in the right cerebral hemisphere that are no longer needed for the processing of simple language functions may become specified for other late-developing functions, such as music learning. Studies have shown that left-sided lateralization of language for the simple word recognition task occurred quite early at about the age of 20 months, long before the end of the period of plasticity in language functions that is thought to depend on the ability to organize these functions in the right hemisphere, which has been estimated to occur between the age of 8 years and puberty. What is the explanation of this discrepancy? It is likely that localization of language on the left side is a gradual process and that more difficult language tasks lateralize to the left hemisphere at later ages. Evidence from imaging suggests that some right cortical activation during processing of language tasks persists in normal adults.

The clinical and evoked potential studies provide confirmation that cortical representation at first tends to be diffuse, with overlapping functions rather than with strict cortical localization. As development progresses, there is increasing restriction of cortical representation, leading to specification of cortical regions for single functions. In other words, during development, the cerebral cortex appears to shift from a distributed system to a more modular one. Development may bring more efficient processing by functional specification of cortical areas, but this may be at the expense of elimination of alternate routes of processing. Such alternate routes (e.g., right hemisphere pathways for language processing) may be an important substrate for plasticity of the immature brain. Increased efficiency of processing in the adult may be bought at the expense of decreased plasticity (Huttenlocher, 2002).

Contrary to age-old assumptions that changes in neural pathways are possible only during critical periods of development, modern neuroscience views the brain as a dynamic structure throughout life. Throughout the past few decades, there has been an abundance of research on neuroplasticity. However, it was not until the development of noninvasive functional neuroimaging in the 1990s that the scientific community really began to embrace the concept of an adult plastic brain. In the past decade, there has been a paradigm shift in neurorehabilitation due to an increased understanding of the brain's striking capacity for reorganization (Huang, 2009).

Neuroscience and, indeed, observation of human behavior leave little doubt that the brain must be fundamentally altered by experience. The notion of neuroplasticity—the brain's capacity to change and alter its structure and function—is particularly relevant to rehabilitation (Sohlberg, McLaughlin, Pavese, Heidrich, & Posner, 2000). The purpose of the activities in this book are to give the brain experiences so that a child's functions, especially attention, can be improved. If neuroplasticity did not exist, this would be impossible; however, we know that experience can alter the brain.

The world's leading researcher on brain plasticity, Michael Merzenich, specializes in improving people's ability to think and perceive by redesigning the brain by training specific processing areas called brain maps, so that they do more mental work. He argues that practicing a new skill under the right conditions can change hundreds of millions and possibly billions of the connections between nerve cells in our brain maps. It seems that each neural system has a different critical period or window of time, during which it was especially plastic and sensitive to the environment and during which it had rapid, formative growth. We have discussed language development as an example. It has a critical period that ends between 8 years and puberty. After this critical period closes, a person's ability to learn a second language without an accent is limited. In fact, second languages learned after the critical period are not processed in the same part of the brain as the native tongue. The more we use our native language, the more it comes to dominate our linguistic map space. Thus, it is also because our brain is plastic—and because plastic is competitive—that it is so difficult to learn a new language.

But why, if this is true, is it easier to learn a second language when we are young? Is there not competition then, too? Not really. If two languages are learned at the same time, during the critical period, both get a foothold. In a bilingual child, all the sounds of the two languages share a single large map, a library of sounds from both languages. It is plasticity that explains why our bad habits are so hard to break or, for lack of a better word, "unlearn." Most of us think of the brain as a container and learning as putting something in it. When we try to break a bad habit, we think the solution is to put something new into the container. But when we learn a bad habit, it takes over a brain map, and each time it is repeated, it claims more control of that map and prevents the use of that space for "good" habits. That is why "unlearning" is often a lot harder than learning and why early childhood education is so important. It is better to get it right early, before the bad habit gets a competitive advantage and controls a brain map.

One of the most famous experiments among neuroscientists concerned the one that mapped a monkey's hand in the brain. Then, the monkey had the middle finger amputated. After a number of months, they remapped the monkey and found that the brain map for the amputated finger had disappeared and that the maps for the adjacent fingers had grown into the space that had originally been mapped for the middle finger (Doidge, 2007).

It appears that it is not the problem of finding new space in the brain for a particular skill to be learned; rather, it has to do with getting that skill learned early enough before something else occupies that space. This has also been shown with amblyopia. If a child does not use an eye due to strabismus or a cataract, then the other eye occupies the brain area of the eye that is not used.

One of the most critical points that needs to be stressed with plasticity is that paying close attention is essential for long-term plastic changes. In numerous experiments, it has been found that lasting changes occurred only when the monkey used in the experiment paid close attention. When the animals performed tasks automatically without paying attention, they changed their brain maps, but the changes did not last (Doidge, 2007). We often use the phrase *the ability to multitask*. While a child can learn with partial attention, the learning does not last. Another indication that multitasking is not always good is the following example. If we are performing a task in which we want to watch TV and ignore voices that are coming from our children nearby, our frontal region of the brain may configure the brain to prioritize visual information and damper down auditory information. Also, the brain's executive will keep us in that mode until we hear, say, one of our children screaming (Hamilton, 2008).

While change can be made even in the adult brain, it is critical that we start with children at an early age to improve attention. For example, a child who is 3 years old with an acute left hemisphere lesion that destroys the major speech areas and even a child with the entire dominant cerebral hemisphere surgically removed will be mute for a few days but will then regain language very rapidly almost to a normal level. An adult with a similar lesion will lose all or most of his or her speech comprehension and production and often has little or no return of language functions, even with intensive speech therapy (Huttenlocher, 2002).

I think we have to remember that, in this book, we are mainly talking about children. Even though these activities can help at any age, it is the child's brain we are talking about, and mainly before adolescence. It also needs to be stressed that the main area of our training is attention, and we must remember that attention and memory go hand in hand. You cannot develop memory without attention, and also memory is critical for attention. For example, the four attentional factors that we are dealing with—(1) focused, (2) sustained, (3) selected, and (4) shifted—all are critical for memory and all need memory (except in bottom-up functions) to function properly. It is not only memory but mostly working memory that is critical for a child to develop to be successful in school and everyday life.

There have been studies with the parietal reach region (PRR) in monkeys and humans that indicate a highly plastic area of the brain. In these studies, human subjects performed delayed saccades and delayed pointing similar to delayed saccade and reach experiments that have been preferred in monkeys. Using event-related functional MRI, they were able to localize an area in the parietal cortex that responded preferentially during memory delay trials for planning pointing movements compared to saccades.

The PRR in humans has attributes that are different from the motor cortex, which may be useful for deriving control signals for neural prosthetics. The main sensory feedback to the motor cortex is from somatosensory inputs, whereas the major sensory feedback for PRR appears to be visual. Often, somatosensory feedback is lost with paralysis, whereas vision is not. This feedback for evolutionary terminal movement errors may be more naturally conveyed to PRR. In addition, the remarkable plasticity seen in PRR during cursor central tasks bodes well for this region's ability to learn to control external devices. PRR is also more removed from motor areas, which undergo pathological changes with paralysis. Thus, it is possible that PRR will be more resilient to the changes that result from disuse following direct damage to corticospinal projections (as in spinal cord injury) (Gazzaniga, 2004). What was encouraging in these studies was how quickly the monkeys who were used in these experiments learned the cursor-controlled tasks, which indicates the plasticity in this region.

Most agree that the stages in memory are attention, encoding, storage, and retrieval with the first one—attention—being the most important. We learned that there is no one brain area that deals with attention; however, the most important appear to be the frontal cortex and the posterior parietal lobe.

The frontal cortex comprises a third of the human brain. It is the structure that enables us to engage in higher cognitive functions. Little is known about cortical representation and plasticity of the so-called higher functions, including abstract reasoning, such as is needed for understanding mathematics, physics, and the executive functions. Even less is known of the anatomical substrate of creativity, the creation of new knowledge and works of art. These as a group represent "elective brain functions." They differ from the basic or obligatory cortical function such as vision, hearing, and locomotion in that they depend completely on specialized teaching and learning. Two of these are reading and learning a musical instrument. Higher cortical functions are represented primarily in two cortical areas: the prefrontal cortex and the posterior parietal cortex. These two cortical regions develop slowly and have the highly complex dendritic development that appears to be necessary for the processing of complex information. The child acquires oral language in the second year of life at a time when language areas of the brain mature and when synaptic density in these cortical areas approaches the maximum. On the other hand, reading is not acquired until the age of 6 or 7 years in most children. This is several years after the occurrence of synaptogenesis, which correlates well the emergence of basic cortical functions, such as the processing of sensory stimuli voluntary motor activities, and oral language, but not with the development of elective functions such as reading. The data show no evidence that the left angular gyrus, or the other brain areas that are thought to be important for reading, develop later than other language areas. We do not know what the function of these cortical areas is prior to school age. An attractive hypothesis is that the angular gyrus is required for other language functions prior to the age of 5. The likelihood of this is increased by the fact that the angular gyrus abuts Wernicke's sensory speech area (Huttenlocher, 2002).

Music ability requires early input. An example is the intense practice of a concert violinist who has developed the drive to perfection in performance. The violinist is able, through his or her own actions, to change the anatomy and function of his or her own cerebral cortex. Research for the first time has demonstrated brain plasticity as a result of music instruction. It shows that children who receive music instruction and practice regularly perform better on sound discrimination and fine motor tasks. Furthermore, brain imaging shows changes to the networks associated with these abilities. Arts training, it seems, helps other areas of cognition, including a study of attention, whose results found evidence of brain plasticity in children who received instruction. Another study found tight correlations between music training and mathematical reasoning. Years of neuroimaging have now given us a plausible or putative mechanism by which arts training could influence cognition, including attention. The training strengthens regions of the brain linked to attention, self-control, and general intelligence. This study focused on the executive attention network. It found that controlled training on attention-related tasks increased the effectiveness of the attention network and also improved far transfer domains.

If controlled training can increase attention, then perhaps arts training, which involves sustained focus and control, also has a far transfer effect in improving cognition in general (Bakalar, 2008; Mauk, 2009).

There is no doubt that training in attention and memory-related areas affects brain development. One study found an increase of 20% in the number of synapses in a section of cortical tissue enriched by experience compared to animals that did not receive the same training. Not only are there more synapses per neuron, there is also more astrocytic material, more blood capillaries, and a higher mitochondria volume in all animals involved in memory and learning (Kolb, 1998).

Another way to say "working memory" is "working attention." They go together. Intervention based on a cognitive neuropsychological model of working memory appears to be an effective way of training attention (Cicerone, 2002). In fact, working memory training can improve this function and motor activity in attention deficit/hyperactivity disorder (AD/HD) students (Klingberg, Forssberg, & Westerberg, 2002). The parietal cortex and working memory training increased brain activity in the middle gyrus and superior and inferior parietal cortices. The changes in cortical activity after working memory training are evidence of training-induced plasticity in the neural systems that underlie working memory (Olesen, Westerberg, & Klingberg, 2004).

There have been several studies that evaluated the results in specifically training the executive function and attentional system. Some of these worked with traumatic brain injury (TBI) patients but could also be used with children who have executive function difficulties. One is called Goal Management Theory (GMT) developed by I. H. Robertson and based on J. Drienean's theory of disorganized behavior following frontal lobe lesions. Many patients with frontal lobe impairments demonstrate problems with attention and concentration. They often demonstrate problems with sustained attention to tasks and are likely to have difficulty with distractibility and with the smooth and effective allocation of attentional resources on more complex tasks. They are also likely to have difficulty shifting and dividing attention. Many brain-injured individuals, including those with significant frontal lobe impairment, have been shown to benefit substantially from exercises and training of attentional skills (Sohlberg, 1993). Sohlberg and Mateer developed and evaluated the efficacy of a package of attention training materials (Attention Process Training [APT]), which is based on a hierarchical model with five levels of attention: focused, sustained, selective, alternating, and divided. A large set of both auditory and visual tasks designed to exercise and challenge different aspects of attention were used in treatment sessions over periods of 6 to 8 weeks in length. Several large-scale studies have shown the gains from this program. They show that attentional training improves working memory (Mateer, 1989 Park, 1999; Sohlberg & Mateer, 1987; Sohlberg et al, 2000).

Another program by Von Cramon (1991), problem-solving training (PST), which contains five stages very similar to GMT stages, showed that participants made significant gains in both laboratory tasks and real-life behavioral ratios in comparison to a control group receiving memory training. This is another example of clinical support for the treatment of executive functioning deficits (Levine et al., 2000).

Many of the training studies deal with acquired brain injuries (ABIs). In fact, the concept of ABI is used for conditions arising postnatally occurring due to trauma, infections, vascular catastrophes, or malignancy. Up to 50% of patients with ABI have been reported to have neuropsychological sequelae (a lesion caused by disease). Deficits in attention and memory are the most common cognitive dysfunctions of ABI and often contribute to significant disability in both children and adults. Brain injury in children also affects functions that are in the process of developing and those that are set to emerge. However, it is the attention and memory functions that cause a major negative effect in academic and social adjustment. Another major difficulty frequently reported in ABI is decreased speed of information processing. It has been suggested that slow processing speed limits attention capacity. Problems with working memory also have been described following injury to frontal systems. A study was conducted at the Amsterdam

Academic Hospital based on the research of Sohlberg and Mateer (1987). It trained three levels: sustained attention, selective attention, and mental tracking. It also worked on three levels of memory function: the sensory register, working memory, and long-term memory. The results showed improved performance in school children aged 9 to 16. Improvement was noted in measures assessing sustained attention and selective attention. Performance on memory tests also improved but this was less marked (van't Hooft, Andersson, Sejersen, Bartfai, & von Wendt, 2003).

AD/HD children have also shown marked improvements with attention training. In fact, these results show that direct interventions aimed at improving attention may be a valuable treatment option for improving cognitive efficiency in children with AD/HD (Kerns, 1999; Semrud-Llikeman et al., 1999).

THE ADULT BRAIN

"You can teach an old dog new tricks." The adult brain can potentially grow new cells and make new connections (Steed, 2008). So, can adult brain neurons actually exhibit neuroplasticity? The short answer is yes. Adult neural stem and/or progenitor cells are now known to continually generate new neurons throughout life in various areas of the mammalian central nervous system. Neurogenesis is necessary for some forms of adult learning memory and mood regulation to occur (Maino, 2009).

There is abundant evidence to show that normal associative learning and experience evoke change in cortical sensory and motor representational fields, and it has been argued that the mechanisms underlying such normal learning may be fundamental to the mechanisms involved in recovery of function following acquired brain damage. There is also evidence interpreted as experience-dependent changes in dendritic sprouting beyond the somatosensory cortex as well as behavioral evidence of experience-dependent improvements in certain linguistic abilities that may be underprimed by changes in synaptic connectivity in the relevant language areas of the cortex. Recent research also shows the possibility of brain cell regeneration in the adult hippocampus and in mice. Such regeneration can be influenced by experience (Eriksson et al., 1998; Gould et al., 1999; Lie et al., 2002; Mesulam, 1990; Palmer, Markakis, Willhoite, Safar, & Gage, 1999). The evidence for experience-dependent synaptic changes should not be surprising given the evidence that synapses in both the peripheral and central nervous system are subject to ongoing turnover in the absence of damage of the tissues and, in some cases, under natural environmental conditions. Such a view is also supported by data for dorsal root ganglion of mice. Many other reviews support the view that a number of experience-dependent changes occur in adult brains including modification of synaptic connectivity.

There are five assumptions concerning the brain and plasticity:

1. The brain is capable of a large degree of self-repair through synaptic turnover and may in fact continuously be engaged in this, even in the absence of overt damage.

2. This synaptic turnover is to some extent experience-dependent and is a key mechanism underlying both learning and recovery of function following brain damage.

3. Recovery processes following brain damage show a common mechanism with normal learning and experience-dependent plasticity processes.

4. Variations in experience and inputs available to damaged neural circuits will shape synaptic interconnections and hence influence recovery.

5. An analysis of the determinants of normal short- and long-termed plasticity in the undamaged central nervous system will yield useful guides to the key variables determining whether and how recovery of functions can be guarded and shaped by rehabilitation methods (Robertson & Murre, 1999). Very significant recovery of function following lesions has been documented in many types of disorders. These include acquired language disorders, perceptual deficits (Wilson & Davidoff, 1993), unilateral neglect (Stone, Patel, Greenwood, & Halligan, 1992), attentional deficits (Van Zomeren & van den Burg, 1985), and tactile discrimination (Weder et al., 1994). There have also been studies that showed phonemic discrimination improvements thought to be strengthened by training-induced changes in cortical reorganization observed in children suffering from specific language impairment.

When we deal with rehabilitation, the executive function is less straightforward. The area of cognitive function is the least well-understood in the brain; however, parietal lobe involvement is common in one reputed executive function—sustained attention. Therefore, if this area can be improved through training, then possibly the executive function can be improved as well. Sustained attention is a system located frontoparietally in the right hemisphere of the brain and is known to be involved in the maintenance of the alert state under conditions of monotony. Also, the rehabilitation of sustained attention results in increased activity in the right frontoparietal network (Robertson, 1996).

There is abundant evidence that attention can go to the processing of information in primary as well as secondary sensory areas of the brain, and it is assumed that attentional circuits argued to be based at least in part on the frontal lobes are the source of such gating. Drevets et al. (1995) showed that blood flow to the primary sensory cortex can be modified by attentional-expecting variables, such that blood flow decreases in those somatic areas where stimulation is not expected. In another study, when participants paid attention to vibration on their fingertips, functional imagery showed 13% more activation in the equivalent sensory area of the brain than when they received the same stimulation but did not attend to it.

Attention can modulate synaptic activity in posterior circuits as well. Attention also influences synaptic connectivity in animals, and direct evidence for this attention-mediated plasticity in humans comes from a study by Pascual-Leone et al. (1995). They showed that purely mental practice of fine motor skills enlarged the area of the motor cortex activated by enactment of the learned skills. This enlargement of the neural circuits subserving the skilled behavior was measured by transcranial magnetic stimulation and was the first demonstration that purely mentally rehearsed training could influence synaptic connectivity in this way, although functional MRI has also shown enlargement after physical practice of a fine motor skill (Robertson, 1996).

One of the principal functions of the frontal cortex is attention control; hence, it is a plausible hypothesis that mental rehearsal (sustained attention) effects on synaptic connectivity are attributable to top-down effects of anterior attentional systems in more posterior neural circuits of the brain. This hypothesis is strengthened by the evidence that frontally based attentional circuits can go to processing in posterior sensory circuits of the brain. Support also comes from activations in the human brain during visual tasks where passive viewing was compared with active attention to the identical visual array. The observed attentionally gated changes in occipital and parietal cortex were found to lose their modulatory source in the prefrontal cortex (Buchel & Friston, 1997), supporting the view that synaptic activity and, hence, plasticity can be modulated in a top-down way by attentional circuits partly based on the prefrontal cortex.

This information is very exciting in that it seems possible that a wide range of neural circuits in the brain can be influenced by the integrity of the attentional systems of the brain.

One of the most interesting examples of plasticity is the work done by Michael Merzenich with learning disabled children. In the mid-1990s, he joined forces with Paula Tallal of Rutgers University to form Scientific Learning, a company that produces and sells a computer-based program called Fast-For-Word. The idea is based on research that by slowing down certain sounds such as "ba" and "da," children who were having trouble processing language could quickly begin to hear the distinct sounds, the "b" separated from the "oh." Over hundreds of repetitious training sessions, during games that can last for 20 hours a week for months, these sounds could gradually be sped up, and, in time, the child would learn to hear and process the sounds at normal speed. According to a research study, a group of dyslexic children participating in Fast-For-Word not only improved in their reading skills but their brains changed—different regions were processing language (Ellison, 2007; Holloway, 2003).

TELEVISION AND VIDEO GAMES

Is all plasticity good for us? I think the jury is still out on this question.

Normal human brains have at their disposal two complimentary methods of processing information: sequential and simultaneous (parallel). Sequential processing takes one bite at a time. The opposite is simultaneous processing, which requires many associations to be processed at the same time. Human brains continually blend simultaneous and sequential processing. The way the brain is trained helps to determine the balance between the two processes. Computers, however, are locked into a mentality that takes sequential processing to the extreme. Because humans have two hemispheres cushioned by emotional centers, we are able to look at the big picture, whereas computers only have a left hemisphere (Healy, 1999). We do not want our children to think like this. An English teacher commented that she has had no trouble telling which of her students started life on a computer. "They don't link ideas—they just write one thing and then they write another one, and they don't seem to see or develop the relationship between them" (Healy, 1999, p. 326).

It is not all bad concerning computers. There is some evidence that extensive work with programs that relate visuospatial activity on the screen to the child's own physical movements in space may improve at least some types of visuospatial reasoning.

Studies have shown that games such as Tetris, in which players have to rotate and direct rapidly falling blocks, alters the brain. It showed that after 3 months of Tetris practice, teenage girls not only played the game better, but their brains became more efficient. A scan that illuminates brain activity showed that at the end of 3 months, the girls' brains were working less hard to complete the games' challenges. What's more, parts of the cortex actually got thicker. The regions that got thicker dealt with visuospatial abilities, planning, and integration of sensory data (Anthes, 2009).

There has also been some improvement in adults' brains using computers. Most mental training programs emphasize the learning of mnemonic tricks. These may be useful for younger children, but, for the older person, they do not work very well. The major reason is that cognitive function declines with age. The brain's decoding process is degraded, and if you cannot fix that, then you cannot restore memory. A young person processes about eight to 10 auditory samples per syllable. An 80 year old processes fewer than two samples per syllable. That is why older individuals' understanding of speech and verbal memory are so fuzzy, and the same is true of the visual system. The only way to remedy the situation is to speed up neural processing by challenging the brain with increasingly difficult stimuli. There is a program called Brain Fitness that does this. This also works on the visual system. It seems that, as we get older, our ability to pay attention to things in the periphery declines. At the same time, the aged brain processes the stream of visual data much more slowly. Any activity that keeps these visual circuits in better working order may improve overall cognitive functioning.

The best way to sum up this section on computers is to mention a section from the book, *Endangered Minds*, by Jane Healy (1999). This section deals with a conversation Healy had with a brain scientist while they were dining.

The scientist was bragging on his daughter's intellectual exploits. He mentioned that she can recite all the dinosaurs' names when she sees their pictures on the computer. He was excited because his daughter loves her computer and spends a lot on time it. The question was asked: "Does you little girl ever just play—by herself or with other little kids?"

"Oh sure." He thought for a moment. "But she really loves that computer! Isn't wonderful how much they can learn at this age?"

"What do you think that computer is doing to her brain?" I asked.

He paused. "You know," he said slowly. "I never thought about it. I haven't a clue."

"I think that the preschool brain's main job is to learn the principals by which the real world operates and then organize and integrate sensory information with body movement 'touch' and 'feel.' It needs much more emphasis on laying the foundation of control systems for attention and motivation than on jamming the store house full of data that makes it look 'smart' to adults" (Healy,1990).

The jury may still be out concerning computers but there seems to be a lot of agreement concerning TV. Television, music videos, and video games, all of which use television techniques, unfold at a much faster pace than real life, and they are getting faster, which causes people to develop an increased appetite for high-speed transitions in those media. It is the form of the television medium—cuts, edits, zooms, pans, and sudden noises—that alters the brain, by activating what Pavlov called the "orienting response," which occurs whenever we sense a sudden change in the world around us, especially a sudden movement. We instinctively interrupt whatever we are doing to turn, pay attention, and get our bearings. The orienting response

evolved, no doubt, because our forbearers were both predators and prey and needed to react to situations that could be dangerous or could provide sudden opportunities for such things as food or sex, in simple to novel situations. The response is physiological: the heart rate decreased for 4 to 6 seconds. Television triggers this response at a far more rapid rate than we experience it in life, which is why we cannot keep our eyes off the TV screen, even in the middle of an intimate conversation, and why people watch TV a lot longer than they intend. Because typical music videos, action sequences, and commercials trigger orienting responses at a rate of one per second, watching them puts us into continuous orienting response with no recovery. No wonder people report feeling drained from watching TV. Yet, we acquire a taste for it and find slower changes boring. The cost is that such activities as reading, complex conversation, and listening to lectures become more difficult (Doidge, 2007).

An article in the *Fort Worth Star* on 04/05/04 mentioned the same concerns. For every hour of TV watched daily, two groups of children aged 1 and 3 faced a 10% increased risk of having attention problems by age 7 (Tanner, 2004). The American Academy of Pediatrics recommends that youngsters under age 2 not watch TV. In the United States, about 36% of 1 year olds watch no TV, while 37% watch 1 to 2 hours daily and had a 10% to 20% increased risk of attention problems. Fourteen percent watched 3 to 4 hours daily and had a 30% to 40% increased risk compared with children who watched no television. The rest watched at least 5 hours daily. Among 3 year olds, only 7% watched no TV, 44% watched 1 to 2 hours daily, 27% watched 3 to 4 hours daily, almost 11% watched 5 to 6 hours a day, and about 10% watched 7 to 9 hours daily.

The problem is that unrealistically fast-paced visual images typical of most TV programming may alter normal brain development. The newborn brain develops very rapidly during the first 2 to 3 years of life. Studies have shown that newborn rats exposed to different levels of visual stimuli have a brain that architecturally looks very different depending on the amount of stimulation (Tanner, 2004).

The fear most often expressed about extended television viewing is that it robs the left hemisphere of development time and space. It has been suggested that nonverbal systems in the right brain were being overstimulated by TV and that even advantaged children would be harmed of neural pathways essential to the development of spoken and written language and critical thoughts were not fully developed (Emery, 1980).

SUMMARY AND ATTENTION TIPS

1. A child, aged 7, can still be helped with eye patching if amblyopia is discovered. If you suspect one of your children is not seeing well in either or both eyes, refer to an optometrist as soon as possible.

2. A child cannot learn with partial attention. The learning activity will not be stored if he or she does not pay full attention to your instructions.

3. If you train memory, you are also training attention. Try to use memory activities in your training program.

4. Learning a musical instrument has been shown to help areas of cognition and attention in young children.

5. Training working memory helps to train attention.

6. TV is not good for children before the age of 2. Parents must limit TV viewing.

REFERENCES

Anthes, E. (2009). How video games are good for the brain. *Brain in the News, Nov,* 2-3.

Bakalar, N. (2008). Memory training shown to turn up brain power. *Brain in the News, May,* 6.

Buchel, C. & Friston, K. J. (1997). Modulation of connectivity in visual pathway by attention: cortical interactions evaluated with structural equation modelling and fMRI. *Cerebral Cortex, 7*(8), 768-778.

Cicerone, K. D. (2002). Remediation of "working attention" in mild traumatic brain injury. *Brain Injury, 16*(3), 185-195.

Daily Mail. (2009). Girl born with half a brain is only person in world to see both fields of vision through one eye. *Brain in the News, August,* 5.

Doidge, N. (2007). *The brain that changes itself.* New York, NY: Penguin Group (USA), Inc.

Drevets, W. C., Burton, H., Videen, T. O., Snyder, A. Z., Simpson, J. R. Jr, & Raichle, M. E. (1995). Blood flow changes in human somatosensory cortex during anticipated stimulation. *Nature, 373,* 249-252.

Eliot, L. (1999). *What's going on in there?* New York, NY: Bantam Books.

Ellison, K. (2007). The plastic brain. *Discover, May,* 47-52.

Emery, M. (1980). The vacuous vision: the TV medium. *Journal of the University Film Association, 32*(30).

Eriksson, P. S., Perfilieva, E., Björk-Eriksson, T., Alborn, A. M., Nordborg, C., Peterson, D. A., & Gage, F. H. (1998). Neurogenesis in the adult human hippocampus. *Nature Medicine, 4*(11), 1313-1317.

Gazzaniga, M. (2004). *The cognitive neurosciences iii.* Cambridge, MA: MIT Press.

Gould, E., Reeves, A. J., Fallah, M., Tanapat, P., Gross, C. G., & Fuchs, E. (1999). Hippocampal neurogenesis in adult old world primates. *Neurobiology, 96*(9), 5263-5267.

Hamilton, J. (2008). Think you're multitasking? Think again. *Brain in the News, Nov,* 4.

Healy, J. (1999). *Endangered minds.* New York, NY: Simon & Schuster.

Holloway, M. (2003) The mutable brain. *Scientific American, Sept,* 79-84.

Huang, J. (2009). Neuroplasticity as a proposed mechanism for the efficacy of optometric vision therapy & rehabilitation. *Journal of Behavioral Optometry, 20*(4), 95-99.

Huttenlocher, P. (2002). *Neural plasticity.* Cambridge, MA: Harvard University Press.

Kerns, K. (1999). Investigation of a direct intervention for improving attention in young children with ADHD. *Developmental Neuropsychology, 16*(2), 273-295.

Klingberg, T., Forssberg, H., & Westerberg, H. (2002). Training of working memory in children with ADHD. *Journal of Clinical and Experimental Neuropsychology, 24*(6), 781-791.

Kolb, B. (1998). Brain plasticity and behavior. *Annual Review of Psychology, 49,* 43-64.

Levine, B., Robertson, I. H., Clare, L., Carter, G., Hong, J., Wilson, B. A., . . . Stuss, D. T. (2000). Rehabilitation of executive functioning: an experimental-clinical validation of goal management training. *Journal of International Neuropsychological Society, 6*(3), 299-312.

Lie, D. C., Dziewczapolski, G., Willhoite, A. R., Kaspar, B. K., Shults, C. W., & Gage, F. H. (2002). The adult substantia nigra contains progenitor cells with neurogenic potential. *The Journal of Neuroscience, 22*(15), 6639-6649.

Maino, D. (2009) Neuroplasticity teaching an old brain new tricks. *Review of Optometry, January,* 62-67.

Mateer, C. (1989). *Training executive function skills.* Puyallup, WA: Good Samaritan Hospital, 1989 Workbook.

Mauk, B. (2009). Music training changes brain networks. *Brain in the News, May,* 1-2.

Mesulam, M. M. (1990). Large scale neurocognitive networks and distributed processing for attention language and memory. *Annals of Neurology, 28,* 597-613.

Olesen, P. J., Westerberg, H., & Klingberg, T. (2004). Increased prefrontal and parietal activity after training working memory. *Nature Neuroscience, 7*(1), 75-79.

Palmer, T. D., Markakis, E. A., Willhoite, A. R., Safar, F., & Gage, F. H. (1999). Fibroblast growth factor–2 activates a latent neurogenic program in neural stem cells from diverse regions of the adult CNS. *The Journal of Neuroscience, 19*(19), 8487-8497.

Park, N. (1999). Evaluation of the attention process training programme. *Neuropsychological Rehabilitation, 9*(2), 135-154.

Pascual-Leone, A., Nguyet, D., Cohen, L. G., Brasil-Neto, J. P., Cammarota, A., & Hallett, M. (1995). Modulation of muscle responses evoked by transcranial magnetic stimulation during the acquisition of new fine motor skills. *Journal of Neurophysiology, 74,* 1037-1045.

Robertson, J. (1996). *Goal management training: a clinical manual.* Cambridge, UK: Psyconsult.

Robertson, I. H. & Murre, J. M. (1999). Rehabilitation of brain damage: brain plasticity and principles of guided recovery. *Psychological Bulletin, 125*(5), 554-575.

Semrud-Llikeman, M., Nielsen, K. H., Clinton, A., Sylvester, L., Parle, N., & Connor, R. T. (1999). An intervention approach for children with teacher and parent-identified attention difficulties. *Journal of Learning Disabilities, 32*(6), 581-590.

Small, G. (2008). *iBrain: Surviving the technological alteration of the modern mind.* New York, NY: Collins Living Publishers.

Sohlberg, M. (1989). *Introduction to cognitive rehabilitation.* New York, NY: The Guilford Press.

Sohlberg, M. (1993). Contemporary approaches to the management of executive control dysfunction. *The Journal of Head Trauma Rehabilitation, 8*(1), 45-50.

Sohlberg, M. (2001). *Cognitive rehabilitation*. New York, NY: The Guilford Press.

Sohlberg, M. & Mateer, C. A. (1987). Effectiveness of an attention training program. *Journal of Clinical and Experimental Neuropsychology, 9*(2), 117-130.

Sohlberg, M., McLaughlin, K. A., Pavese, A., Heidrich, A., & Posner, M. I. (2000). Evaluation of attention process training and brain injury education in persons with acquired brain injury. *Journal of Clinical and Experimental Neuropsychology, 22*(5), 656-676.

Steed, J. (2008). It's never too late to grow your brain. *Brain in the News, Dec, 8.*

Stone, S.P., Patel, P., Greenwood, R. J., & Halligan, P. W. (1992). Measuring visual neglect in acute stroke and predicting its recovery: the visual neglect recovery index. *Journal of Neurology, Neurosurgery and Psychiatry, 55*(6), 431-436.

Tanner, L. (2004). Children's TV habits may lead to attention problems. *Fort Worth Star,* 04/05/04.

van't Hooft, I., Andersson, K., Sejersen, T., Bartfai, A., & von Wendt, L. (2003). Attention and memory training in children with acquired brain injuries. *ACTA Paediatrica, 92,* 935-940.

Van Zomeren, A. H. & van den Burg, W. (1985). Residual complaints of patients two years after severe closed head injury. *Journal of Neurology, Neurosurgery and Psychiatry, 48,* 21-28.

Von Cramon, D. (1991). Problem-solving deficits in brain-injured patients: a therapeutic approach. *Neuropsychological Rehabilitation, 1,* 45-64.

Weder, B., Knorr, U., Herzog, H., Nebeling, B., Kleinschmidt, A., Huang, Y., . . . Seitz, R. J. (1994). Tactile recognition of shape after subcortical ischaemic infarction studied with pet. *Brain 117,* 593-605.

Wilson, B. A. & Davidoff, J. (1993). Partial recovery from visual object agnosia. a 10 year follow up study. *Cortex, 29*(3), 529-542.

SUGGESTED READING

Duncan, J. (1986). Disorganization of behavior after frontal lobe damage. *Cognitive Neuropsychology, 3,* 271-290.

McAuliffe, K. (2008). Mental fitness. *Discover, Sept,* 56-60.

Cerebrovascular Accident and Traumatic Brain Injury

CEREBROVASCULAR ACCIDENT

On December 10, 1996, Jill Bolte Taylor, a 37-year-old Harvard-trained brain scientist, experienced a massive stroke in the left hemisphere of her brain. As she observed her mind deteriorate to the point that she could not walk, talk, read, write, or recall any of her life—all within 4 hours—Taylor alternated between the euphoria of the intuitive and kinesthetic right brain, in which she felt a sense of complete well-being and peace, and the logical, sequential left brain, which recognized she was having a stroke and enabled her to seek help before she was completely lost. It would take 8 years to fully recover (Taylor, 2009).

Cerebrovascular accidents (CVAs) result in deficits of varying severity. The presentation of cerebral ischemia with signs and symptoms that pass in 24 hours is considered a transient ischemic attack (TIA).

Interestingly enough, asymptomatic defects are reported in 29% of patients with TIAs and 57% of those with minor strokes. The most commonly exhibited defect is scotoma located solely or predominantly in the upper field (85% of cases). A scotoma is an area of depressed vision within the visual field or a loss of vision in part of a visual field.

Signs and symptoms that last longer than 24 hours but are resolved by 3 weeks are classified as reversible ischemic neurological deficit (RIND). CVAs with lingering involvement (past 3 weeks) are a result of irreversible brain damage and are then considered a stroke (Optom, 2010).

Stoke is the number one disabler in our society and the number three killer. Because neurological disease often involves the higher cognitive layers of our cerebral cortex, and because stroke occurs four times more frequently in the left cerebral hemisphere, our ability to create or understand language is often compromised. The term *stroke* refers to a problem with the blood vessels carrying oxygen to the cells of the brain, and there are basically two types: ischemic and hemorrhagic (Taylor, 2009). Strokes due to thrombus or embolus cause some 65% to 80% of all CVAs and are considered primary ischemic events. The remaining 20% to 35% are considered primary hemorrhagic events. These can be caused by spontaneous subarachnoid hemorrhage (Optom, 2010).

With ischemic stroke, a blood clot travels into the artery until the tapered diameter of the artery becomes too small for the clot to pass any further. The blood clot blocks the flow of oxygen-rich blood to the cells beyond the point of obstruction; consequently, brain cells become traumatized and often die.

The hemorrhagic stroke occurs when blood escapes from the arteries and floods into the brain. Blood is toxic to neurons when it comes in direct contact with them, so any leak can have devastating effects on the brain.

Lane, K. A. *Visual Attention in Children: Theories and Activities* (pp. 119-130).

WARNING SIGNS OF STROKE

S = Speech, or any problem with language

T = Tingling, or any numbness in the body

R = Remember, or any problems with memory

O = Off balance, problems with coordination

K = Killer headache

E = Eyes, or any problems with vision (Taylor, 2009).

ACQUIRED BRAIN INJURY

Acquired brain injury (ABI) refers to sudden neurologic changes secondary to head trauma, CVA, or postsurgical complications. Patients with ABI manifest a spectrum of sensory, motor, language, and perceptual deficits, many of which are amenable to rehabilitation. The natural recovery from an ABI can be up to 1 year postinjury and can be incomplete, with many patients eventually being left with multiple residual deficits including reading and visual scanning dysfunctions relating to the oculomotor dysfunction. These residual deficits, including vision deficits, may adversely affect their rehabilitation as well as other avocational and vocational goals.

The prevalence of oculomotor deficits in the ABI population ranges from 40% to 85%, depending on the literature source. Basic oculomotor deficits include jerk and pendular nystagmus, increased fixational drift, saccadic dysmetria, increased saccadic latency, and reduced pursuit gain. These oculomotor signs translate into symptoms while reading, resulting in loss of place, reduced speed, and the sensation of visual motion (Kapoor, Ciuffreda, & Han, 2004).

Patients with ABI report problems with concentration, distractibility, forgetfulness, and difficulty doing more than one thing at a time. Even small decrements in an individual's attention ability may significantly reduce the capacity for new learning and may affect academic performances. Attention impairments frequently accompany executive dysfunction. Patients have problems with the allocation of the attentional resources, switching between tasks with different cognitive requirement and time-sharing processing resources and overcoming automatic responses when faced with nonroutine situations (Sohlberg, 2001).

Deficits in attention and memory are the most common cognitive dysfunctions in ABI and often contribute to significant disability both in adults and children. Brain injury in children not only disrupts established functions but also affects functions that are in the process of developing and those that have yet to emerge (Boll & Barth, 1981). Children who appear to have fully recovered from brain injury may, over time, demonstrate deterioration in cognitive behavioral and/or socioemotional functioning.

Memory and attention are crucial for learning; deficits in these functions have a major negative influence on academic and social adjustment. Another major difficulty frequently reported following ABI is decreased speed of information processing. It has been suggested that slow processing speed limits attention capacity. Problems with working memory have also been described following injury to frontal brain systems (van't Hooft, Andersson, Sejersen, Bartfai, von Wendt, 2003).

TRAUMATIC BRAIN INJURY

Children and adults acquire traumatic brain injury (TBI) when they experience an acute external force to the skull. Many cases of childhood TBI are preventable, but, unfortunately, various potentially effective protective measures such as bicycle helmets and car seats are not always used appropriately or consistently. About 180 per 100,000 children incur TBI every year, accounting for approximately 30% of all childhood injury deaths. There is considerable long-term morbidity in the survivors of those with relatively severe injuries. Rates are higher for boys than girls, and whereas falls are the most common cause for young children, motor vehicle accidents become increasingly prevalent in older children (Donders, 2007).

It has been noted that 100,000 deaths per year in the United States result from head injury, with 400,000 to 700,000 nonfatal head injuries being severe enough to require hospitalization. Head injury is the fourth leading cause of death in this country (1 in 16 deaths attributable to head trauma alone). In addition, some 50,000 to 70,000 of these patients will retain varying levels of impairment. Only 20% of patients who survive head trauma regain enough function to return to some form of work. Approximately 60% do not return to the competitive work force, and 5% do not recover from coma. The economic loss from this has been estimated to be $4 billion per year. Perhaps more devastating is the loss of personal productivity and the disruption of lives of family and friends of the patient with cerebral injury (Optom, 2010).

The brain is often viewed as a rigid mass when in fact it is more a firm jellylike substance. It floats within the hard bony skull completely enveloped by the cerebrospinal fluid. Closed head trauma (the most common form of head injury) leaves the dura intact. The dura is the outermost, toughest, and most fibrous of the three membranes covering the brain and spinal cord. Even though the dura may be intact, cranial bones may be fractured, and forces sufficient to fracture the skull are also likely to cause brain injury.

Disruption of the visual system results from injury to the optic nerve, chiasm, tracts, radiations, or primary and associated visual cortical areas. Optic nerve injury alone occurs in 1% to 2% of all closed head trauma cases. Complete optic nerve dysfunction occurs in 0.5%. Supraorbital and frontal head injuries are most likely to cause optic nerve dysfunction; injury to the temporal, parietal, and occipital regions is less likely to damage the nerve. In all cases, however, it is important to remember that even minor head injuries are capable of causing severe vision loss (Optom, 2010).

In general, children with mild head injuries show good recovery, and only few have any long-term sequelae. On the other hand, children with severe injuries often show neurological impairments, lowered intelligence, slowed motor speed, memory problems, expressive language difficulties, reading problems, and behavioral disorders (Brown, Chadwick, Shaffer, Rutter, & Traub, 1981).

GLASGOW COMA SCALE

The Glasgow Coma Scale is often used to describe the severity of head injuries. The scale rates the head injury as mild with a score 13 or over, moderate with 8 to 12, and severe with score of 7 or less. The scores are based on loss of consciousness and other neurological findings.

In general, it is not clear whether younger children recover faster or more completely than older counterparts. Post-traumatic improvement in IQ scores is not significantly different for children aged less than 10 years than for those over age 10 at the time of their injuries; however, the data tend to suggest the younger group improves more. Clinical observation would suggest that the younger children do make a more rapid and complete recovery. This statement agrees with the "Kennard principle," which is that brain injury sustained early in life results in less impairment than later injury.

It appears that the most sensitive functions affected by head injury are those with heavy visuomotor speed and coordination components. A positive finding in the case of the severe group is that despite the duration length of coma and post-traumatic amnesia (PTA), remarkable improvements occur in intellectual functioning. All three groups of severity—mild, moderate, and severe—improve in their IQ scores over a period of time. Nevertheless, the persistence of behavior difficulties such as irritability, inattentiveness, and difficulties with social interaction seem to continue and need intervention strategies (Knights et al., 1991).

Brain injury in children not only disrupts established functions but also affects those functions that are in the process of developing and those that have yet to begin development. Disruption of primary skills may result in changes to the order, rate, and/or level of learning in the child. Higher-order skills, which depend on established primary skills, may later develop incorrectly, incompletely, or not at all. In many cases, children initially appear to have fully recovered from their injuries (with no apparent residual deficits) but, over time, begin to demonstrate deterioration in cognitive behavioral and socioemotional functioning. This process is sometimes referred to as "growing into a deficit" (Mateer, Kerns, & Eso, 1996).

AREAS OF THE BRAIN AND EFFECTS OF TRAUMATIC BRAIN INJURY AND CEREBROVASCULAR ACCIDENT

A good remediation program cannot be effective unless you have a good understanding of the different areas of the brain and the functions they control. By using this information, you will be able to direct your remediation to attain the best results for your patients. The following section of this chapter will talk about visual brain areas, neglect, and specific functions of other areas of the brain that can be affected by TBI and CVA.

VISUAL AREAS OF THE BRAIN

Area 17 (Primary Visual Cortex)

The primary visual cortex (VI) (Figure 8-1), also called Brodmann's area 17, receives visual information as a direct retinotopic map. It is made up of a disproportionately large number of macular fibers that end near the occipital pole. Area 17 is completely specific in its function, being involved only in visual reception. Damage to it results in compromised visual acuity and visual field defects. Because of its proximity to the base of the skull, it is more susceptible to the effects of trauma and subsequent edema than other areas in the visual cortex.

Area 18 (Visual Association Area)

Trauma to areas other than the occipital cortex can lead to visual sensory deficits. The second visual area, Brodmann's area 18, interacts with the language centers of the left hemisphere and with spatial relations and other nonlanguage skills from the right hemisphere. It is critically involved in the interpretation of objects perceived, and it is also where visual perception and differentiation of shape, color, and size take place. Damage to it results in compromised word and letter recognition.

Area 19 (Visual Association Area)

Brodmann's area 19, known as the tertiary zone, is highly multifunctional, the site where visual information is decoded, coded, integrated, and stored. Normal function of this area is also critical to the interpretation of objects perceived. Area 19 is the visual association center responsible for associating and categorizing related visual messages, and, along with area 18, it contributes to saccadic eye movements, which, in turn, provide an afferent (toward the center) feedback to the higher cognitive centers (Optom, 2010).

Area 8 (Frontal Eye Field)

All voluntary eye movements are generated from this area. The extraocular muscles are controlled by both frontal eye field (area 8) and the parieto-occipital eye field (areas 17, 18, and 19). Area 8 is responsible for moving the foveas to an image (saccade), and areas 17 to 19 are responsible for maintaining the fovea in the image (pursuit). Five levels of ocular movement require control by these centers. These movements are as follows:

- Smooth pursuit
- Saccade
- Optokinetic nystagmus
- Vestibular reflex
- Convergence

Ocular dysfunctions will result from injury to these eye movement control centers or to the extraocular muscles themselves. They may also interfere with performance in the visual perceptual areas of closure, figure-ground detection, and visual memory. Therefore, an accurate assessment of visual perceptual skills should not be undertaken without prior knowledge of elementary oculomotor functioning obtained from observation of a patient's scanning movement (Optom, 2010).

The following is a summary that lists visual disturbances with cortical insult:

- Agnosia—Inability to understand or interpret what is meant
- Alexia—Inability to recognize or comprehend written or printed words
- Aghasia—Inability to recognize, comprehend, or express written or printed words
- Color anomia—Inability to name or recognize colors
- Color dischromatopsia—Inability to see colors or achromatopsia
- Prosopagnosia—Inability to recognize a familiar face or complex nonverbal stimuli
- Simultanagnosia—Inability to recognize more than one element at a time
- Optic ataxia—Mislocation when reaching for or pointing at objects (Optom, 2010).

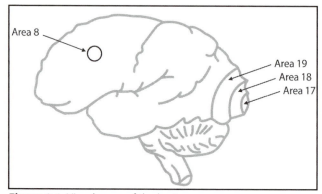

Figure 8-1. Visual areas of the brain.

POST-TRAUMA VISION SYNDROME

Following a brain injury, CVA, multiple sclerosis, cerebral palsy, or autism, to name several, interference with function can often occur with ambient visual processing. When this occurs, information is received by the occipital cortex without spatial preprogramming. The person will often experience a very focalized nature of his or her vision. The visual world in this type of altered state can often cause the person to experience a number of symptoms such as diplopia, seeing words and print move, difficulty shifting gaze, difficulty in adapting to environments where there is movement in the periphery, such as in shopping malls, etc. The ambient process is responsible for stability in the visual spatial world. It enables us to move our eyes from one point to the other without seeing the world shift and jump. The ambient process also enables us to move within the busy moving environment and maintain orientation spatially. Without this process, any movement will appear as detail and not only can become quite disturbing but can interfere with our ability to maintain our spatial orientation. People with ambient visual processing dysfunction will often describe having significant difficulty in a busy supermarket. They may find that movement in their peripheral vision is overwhelming.

Remember that the ambient visual system deals particularly with our peripheral vision. The peripheral vision is matched up with sensorimotor processes for the purpose of developing concepts of midline body posture and orientation. Once this is accomplished, a feed-forward phenomenon occurs. Information is relayed from midbrain up to the occipital cortex where it preprograms the higher-seeing area to know how to look at visual information first spatially before focalizing on detail. This is called the ambient visual process. In this manner, the occipital cortex will organize information first spatially before it looks at the details. In other words, it is as if we know where to look before we know what we are looking at (Padula & Argyris, 1996).

It is extremely important that occupational therapists (OTs) understand how important our ambient visual system is when we remediate children and adults. Earlier in this book, we also called this the M system. In order to shift the position of the eyes from one point to another, we must spatially orient to the next destination "before" shifting the eyes to look at detail. The ambient process is not a conscious process as the focal system is. We subconsciously use motor information to control this system. Without the ambient visual system, not only would we become fragmented in vision, but we will have difficulty in organizing posture and movement.

Patients with post-trauma vision syndrome (PTVS) need help from both OTs and developmental optometrists. A study was conducted to evaluate brainwave responses as measured on visual evoked potentials (VEP) for TBI patients (Padula, Argyris, & Ray, 1994). The experimental group in this study showed increased amplitudes with treatment. The treatment consisted of low levels of prism and binasal occlusion (two vertical bars placed on glasses located on the nasal side of each lens). This indicates that the prism and binasal occlusion acted to re-establish spatial organization on the ambient process, thereby influencing the wave form generated by the occipital cortex. The control group, composed of people who were not brain injured, demonstrated decreased amplitude with the same treatment. This means that binasal occlusion and prism interfere with ambient visual processing for individuals who were not brain injured. This seems to contradict my earlier suggestion of binasal occlusion to improve peripheral vision; however, my earlier suggestion was only for short periods of time (about 10 minutes) not total occlusion, as with the brain-injured individuals.

It has been found that by rebalancing the ambient visual process through use of lenses/prisms and binasal occlusion (all through the supervision of a developmental optometrist), the ambient visual process can be rebalanced, and the relationship to sensorimotor functioning and higher focal processing of the visual system can be re-established (Padula et al., 1994).

The common characteristics of the visual system following a brain injury are exotropia ("eyes turn out"), convergence insufficiency, accommodative dysfunction (difficulty focusing at near), and oculomotor dysfunction. Other symptoms of PTVS include balance and posture difficulties, lowered blink rate, and spatial disorientation (Optom, 2010).

Studies by Padula and Argyris, (1996) have demonstrated that the visual process is involved with organizing concepts of midline related to posture. Through the ambient visual process, information is matched with kinesthetic, proprioceptive, and vestibular information, which is then organized through higher visual perceptual processing as a concept of visual midline. This may be observed by passing an object in front of a person's face and asking him or her to report when the object appears to be directly in front of his or her nose. In the case of a visual field loss, such as a homonymous hemianopsia (loss of vision in the right or left half of the visual field), the person will report the target in front of his or her nose when it is directed to the side away from the visual field loss. An interesting observation occurs when working with patients with hemiparesis or hemiplegia. The person will also project the concept of midline in the majority of cases away from the neurologically affected side. The shift in concept of visual midline away from the side of the hemiparesis (muscle weakness to one side) and/ or hemiparesis homonymous is called visual midline shift syndrome (VMSS) and appears to be a survival mechanism. By doing this, the midline shift will enable the person to weightbear on the side that is more functional. This, however, interferes with aspects of rehabilitation in which the physical therapist will attempt to develop the ability to weightbear on the affected side. In a sense, the shifting concept of visual midline away from the affected side essentially reinforces the neglect. Visual midline shift can also occur with other types of neurological conditions, such as multiple sclerosis, cerebral palsy, Friedreich's ataxia, and autism.

Through a neuro-optometric rehabilitation examination, the optometrist will prescribe prisms that can be used to counter the distortion of space and thereby shift the midline to a more centered position. Placing prisms in the appropriate angle before both eyes with the apex and base end of prism in the same direction (yoked prism) will counter the distortion of space covered by the visual midline shift syndrome. The optometrist will often prescribe yoked prisms in conjunction with physical and occupational therapy. The combination maximizes potential for the individual in rehabilitation (Padula & Argyris, 1996).

UNILATERAL NEGLECT

Neglect is a visuospatial attentional disorder leading to impaired perception of and diminished responses to stimuli presented in one side of space, more commonly the left (Sohlberg, 2001). The key words here are attentional disorder. Patients with spatial neglect often behave as if one side of their world no longer existed. Patients may ignore people, objects, and events toward the contralateral (side opposite the lesion, usually left) side in overt behavior or when describing a scene. Their eyes, head, and trunk may be oriented rightward. They may eat food from only the right side of a plate, shave or apply makeup to just the ride side of their face, dress only the right side of their body, and overlook or forget left turns in routes. Even if their left hand is not paralyzed, they may not use it spontaneously.

Neglect may arise at different spatial degrees within the same person. As well as ignoring stimuli at the extreme left in their environment, patients may neglect a left page when reading a small book or words to the left of the right page, and even letters at one end of each word. Many neglect patients do not realize they are missing information. If their lesion also causes paralysis of contralesional limbs, some patients remain unaware of this. Even when neglect patients are blindfolded, haptic exploration can deviate toward the ipsilesional (same side as lesion) task (Gazzaniga, 2004).

Neglect can be caused by lesions at different cortical sites. The most common location is the right parietal lobe, but a high frequency also exists for anterior (frontal lobe cortex) and posterior (temporal, parietal, and occipital lobe cortical lesions) (Optom, 2010). In both humans and monkeys, cortical lesions that consistently yield neglect have been described in one of the following three areas: (1) the dorsolateral posterior parietal cortex, (2) the dorsolateral premotor prefrontal cortex, and (3) the cingulated gyrus (Mesulam, 1990).

The right side of the human brain is dominant for distributing attention across the extrapersonal world. Consequently, severe leftward neglect after a right hemisphere lesion is far more common than severe rightward neglect following a left hemisphere lesion.

Neglect behavior can be dissociated into perceptual, motor, and limbic components. There is a perceptual component in the sense that sensory events occurring within the neglected hemispace have a diminished impact on awareness, especially when competing sensory events occur in the contralateral hemispace. Sensory extinction and deficits in the covert (internal) shift of the attention focus are major manifestations of this component. A disinclination to direct orienting and exploratory behaviors with the head, eyes, and limbs into the neglected hemispace constitutes the motor component of neglect behavior. There is also a limbic or motivational component reflected by a devaluation of the neglected hemispace so that the patient behaves as if nothing important could be expected to emanate from that side of space (Mesulam, 1990).

An interesting example of neglect is shown in Figure 8-2. The patient can detect not only (A) the right unilateral visual stimulus but also (B) the left unilateral stimulus on the affected side; however, he or she will miss the left side stimulus if there is (C) a competing right side stimulus presented at the same time.

ATTENTION, BRAIN AREAS, AND TRAUMATIC BRAIN INJURY

Clinical research has identified attentional impairments as a major consequence of TBI in adults and children. The attentional system exists within the brain, which relies on the efficient functioning of discrete, but interacting,

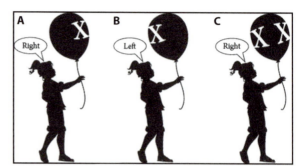

Figure 8-2. Example of neglect.

cerebral regions. Damage or dysfunction within any one of these areas may lead to deficiencies that impact attentional skills in a global way or may impact differentially on specific aspects of attentional processing.

Children appear to be particularly vulnerable to attentional problems, perhaps because these skills are continually developing during childhood. Research demonstrates ongoing maturation of attentional skills through childhood and into adolescence, with focused attention reaching adult levels during midchildhood, and other aspects of attention continuing to progress into adolescence. The emerging nature of these skills renders them at increased risk for disruption in the event of an interruption in development due to cerebral insult. In parallel with this cognitive progression is the process of cerebral maturation. Specifically, cerebral regions thought to subsume attentional skills, such as subcortical and anterior areas, also continue to mature into early adolescence. Further, these areas are particularly susceptible to damage from TBI. Such damage in childhood may not simply interfere with ongoing improvements in attentional skills, but may cause permanent damage (Anderson, Fenwick, Manly, & Robertson, 1998).

This section deals with the consequences of TBI on attention and the brain areas that are involved. The purpose of this section is to make you familiar with symptoms of brain injuries so that you will be better able to help your patients. By knowing what your patients may be experiencing, you will be better able to develop lesson plans, make proper referrals, and, in general, give your patient a better chance for recovery. I will separate this material into the following brain areas:

- Parietal

- Frontal

- Cerebellum

Parietal

Spatial inattention is most commonly reported in patients with damage to the posterior cortex. Many autistic patients appear to focus intensely on some small element of the environment while ignoring surrounding contextual information. This inattention appears similar to that observed in patients with acquired lesions to the posterior cortex and patients with parietal damage. Importantly, these autistic patients with developmental parietal abnormalities perform like patients with acquired parietal damage on spatial tasks.

The parietal cortex is involved in the distribution of visual attention at both attended and unattended (or less attended) locations. In the case of unilateral parietal damage, the sensory maps most affected would be in contralateral sensory space. Among the most prominent of current hypotheses regarding the role of the parietal cortex in spatial attention is that a damaged cortex leads to difficulties in the disengagement of attention (Posner, Walker, Friedrich, & Rafal, 1984).

Also, the parietal cortex may maintain an internal representation of sensory space and play a critical role in the allocation of attentional resources across that space. A damaged cortex would have a constricted sensory map that would result in a narrowed distribution of spatial attention (Townsend, 1994). In fact, posterior parietal lesions, in particular, seem to affect the ability to disengage from stimuli in the ipsilesional (same) side, when attention must be shifted contralesionally. It is also noted that superior parietal cortex controls lateralized shifts of attention in visual field coordinates but asymmetrically for the two hemifields. Attention to the left field is mostly controlled by one region in the right parietal cortex, while attention to the right field is controlled more bilaterally by a left parietal and a distinct right parietal region. The right parietal cortex may then contain the neural hardware to direct attention contralaterally and ipsilaterally (Corbetta, Miezin, Shulman, & Petersen, 1993).

In addition to being extremely important in spatial tasks, parietal regions are also involved in the storage of verbal information in working memory. There is evidence that left posterior parietal lesions can impair verbal short-term memory (Cabeza & Nyberg, 2000) and that the left parietal cortex also has neural network involvement in the phonological loop component of working memory. It, therefore, seems that the right frontoparietal network is involved in sustained and possibly selective attention (Coull, Frith, Frackowiak, & Grasby, 1996).

In summary, it is the right hemisphere that is needed to maintain an alert state and controls most of our attention. Any lesion to the parietal cortex, especially the right parietal cortex, will affect your patient's attention, and right parietal damage will have more of an effect in the left field compared to the right field. The parietal lobe is central to spatial attention to external locations. It is critical for maintaining an alert state (Posner & Petersen, 1990), visual imagery, performance of vigilance tasks, spatial working memory, disengagement of attention, and our ability to select information for the highest levels of conscious integration, especially spatial information.

Frontal

Prefrontal Cortices

The prefrontal lobes are those parts of the frontal lobes that are located anterior to the motor areas of the brain. By virtue of the fact that the prefrontal lobes are capable of storing many pieces of information for temporary periods of time, they are able to consider all relevant information (including past experience) before deciding on the best course of action. To prevent the ideomotor center from making impulsive decisions, the prefrontal lobes normally keep the ideomotor (arousal by an idea or thought) center suppressed until an appropriate course of action has been decided on. One of the characteristics of a person who has lost his or her frontal lobes is the ease with which he or she can be distracted from a sequence of thoughts. The human being without frontal lobes is still capable of performing many intellectual tasks, such as answering short questions, performing simple arithmetic computations, and so forth, thus illustrating that the basic intellectual activities of the cerebral cortex are still intact without the frontal lobes. Yet, if concerted sequences of cerebral functions are required of the person, he or she becomes completely disorganized. Therefore, the frontal lobes seem to be important in keeping the mental functions directed toward goals (Optom, 2010). The prefrontal lobes are concerned with planning for the future, solving complex mathematical and/or logical problems, anticipating the consequences of motor actions even before they are performed, and controlling one's activities in accordance with moral laws (Guyton, 1963). Surgical intervention in the prefrontal lobes leads to definite personality changes (Optom, 2010).

Cognitive neuroscientists have come to realize that the frontal lobes—more specifically, the prefrontal cortices—contribute to a wide array of cognitive functions, including aspects of attention, language, memory, and problem solving. The prefrontal region comprises about 28% of the cortical mantle in humans and is intricately connected to many other neocortical as well as subcortical regions. Patients with frontal lobe lesions exhibit impairment in memory for the temporal order in which stimuli are presented. This area of the brain is also important for working memory or executive control (Sohlberg, 1993). Frontal lobe lesions appear to affect the ability to gate or inhibit irrelevant stimulus information (Shimamura, 1995).

Hemispheric Differences

A difference between elementary sensory and motor processes and higher-order mental functions concerns the hemispheric lateralization of their neural basis. The cerebral correlates of language and visuospatial processing are largely asymmetric, with the well-known specialization of the left hemisphere for many linguistic processes and the right hemisphere for a variety of spatial processes. In contrast, the neurological organization of sensorimotor systems has a contralateral architecture, so that each hemisphere is primarily concerned with the opposite side of personal (i.e., the body) and extrapersonal space (e.g., visual or auditory objects). This state of affairs has implications in the domain of clinical neurology. It is a current view that damage to specifically committed regions of each cerebral hemisphere brings about somatosensory, visual, and motor deficits, contralateral to the side of the lesion with no relevant left-right asymmetries (Rowland, 1995).

There is also, however, some evidence of such asymmetries for sensory and motor deficits associated with unilateral lesions. A community-based epidemiological survey has shown that somatosensory, visual half-field, and motor deficits are more frequent after lesions in the right hemisphere, compared with left brain damage (Sterzi et al., 1993). In a study of 154 left and 144 right brain-damaged stroke patients, the incidence of contralateral somatosensory deficits (position sense) was 37% after damage to the left hemisphere. The incidence of deficits of sense of pain was 57% in right and 45% in left brain-damaged patients. Similarly, the incidence of contralesional visual half-field deficits was 18% in right brain-damaged and 7% in left brain-damaged patients. Finally, 95% of right brain-damaged patients exhibited motor deficits, which were found in only 85% of left brain-damaged patients (Burgess, 1999).

Cerebellum

The human cerebellum has more neurons than the remainder of the brain combined. It is physiologically connected by monosynaptic or multisynaptic pathways with all of the major subdivisions of the central nervous system (CNS), including the cerebrum, basal ganglia, diencephalon, limbic system, brainstem, and spinal cord. It is, therefore, one of the busiest intersections in the human brain. Nonetheless, for more than a century, neurologists and neuroscientists alike have held the view that the singular function of the human cerebellum is to help coordinate movement. New studies show that the cerebellum may be involved in a variety of nonmotor functions, including sensory discriminations, attention, working memory, semantic association, verbal learning, and complex problem solving (Schmahmann, 1997). In the face of such critical confounding factors, the cerebellum is still a device whose function is motor controlled. We now have found evidence of a classic double dissociation in structure and function between areas of the cerebellum. Visual attention activates one anatomic location within the cerebellar cortex, whereas motor performance activates a distinctly different location. Moreover, attention activation can occur independently of motor development (Allen, Buxton, Wong, & Courchesne, 1997).

The neocerebellum is necessary to rapidly shift the mental focus of selective attention between sensory modalities. A damaged cerebellum significantly impairs patients in the ability to respond rapidly and shift their attention from one sensory domain, such as visual and auditory, to another. It appears that the neocerebellum may be involved in any type of task that requires rapid sequential changes and adjustments of neural activity in order to proceed from one motor or cognitive condition to another (Akshoomoff & Courchesne, 1992).

The cerebellum serves an important role in maintaining balance and postural control and in coordinating voluntary movements. Like the basal ganglia, the cerebellum does not connect directly with the spinal cord. Rather, its elaborate interconnections, which include projections to and from subcortical regions and the prefrontal cortex, make it possible to assemble separate motor acts into complex, unitary behaviors and to ensure precision timing and accuracy of movements. Also involved with motor and cognitive learning, the cerebellum is part of a coordinated circuit that includes the prefrontal cortex and is active when confronting activities that are unfamiliar or difficult, that require rapid responding and concentration, or that involve changing conditions and parameters. Cerebellum damage is typically associated with tremor and incoordination during intentional movement (ataxia), impaired rapid alternating movements, overshooting when reaching for an object (dysmetria), nystagmus, or awkward posture and gait (Hunter, 2007).

MECHANISMS OF RECOVERY

The most commonly cited CNS mechanisms of recovery include the following:

- Diaschsis—A term originally used in early studies to describe recovery following temporary disruption of functioning in areas adjacent to the primary damage. Brain trauma may result in such factors as edema, metabolic changes, intracranial pressure changes, and modification of blood flow, all of which can render otherwise intact brain regions temporarily dysfunctional. Following a reduction of these "shock" effects, the functions that were inhibited in the affected but undamaged brain tissue slowly re-emerge. Diaschsis may be differentiated from the other mechanisms of recovery by the fact that it refers to the re-establishment of unimpaired neurologic systems.

- Axonal growth—Some forms of damage do not necessarily completely destroy neurons, and there may be regeneration of neural elements following injury. Axonal sprouting, including growth from damaged axons as well as collateral sprouting from intact axons, is a frequently cited recovery mechanism.

- Denervation supersensitivity—In the peripheral nervous system, it has been documented that postsynaptic receptor sites not only proliferate but also become more sensitive to neurotransmitter agents in denervated neurons. It is usually assumed that areas of the brain that are partially denervated by the lesion become hypersensitive to the remaining input, thus permitting a more rapid return of function.

- Substitution—This refers to the notion that existing intact brain structures can assume functions previously held by the lesioned areas. This might be responsible for recovery of functions such as language, visuospatial skills, and abstract thinking in which there is an overlap of corresponding brain territory (Sohlberg & Mateer, 1989).

REHABILITATION

Among the more consistent findings in individuals with brain injury are decreased reaction time; reduced speed of information processing; problems with concentration, distractibility, and forgetfulness; and the ability to do more than one thing at a time (Sohlberg, 2001). These observations are consistent with the different models of attention that are discussed in this book, which are sustaining attention over time (sustained attention), capacity of holding and working with information in mind (working memory), shifting attention, divided attention, and screening out nontarget information (selective attention). All of these are part of a program that can be used to train attention. In addition to training attention, there are other things that can be done to manage attention problems. These include the following:

- Environmental modifications—These procedures are used to reduce distractions. A common example of an attention problem is difficulty attending in distracting environments. The clinician and patient might make a list of "difficult" and "helpful" environments. This could result in a list of restaurants that are "noisy" or "busy" and those that are "quiet." Other strategies include reducing or eliminating distractions by turning off the TV or computer.

- Self-regulatory strategies—An example of this is pacing. Patients with attention problems often experience difficulty with fatigue or maintaining concentration over an extended period of time. It can be helpful to teach them pacing strategies (Sohlberg, 2001).

- External aids—Teach the patient to develop the use of lists, calendars, and organizers.

- Psychosocial support—This can be done by relaxation training, psychotherapy, or biofeedback.

- Attention training—This involves the use of specific exercises to train specific levels of attention such as the ones listed in this book: focused attention, sustained attention, selective attention, shifting attention, and divided attention.

ATTENTION TRAINING

The first two areas of attention that are critical for an attention training program are focused attention and sustained attention.

Focused attention is the ability to respond discretely to specific visual, auditory, or tactile stimuli. Although almost all patients recover this level of attention, it is often disrupted in the early stages of emergence from coma. The patient may initially be responsive only to internal stimuli (e.g., pain, temperature) (Sohlberg, 2001). In this book, I use focused attention to include the ability to quickly scan the environment and find the visual target.

Sustained attention is also called vigilance and is the ability to maintain a consistent behavioral response during continuous and repetitive activity. A disruption of this area of attention would be observed in a patient who can only focus on a task for a brief period (i.e., seconds to minutes) or who fluctuates dramatically in performance over even brief periods. It also incorporates the notion of mental control or working memory with tasks that involve manipulating information and holding it in the mind (Sohlberg, 2001). The control of sustained attention is known to be more strongly represented in the right compared to the left hemisphere of the brain. Unilateral neglect, as well as sustained attention, has been shown to improve with specific activities designed to improve sustained attention (Robertson, Tegnér, Tham, Lo, & Nimmo-Smith, 1995).

Working memory is the ability to retain information during short periods of time. Regions in frontal and parietal cortices are important for working memory. Studies have found that working memory can be improved through training. A study showed that after training, brain activity that was related to working memory increased in the middle frontal gyrus and superior and inferior parietal cortices. This shows evidence of training-induced plasticity in the neural systems that underlie working memory (Cicerone, 2002; Olesen, Westerberg, & Klingberg, 2004).

The three main attention areas to train after focused and sustained attention are selective, shifting (alternating), and divided attention.

Selective attention refers to the ability to maintain a behavioral or cognitive set in the face of distracting or competing stimuli. An example of this ability is trying to prepare a meal with children playing in the background or trying to study with the TV on.

Shifting attention refers to the capacity of mental flexibility that allows individuals to shift their focus of attention and move between tasks having different cognitive requirements, thus controlling which information will be selectively processed. An example of this would be a secretary who must continuously move between answering the phone, typing, and responding to inquires (Sohlberg, 2001).

The last area is divided attention. This involves the ability to respond simultaneously to multiple tasks or multiple task demands. An example of this would be driving a car while listening to the radio.

The March 2011 issue of *Discover Magazine* shows how some patients who have had severe TBI accidents are now making incredible comebacks due to modern science and the brain's ability to repair itself.

Some subjects have unbelievable Rip Van Winkle stories. An Arkansas man named Jerry Walles spent 19 years in a minimally conscious state after a car accident and then abruptly woke up in 2003. He said, "Mom" and then "Pepsi." Within days, he was speaking fluently. Later, scientists brought Walles to a neuroimaging specialist who caught Walles' brain in the act of rewiring itself. Using diffusion tensor imaging, which can depict axonal fibers, they found a thick cable of what looked like new axons sprouting at the back of the patient's brain. This study was extremely important, as it showed that the brain can reconnect itself decades after it was injured.

It is the plasticity of the human brain that gives us the success we have with TBI patients. The next chapter will discuss training activities you can use to help your patients develop attentional skills that will benefit their lives. They do not have to be TBI patients. All of your patients, regardless of the nature of their disorders, can benefit by having their ability to pay attention improved.

SUMMARY AND ATTENTION TIPS

1. Common deficits with ABI include attention, memory, and decreased speed of information processing.

2. Frontal brain injury can affect working memory.

3. All groups of head injuries improve in IQ scores over a period of time, but behavioral difficulties such as irritability and inattentiveness seem to continue.

4. Ocular motor dysfunction can interfere with closure, figure-ground, and visual memory. Therefore, do not do an assessment of perceptual skills until you have tested oculomotor skills first.

5. People with ambient visual processing dysfunction may find that movement in their peripheral vision is overwhelming.

6. The occipital cortex will organize information first spatially before it looks at detail.

7. Common characteristics of the visual system following a brain injury are exotropia, convergence insufficiency, accommodative dysfunction, and oculomotor dysfunction.

8. Visual midline shift will cause the person to project the concept of his or her midline away from the neurologically affected side. By doing this, the person will be able to weightbear on the side that is more functional.

9. Spatial inattention is most commonly reported in patients with damage to the posterior cortex.

10. The parietal cortex is involved in the distribution of visual attention at both attended and unattended (or less attended) locations.

11. The parietal cortex is involved in the disengagement of attention.

12. Attention to the left visual field is mostly controlled by one region in the right parietal cortex, while attention to the right is controlled by both the right and left parietal cortices.

(continued)

SUMMARY AND ATTENTION TIPS (CONTINUED)

13. Frontal lobe damage causes a patient to be easily distracted from a sequence of thoughts. This area of the brain is important in keeping the mental functions directed toward a goal.

14. Surgical intervention in the prefrontal lobes leads to definite personality changes.

15. Frontal lesions cause impairment in memory for temporal order and working memory or executive control. Frontal lobes are also important in inhibiting irrelevant stimulus information.

16. Left hemisphere involves language. Right hemisphere involves spatial processes.

17. Neurological organization of sensorimotor systems has a contralateral architecture so that each side is primarily concerned with the opposite side of the body.

18. A damaged cerebellum impairs a patient's ability to rapidly shift his or her attention from one sensory domain, such as visual to auditory, to another.

19. Cerebellum damage is typically associated with tremor and poor coordination during intentional movement (ataxia).

20. The more consistent findings in individuals with brain injury are as follows:

    a. Decreased reaction time

    b. Reduced speed of information processing

    c. Problems with concentration

    d. Distractibility

    e. Forgetfulness

    f. The ability to do more than one thing at once

REFERENCES

Akshoomoff, N. A. & Courchesne, E. (1992). A new role for the cerebellum in cognitive operations. *Behavioral Neuroscience, 106*(5), 731-736.

Allen, G., Buxton, R. B., Wong, E. C., & Courchesne, E. (1997). Attentional activation of the cerebellum independent of motor involvement. *Science, 275,* 1940-1943.

Anderson, V., Fenwick, T., Manly, T., & Robertson, I. (1998). Attentional skills following traumatic brain injury in childhood: a componential analysis. *Brain Injury, 12*(11), 937-949.

Boll, T. & Barth, J. (1981). Neuropsychology of brain damage in children. In S. B. Filskov & T. J. Boll (Eds.), *Handbook of clinical neuropsychology,* New York, NY: Wiley, 418-452.

Brown, G., Chadwick, O., Shaffer, D., Rutter, M., & Traub, M. (1981). A prospective study of children with head injuries: Psychiatric sequelae. *Psychological Medicine, 11*(1), 63-78.

Burgess, N. (1999). *The hippocampal and parietal foundations of spatial cognition.* New York, NY: Oxford University Press.

Cabeza, R. & Nyberg, L. (2000). Imaging cognition ii: an empirical review of 275 PET and fMRI studies. *Journal of Cognitive Neuroscience, 12*(1), 1-47.

Cicerone, K. D. (2002). Remediation of "working attention" in mild traumatic brain injury. *Brain Injury, 16*(3), 185-195.

Corbetta, M., Miezin, F. M., Shulman, G. L., & Petersen, S. E. (1993). A PET study of visuospatial attention. *The Journal of Neuroscience, 13*(3), 1202-1226.

Coull, J. T., Frith, C. D., Frackowiak, R. S., & Grasby, P. M. (1996). A fronto-parietal network for rapid visual information processing: a PET study of sustained attention and working memory. *Neuropsychologia, 34*(11), 1085-1095.

Donders, J. (2007). *Pediatric neuropsychological intervention.* Cambridge, UK: Cambridge University Press.

Gazzaniga, M. (2004). *The cognitive neurosciences iii.* Cambridge, MA: MIT Press.

Guyton, A. (1963). *Textbook of medical physiology, 2nd ed.* Philadelphia, PA: W.B. Saunders Co.

Hunter, S. (2007). *Pediatric neuropsychological intervention.* Cambridge, UK: Cambridge University Press.

Kapoor, N., Ciuffreda, K. J., & Han, Y. (2004). Oculomotor rehabilitation in acquired brain injury: a case series. *Archives of Physical Medicine and Rehabilitation, 85*(10), 1667-1678.

Knights, R., Ivan, L. P., Ventureyra, E. C., Bentivoglio, C., Stoddart, C., Winogron, W., & Bawden, H. N. (1991). The effects of head injury in children on neuropsychological and behavioural functioning. *Brain Injury, 5*(4), 339-351.

Mateer, C. A., Kerns, K. A., & Eso, K. L. (1996). Management of attention and memory disorders following traumatic brain injury. *Journal of Learning Disabilities, 29*(6), 618-632.

Mesulam, M. M. (1990). Large-scale neurocognitive networks and distributed processing for attention, language and memory. *Annals of Neurology, 28*(5), 597-612.

Olesen, P. J., Westerberg, H., & Klingberg, T. (2004). Increased prefrontal and parietal activity after training working memory. *Nature Neuroscience, 7*(1), 75-79.

Optom, S. (2010.) *Interdisciplinary perspectives and clinical applications.* Optometric Extension Program.

Padula, W. V. & Argyris, S. (1996). Post trauma vision syndrome and visual midline shift syndrome. *Neurorehabilitation, 6*(3), 165-171.

Padula, W. V., Argyris, S., & Ray, J. (1994). Visual evoked potentials (VEP) evaluating treatment for post-trauma vision syndrome (PTVS) in patients with traumatic brain injuries (TBI). *Brain Injury, 8*(2), 125-133.

Posner, M. I., Walker, J. A., Friedrich, F. J., & Rafal, R. D. (1984). Effects of parietal injury on covert orienting of attention. *The Journal of Neuroscience, 4*(7), 1863-1874.

Posner, M. I. & Petersen, S. E. (1990). The attention system of the human brain. *Annual Review of Neuroscience, 13,* 25-42.

Robertson, I. H., Tegnér, R., Tham, K., Lo, A., & Nimmo-Smith, I. (1995). Sustained attention training for unilateral neglect: the theoretical and rehabilitation implications. *Journal of Clinical and Experimental Neuropsychology, 17*(3), 416-430.

Rowland, L. (1995). *Merritt's textbook of neurology.* 9th *edition.* Baltimore, MD: Williams and Wilkins.

Schmahmann, J. (1997). *The cerebellum and cognition.* Philadelphia, PA: Elsevier.

Shimamura, A. (1995). Susceptibility to memory interference effects following frontal lobe damage: findings from tests of paired-associate learning. *Journal of Cognitive Neuroscience, 7*(2), 144-152.

Sohlberg, M., & Mateer, C. (1989). *Introduction to cognitive rehabilitation: theory and practice.* New York, NY: The Guilford Press, 3–17.

Sohlberg, M. (1993). Contemporary approaches to the management of executive control dysfunction. *The Journal of Head Trauma Rehabilitation, 8*(1), 45-58.

Sohlberg, M. (2001). *Cognitive rehabilitation. An integrative neuropsychological approach.* New York, NY: The Guilford Press.

Sterzi, R., Bottini, G., Celani, M. G., Righetti, E., Lamassa, M., Ricci, S., & Vallar, G. (1993). Hemianopsia, hemianaesthesia, and hemiplegia after left and right hemisphere damage: a hemispheric difference. *Journal of Neurology, Neurosurgery & Psychiatry, 56*(10), 308-310.

Taylor, J. B. (2009). *My stroke of insight: A brain scientist's personal journey.* New York, NY: Penguin Group (USA), Inc.

Townsend, J. (1994). Parietal damage and narrow "spotlight" spatial attention. *Journal of Cognitive Neuroscience, 6*(3), 220-232.

van't Hooft, I., Andersson, K., Sejersen, T., Bartfai, A., von Wendt, L. (2003). Attention and memory training in children with acquired brain injuries. *ACTA Paediatr, 92*(8), 935-940.

SUGGESTED READING

Sohlberg, M., McLaughlin, K. A., Pavese, A., Heidrich, A., & Posner, M. I. (2000). Evaluation of attention training and brain injury education in persons with acquired brain injury. *Journal of Clinical and Experimental Neuropsychology, 22*(5), 656-676.

The Training Program

The following is a list of the areas of attention that we will be training. They are listed from the most basic to the most complex, and they should be remediated with this in mind. Always train the most basic first and then move on to the most complex. For example, you do not start your training program by doing divided attention activities before having spent time on the more basic areas, such as focused and sustained attention. With that in mind, the following are the areas of attention we will work on.

FOCUSED ATTENTION

This is the ability to respond discretely to specific visual, auditory, or tactile stimuli. The most basic form of focused training is a patient rapidly turning his or her head to a visual or auditory stimulus. Focused training also involves training the patient to quickly identify a visual target in a crowded background, such as the visual search activities in this book. Activities under other areas of attention, such as sustained attention, can be changed to a focused activity. For example, having the child follow the Marsden ball is a pursuit activity and is considered a sustained attention area; however, having the child identify specific visual targets in the pursuit movement would make it a focused activity. For young patients or patients with severe attention problems, like some autistic children, the focused activities should consist more of alertness-type training by having the child quickly respond to a light or sound. The goal would be to try to increase the speed of responding to the stimulus.

SUSTAINED ATTENTION

This refers to two aspects of performance relating to time. The first involves the duration of time over which a given level of performance can be maintained, and the second involves the consistency of performance over that period. Periods of poor performance, alternating with normal or near-normal performance, may imply lapse of attention (Sohlberg & Mateer, 1989).

The developmental changes in pursuit eye movements occur primarily in conjunction with sustained attention development (Richards & Holley, 1999). It is unrealistic to expect a young child or a child with very poor attention to do the same sustained training activities that an adult will do. Smooth pursuit training is a very good way to train sustained attention in a child. Observing a child's smooth pursuit eye movements is also a good way to see if the child has sustained attention problems. It is best to train and test smooth pursuit monocularly and in the horizontal direction. Attention during stimulus tracking affects horizontal eye movements to a much larger degree than vertical eye movements (Richards & Holley, 1999).

Patients who have sustained difficulties can only focus on a task or maintain responses for a brief period (i.e., seconds to minutes) or will fluctuate dramatically in performance over even brief periods. It also incorporates the notion of mental control or working memory on tasks that involve manipulating information and holding it in the mind (Sohlberg, 1989). Just as sustained activities can be changed to focused activities, so can activities be changed to sustained by incorporating the addition of working

Lane, K. A. *Visual Attention in Children: Theories and Activities* (pp. 131-134).
© 2012 SLACK Incorporated.

memory. For example, having the patient recall a list of numbers in reverse order adds a working memory component to the exercise.

SHIFTING ATTENTION

This is the ability to rapidly shift your visual attention from one target to another. This is also called saccadic fixations, which are critical for such skills as reading or copying from the board or a text. This area of attention is often very poor in children who have reading problems. They will often lose their place when they read or have to use their fingers to keep from losing their place as they read. Young children often have difficulty in this area. To train a young child, you may have to give him or her a clue when you want him or her to quickly move his or her eyes: "Are you ready?" You may have to say, "On 2, move your eyes to the target," or you may have to use a metronome and at each beat of the metronome, the child will move his or her eyes to the next target. The shifting of attention in this book is different from alternating attention that you find in other attention programs. This type of attention refers to the capacity for mental flexibility to shift focus of attention and move between tasks having different cognitive requirements. An example of this would be the secretary who must continuously move between answering the phone, typing, and responding to inquiries.

These areas of attention—focused, sustained, and shifting—need to be trained first in any attention training program before going on to the next two areas—selective attention and divided attention—which are on a much higher level.

SELECTIVE ATTENTION

This level of attention refers to the ability to maintain a behavioral or cognitive set in the face of distracting or competing stimuli. It thus incorporates the notion of freedom from distractibility. Individuals with deficits at this level are easily drawn off-task by extraneous, irrelevant stimuli. These can include external sights, sounds, or activities as well as internal distractions (worry, etc.). Examples of problems at this level include an inability to perform therapy tasks in a stimulating environment (e.g., an open treatment area) or to prepare a meal with children playing in the background (Sohlberg, 2001).

DIVIDED ATTENTION

This level involves the ability to respond simultaneously to multiple tasks or multiple task demands. Two or more

behavioral responses may be required, or two or more kinds of stimuli may need to be monitored. This level of attentional capacity is required whenever multiple simultaneous demands must be managed. Performance under such conditions (i.e., driving a car while listening to the radio or holding a conversation) may actually reflect either rapid and continuous alternating attention or dependence on more unconscious automatic processing for at least one of the tasks (Sohlberg & Mateer, 1989).

One of the more demanding tasks is two sequences in the same modality. An example of this is having two pieces of paper in front of you. On the left piece of paper, cross out numbers in ascending order, and on the right, cross out numbers in descending order. The patient must vary from one piece of paper to the other.

MOTOR AND RIGHT HEMISPHERE TRAINING

This is not an area of attention but, because of the importance of the right hemisphere to attention, this section was added to the program. Also, the role of the cerebellum with motor control is well-known. What is not as well-known is that the coordination of the direction of distributing and shifting of attention (the orienting, distributing, and shifting of attention) is an adaptive anticipatory function and may normally be one of the many anticipatory tools under cerebellar control.

Because of the importance of both motor and right hemispheric control, these activities were introduced in addition to the areas of attention.

STARTING THE TRAINING PROGRAM

The success of any training program is not the exercises or special equipment but the therapist. One of the goals I had in writing this book was to give therapists and optometrists all of the information they would need to develop and to have a successful attention training program. This program is not intended to replace the activities you are now doing with your patients, but to enable you to incorporate these activities into your present program. These activities should be used in conjunction with your present sensory integration activities. For example, a simple walking rail procedure can be turned into a procedure that also remediates attention. Let's look at the five areas of attention and see how they can be added to your walking rail activities:

- Focused attention: Have the child scan a chart on the wall and identify certain letters or numbers.

- Sustained attention: Have the child balance in a heel-to-toe manner and follow a swinging Marsden ball. This is pursuit training and develops sustained attention.

- Shifting attention: Hang a letter chart on the wall, and have the child call out all the letters in proper sequence in a left-to-right direction. These are saccadic fixations and train shifting attention.

- Selective attention: Do any of the above activities and also have a CD player playing a story that the child has to listen to and remember for comprehension.

- Divided attention: Have the child walk on the walking rail, and you ask him or her questions that will stimulate his or her working memory (e.g., math questions or repeating a short number sequence in reverse order).

The first thing that the therapist needs to do is to determine the attention areas to focus on based on the needs of the patient.

Past research and experience have enabled us to identify certain areas of attention that go with different conditions. These would include the following:

- Learning disabilities usually fall into either reading or math areas. Children with reading problems would greatly benefit from shifting attention activities to help them to not lose their place when they read. They would also be helped with sustained attention activities. Math disabilities usually involve working memory and would benefit from working memory procedures. The child would also benefit from sustained and focused attention training.

- AD/HD children should receive sustained attention along with selective attention.

- Brainstem injuries would benefit from alertness or focused attention training along with sustained attention.

- Right brain injuries are helped with sustained attention training.

- Left brain injuries are helped by selective attention.

- Right brain injuries are also helped by alertness or focused attention training.

- Neglect patients should receive sustained training because it is usually the result of a right brain injury.

How to Determine Which Attention Area to Train Based on Previous Testing

Many of your patients have had previous testing, especially the Wechsler Adult Intelligence Scale (WAIS-III) or the Test of Variables of Attention (TOVA). These tests can indicate in which areas your patient is deficient. The following is a list of the attention areas and those tests that can be used to identify problem areas:

- Focused attention: The symbol search subtest of the WAIS-III Trail Making Tests

- Sustained attention: The symbol digit coding of the WAIS-III, TOVA

- Shifting attention: The Developmental Eye Movement (DEM) Saccadic Fixation Test from Bernell Corporation

- Selective attention: The Stroop test measures the speed at which an individual can read a set of color names that are printed on letters of a conflicting color (e.g., the word "red" is printed in blue ink (Sohlberg, 1989).

- Divided attention: The Letter-Number Sequencing Subtest of the WAIS-III.

Another way to accomplish this is to take one of the exercises from each of the categories in this book, see how well the patient can perform them, and use this as a baseline. You do not have any statistics, but the patient's performance will give you an idea of how difficult it is for him or her to do each of these categories.

Which Areas Do You Train First or Do You Train All of Them at the Same Time?

A quick answer is no. You do not train all the areas at the same time. By doing this, you may actually make matters worse.

I am listing all the attention areas in their order of simplicity:

- Focused
- Sustained
- Shifting
- Selective
- Divided

A study (Sturm, 1997) showed that with nonspecific training (training all at the same time), there was a high number of patients who either did not show any significant change in performance or even deteriorated significantly. This study supports the hypothesis of a hierarchical organization of attention functions. This was previously listed with focused first and divided last. The lower levels are prerequisite for higher-level functions. Impairments on a given level can only be approached by training in the same or subordinate level. In other words, if you train all the levels at the same time, the higher-level training could interfere with the lower-levels' training. However, if you train the lower levels first, then they are beneficial prerequisites for the higher levels.

Therefore, to start an attention training program:

1. Determine which areas to train.

2. Try to get baseline scores, for example, the TOVA for sustained attention.

3. Have a plan and set goals.

THE TRAINING PROGRAM

The activities in the next section were taken from research studies in various journal articles, were designed by myself, or were taken from three books (Dehn, 2008; Pickering, 2006; Sohlberg, 2001).

The possibility of activities is endless, and a good therapist should be able to develop his or her own. For example, go-no-go activities to help train a child to control his or her impulses should be part of every training program. The best example of this type of activity was the famous "Marshmallow Study" from the 1960s in which a researcher would place a marshmallow in front of a hungry 4 year old and tell the child that he or she could eat the marshmallow right then or have two if he or she waited until the researcher returned. About one-third of the children could distract themselves and wait. Followed for years, these highly disciplined kids had better school outcomes and scored more than 200 points higher on the SAT than the children who shoved the marshmallow into their mouths right away. Children today are in need of this type of training. It is suggested that you modify some of these activities to a go-no-go format.

This type of program can be very effective. This was shown by research studies that found that children who received this type of training 20 minutes a day, compared to a control group who did not, had increases in prefrontal and parietal areas associated with working memory (Olesen, Westerberg, & Klingberg, 2004).

SUMMARY AND ATTENTION TIPS

1. Do not use these activities as a separate program. Add them to your existing program.

2. Identify which areas need to be trained.

3. Do specific training, starting with the lower levels and working up to the more advanced areas, such as divided attention. Do not use a "shotgun" approach and train all of the areas at the same time.

4. Try to get baseline scores from previous testing.

5. Set goals, and then develop your program to achieve these goals.

REFERENCES

Dehn, M. J. (2008.) *Working memory and academic learning.* New York, NY: John Wiley and Sons.

Olesen, P. J., Westerberg, H., & Klingberg, T. (2004). Increased prefrontal and parietal activity after training working memory. *Nature Neuroscience, 7*(1), 75-79.

Pickering, S. J. (2006). *Working memory and education.* Philadelphia, PA: Elsevier.

Richards, J. E. & Holley, F. B. (1999). Infant attention and the development of smooth pursuit tracking. *Developmental Psychology, 35*(3), 856-867.

Sohlberg, M., & Mateer, C. (1989). *Introduction to cognitive rehabilitation: theory and practice.* New York, NY: The Guilford Press.

Sohlberg, M. (2001). *Cognitive rehabilitation: an integrative neuropsychological approach.* New York, NY: The Guilford Press,

Sturm, W. (1997). Do specific attention deficits need specific training? *Neuropsychological Rehabilitation, 7*(2), 81-103.

Attention Training Activities

Lane, K. A. *Visual Attention in Children:*
Theories and Activities (pp. 135-206).
© 2012 SLACK Incorporated.

HOW TO USE THE MASKS

The following two pages show the mask targets. You can also make your own. The purpose of a mask is to delay the child's response to an exercise. Before the child answers, show him or her a mask for a few seconds, and then have him or her answer the specific exercise.

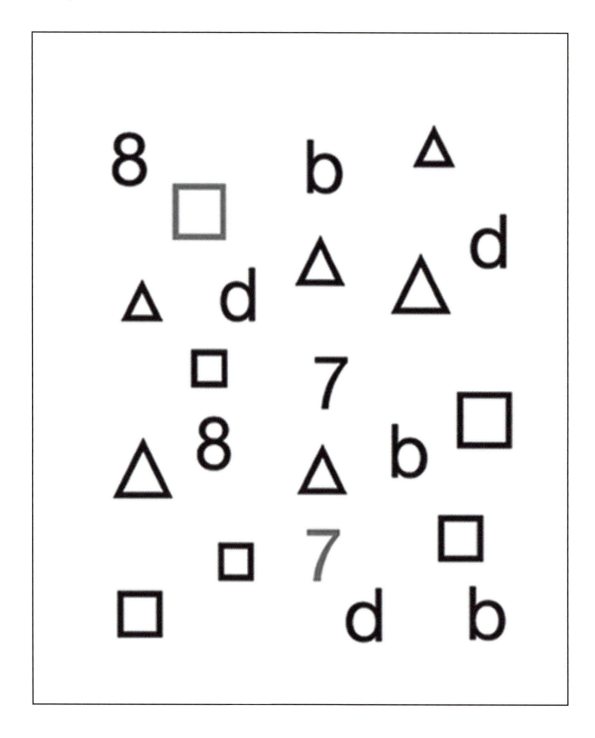

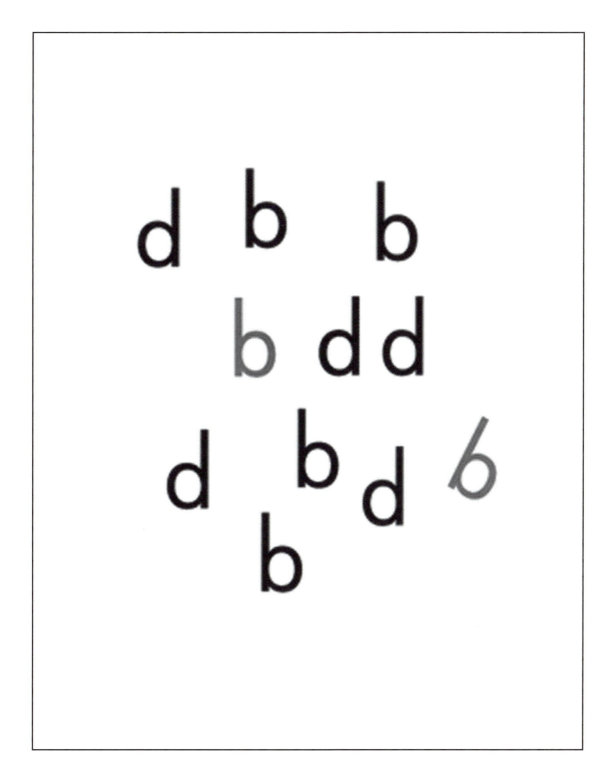

FOCUSED ATTENTION

Pursuits

The next four activities involve pursuits. You will need to laminate the page from this book and attach it to a flat stick (like a paint stirrer) with a small clamp, or hold it with one hand. Sit directly in front of the child, and hold the target about 3 feet in front of him or her. He or she should start these activities with one eye patched. When he or she has successfully done them with one eye, switch to the other eye and then finally both eyes at the same time. He or she is not to move his or her head, only his or her eyes. Move the target in horizontal or small circular directions. Do not move it very fast. Ask questions like the ones provided in the activities.

The masks are to be used directly before the child answers the question. They are only held for a few seconds.

Pencil/Marsden Ball Pursuits

Area of attention: Focused

Materials: Marsden ball, pencil, and eye patch or occluder. This activity must be completed before you go on to the other pursuit activities.

Procedure 1: Sit in front of the child. Start by having the child wear an eye patch. Slowly move the pencil in a left-to-right direction in front of the child at about 3 feet. Do not go more than 2 feet in his or her peripheral vision. The child is to follow the pencil with his or her eye and not move his or her head or body. When the child can do it without any difficulty, put the patch on the other eye and repeat the procedure.

Procedure 2: Have the child lying under the ball that you are holding. Hold it about 3 feet above the child's head. Slowly swing the ball in a left-to-right direction.

Reversals and Pursuits

Area of attention: Focused

Materials: Four rows of letters and numbers reversed and in different colors

Procedure: Have the child seated in front of you with one eye covered. Hold the target about 3 feet in front of him or her and slowly move it in a horizontal left-to-right motion. He or she is not to move his or her head, only his or her eyes. As you move the target, ask him or her questions, such as:

1. Call out all the letters in a left-to-right direction, starting with the top row.

2. Call out all the red letters or red numbers.

3. Call out all the blue numbers.

Ways to modify: Use a figure ground target (a mask) over the target.

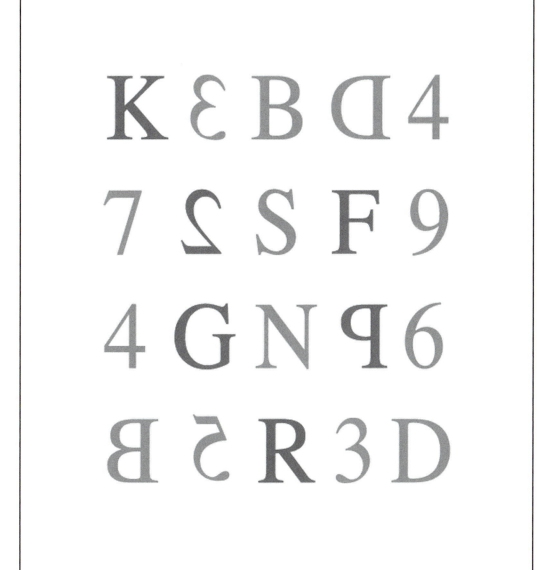

To see this image in color, please see page CA-1.

Pursuit Target

Area of attention: Focused

Materials: Pursuit targets, eye patch, mask target. There are three targets with this activity.

1.   Find R among Ps and Qs.

2.   Find the vertical line among other lines.

3.   Find the circle without a line among circles with lines.

Procedure: Follow the directions for doing pursuit training. Remember the child should not move his or her head or body, only his or her eyes.

Ways to modify: Use the figure ground target (mask) over it or turn the target upside down.

P Q R P P Q Q R P Q P R Q P

R R P P Q P Q P R P Q P P Q

Q Q Q P R P R P Q P R P Q P

P Q P Q P P Q P R P Q P R P

P Q P P Q P R P Q R P P Q P

R R P P Q Q Q R P P P Q P Q

P Q P P P Q P R P P Q P Q P

Pursuit Target *(continued)*

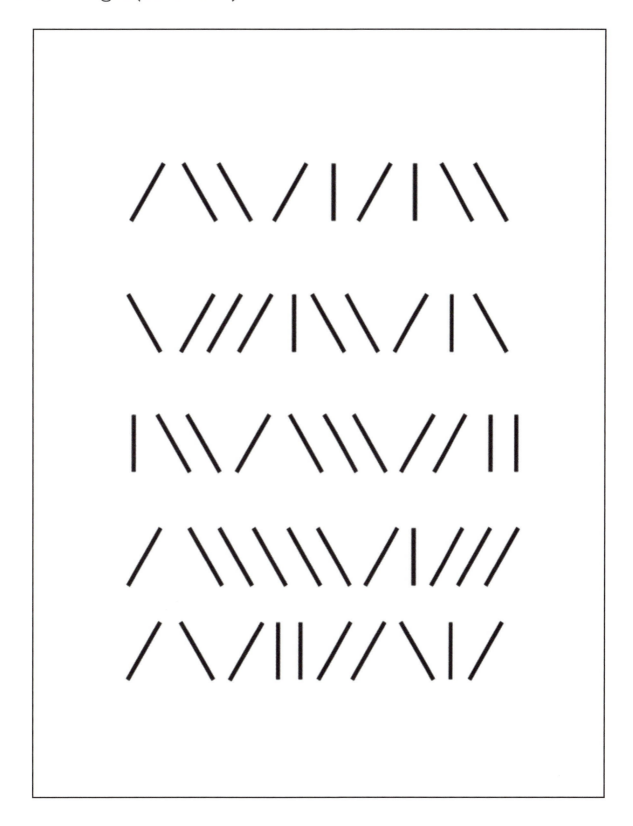

Pursuit Target (continued)

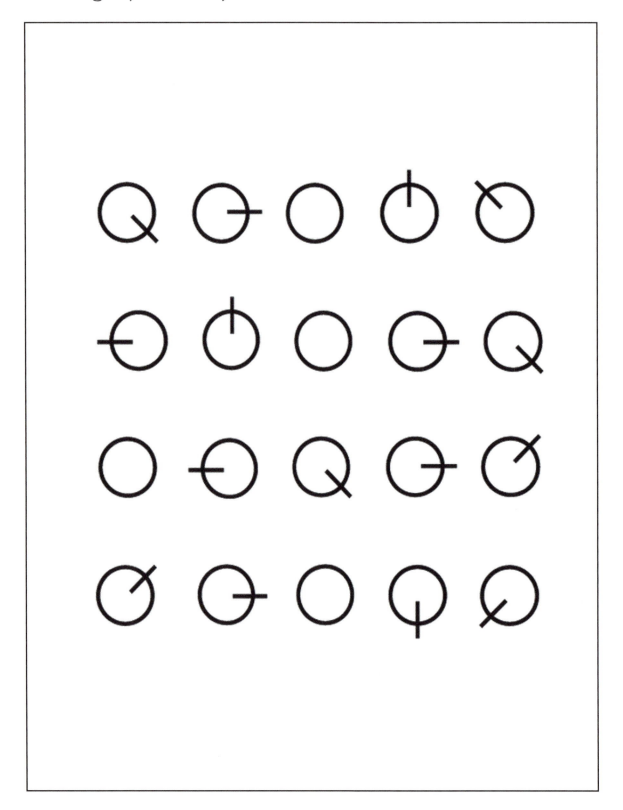

Pursuit

Area of attention: Focused

Materials: Pursuit target with colored figures or shapes

Procedure: Do the pursuits as they were explained at the beginning of this section. Remember, do not move the target too fast or too far away from the patient. Keep it about 3 feet in front of him or her and no more than 2 feet in his or her peripheral vision. Ask him or her questions, such as

1. How many red squares do you see?

2. How many blue triangles, etc.?

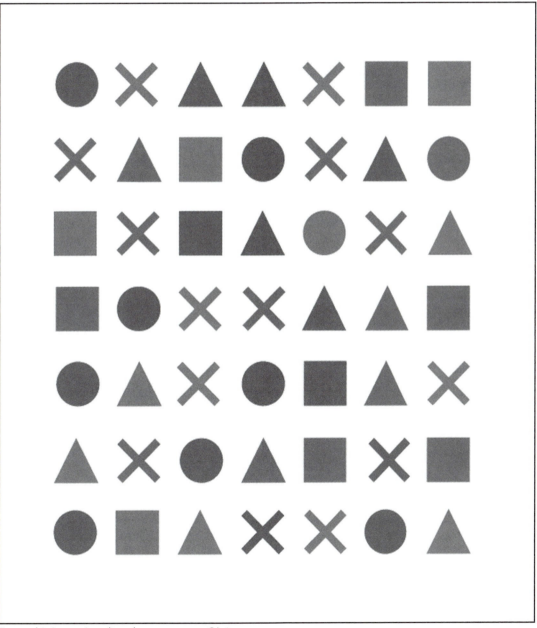

To see this image in color, please see page CA-1.

From Lane, K. A. (2012). *Visual Attention in Children: Theories and Activities*. Thorofare, NJ: SLACK Incorporated. © 2012 SLACK Incorporated.

Two-Colored Letters

Area of attention: Focused

Materials: Targets with colored letters, mask

Procedure: Briefly show the child the target card with the colored letters and then the mask (the H). Ask him or her questions. For example:

1. What was the color of the letter on the top right?

2. What letters were on the card?

3. Name the colors of the two letters.

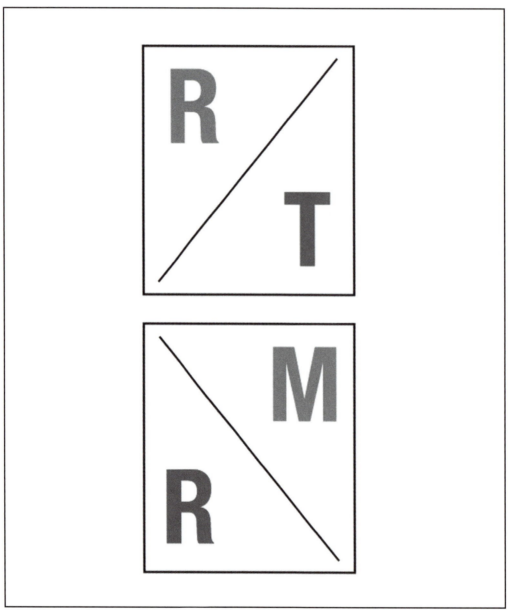

To see this image in color, please see page CA-2.

Two-Colored Letters (continued)

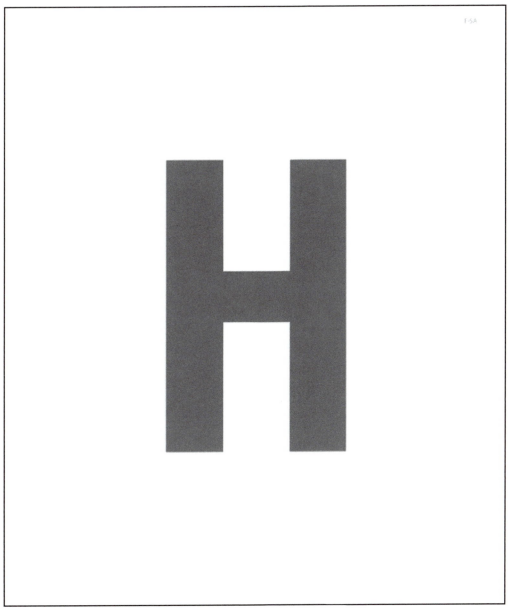

To see this image in color, please see page CA-2.

Delayed Match

Area of attention: Focused

Materials: Crowded target, targets with several letters or numbers

Procedure: Have the child seated in front of you. Show him or her one of the targets. Let him or her look at it for about 3 seconds and then take it away. Then, hold up the crowded target. He is to point out the locations of the letters or numbers in the original target.

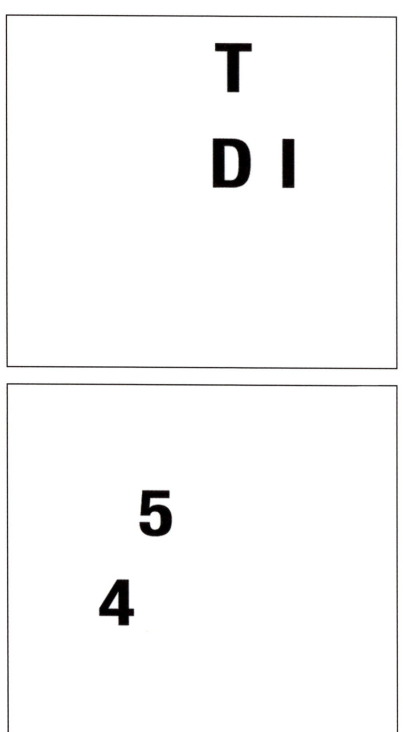

H

D 8

R 3 K T 6 P

J D 5 D I M

W 4 7 H J I

L E 9 D 8 C

Shape and Colors

Area of attention: Focused

Materials: Shape and color worksheet

Procedure: Have the child seated about 3 feet in front of you. Briefly show him or her the target (about 5 seconds), and then ask him or her questions such as the following:

1. Which line was the red C on?

2. What was the location of the black upside down T?

3. Which line had the backward F?

4. How many red letters did you see?

5. How many Ts did you see?

Ways to modify: You can use a mask. You can repeat the 5-second showing when the child cannot correctly give any more responses.

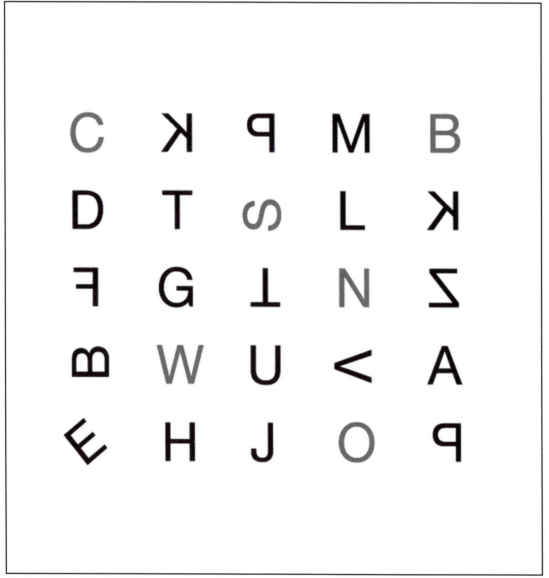

To see this image in color, please see page CA-2.

From Lane, K. A. (2012). *Visual Attention in Children: Theories and Activities.* Thorofare, NJ: SLACK Incorporated. © 2012 SLACK Incorporated.

Go-No-Go

Area of attention: Focused

Materials: Pen light, stopwatch

Procedure: The purpose of this exercise is to teach the child to inhibit his or her responses. Have the child sit across the table from you. You have a pen light and flash it a number of times. The child must tap his or her left hand the same number of times as the flash. However, after you flash the pen light, hold up the number of fingers that you want him or her to wait in seconds before he or she taps the answer. For example, you flash the pen light five times and hold up five fingers. He or she must wait 5 seconds before he or she taps his or her left hand five times.

Ways to modify: Not only must he or she wait until the first tap of his or her left hand, he or she has to wait that period of time between each tap.

Under and Over

Area of attention: Focused

Materials: White board or paper with rows of numbers

Procedure: Tell the child to draw a line over each even number and under each odd number. The patient is to try to not hit any of the numbers.

Ways to modify: You can use letters and numbers and go over the letters and under the numbers.

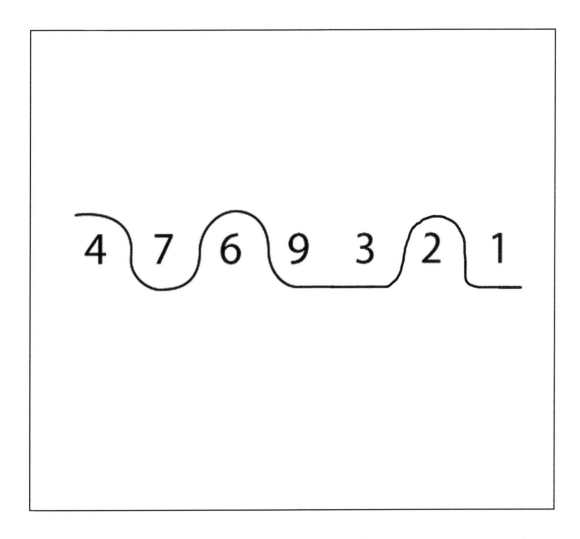

Conjunctions

Area of attention: Focused

Materials: A diamond configuration of colored shapes.

Procedure: Quickly show the patient the target (about 2 seconds), and then take it away. The patient must answer questions concerning the target. For example:

1.   How many red shapes were there?

2.   How many squares were there?

3.   Were there more blue or red shapes?

4.   What was the shape and color of the one on the bottom?

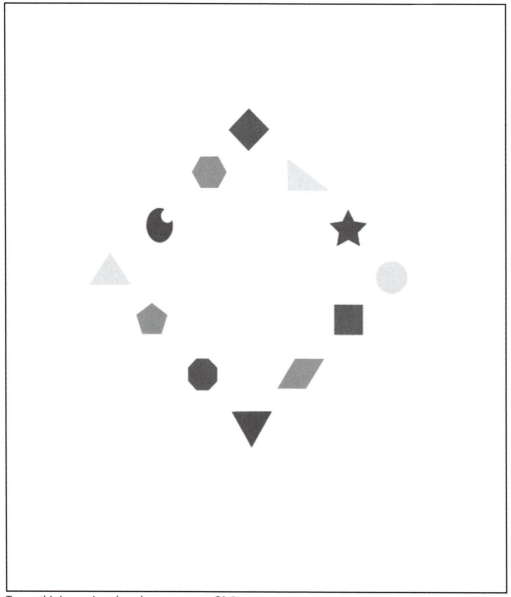

To see this image in color, please see page CA-2.

Reverse Order or Not

Area of attention: Focused

Materials: Numbers in sequence on index cards, 4 to 6 inches in length

    For example: 7   6   9   2   1

Procedure: Show the child the numbers. Then, ask him or her to remember their sequence. The difference in this exercise is that he or she will not know which order (forward or reverse) you want him or her to repeat them until after you take the card away. Because this is difficult, give him or her a little extra time when you show him or her the numbers. Start with just three numbers and work up to five numbers.

Ways to modify: You can use a combination of letters and numbers instead of just numbers.

Letters Up or Down?

Area of attention: Focused

Materials: Flash card with a single letter on it

Procedure: Time the child's response and see how fast he or she can do 10 of these. Make it a contest and keep his or her scores. Show the child one letter at a time, and then say either up or down. Up means that he or she has to name the next letter in the alphabet. Down means that he or she has to name the letter that proceeds the letter in the alphabet. For example, "K" down would be "J."

Ways to modify: Do two up or two down. So, up would be two letters after the letter, and down would be two letters before the letter.

Timed Search

Area of attention: Focused

Materials: Target with random letters and numbers and a metronome

Procedure: Hold the target in front of the child. When he or she hears the beat of the metronome, he or she is to call out one of the letters or numbers for each beat. He or she must not repeat any. You will need to record his or her answers to keep track of his or her responses. If he or she repeats any, start over. You may also have him or her alternate from black to color or just colored targets.

To see this image in color, please see page CA-3.

Arm Angles

Area of attention: Focused

Materials: The patient has a sheet with angles.

Procedure: The therapist goes through a series of arm movements using only his or her right arm. After he or she has completed his or her movements, the child must remember them and find the correct sequence on the sheet in front of him or her. Start with three and try to work up to seven. A dot is your fist held straight out. A dot on top of a line is your arm held straight up, etc.

Ways to modify: You can try using two arms and the child has to remember the correct sequence of both arms at the same time.

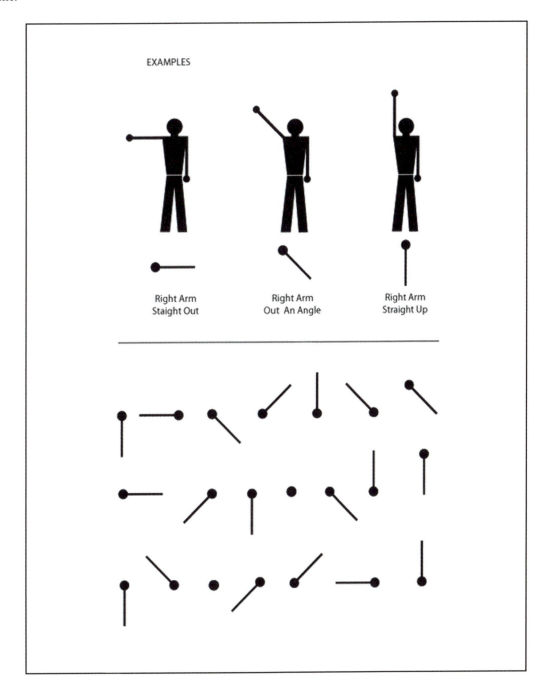

Magazine Picture

Area of attention: Focused

Materials: Full-page picture from a magazine

Procedure: Show the child a picture and let him or her look at for a full minute, and then take it away. Make 10 questions and see how many he or she can correctly answer. For example, "How many people were in the picture? What was the color of the car?"

Ways to modify: Let him or her make notes about the picture before you take it away. He or she can look at his or her notes for help.

Find the "B"

Area of attention: Focused

Materials: Index cards with all "d"s except one "b," and one "d" is red

Procedure: Show the child the card, and see how quickly he or she can find the "b." The chances are he or she will go to the red "d" first. Make several cards to vary the exercises.

Ways to modify: You can use a mask overlay to make it more difficult.

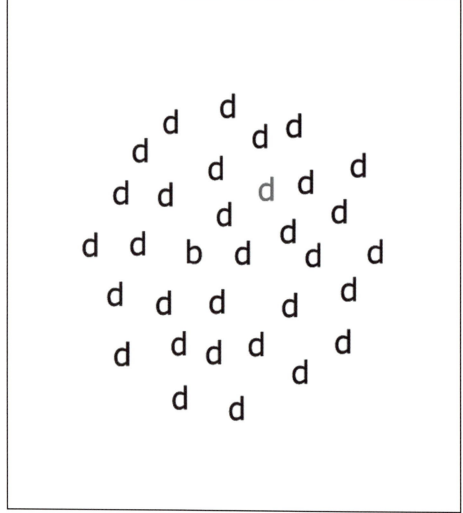

To see this image in color, please see page CA-3.

Size, Position, Orientation, Color

Area of attention: Focused

Materials: Size, position chart. This chart is made of many different figures and shapes of different colors and orientations.

Procedure: Sit across from the patient, and put the worksheet in front of him or her. Call out a specific target, for example, "small green square," and see how long it takes him or her to find it. Make up different choices, for example, "What is the figure to the left of the red triangle?"

Ways to modify: You can use an overlay on this to make it more difficult.

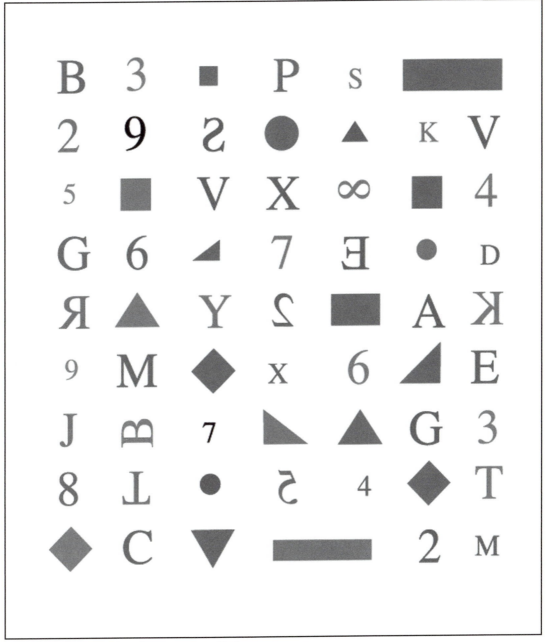

To see this image in color, please see page CA-4.

From Lane, K. A. (2012). *Visual Attention in Children: Theories and Activities.* Thorofare, NJ: SLACK Incorporated. © 2012 SLACK Incorporated.

Dark Rotations

Area of attention: Focused

Materials: Stool that rotates, pen light, laser pointer, or flashlight

Procedure: Have the child on the stool holding a laser pointer straight out in front of him or her. The lights are on. Point out a target such as a lamp, and rotate him or her until the pointer is on it. Now, he or she closes his or her eyes, and you turn the stool. He or she keeps his or her arm and pointer straight ahead. See if he or she can remember how far you rotated the stool. He or she is to slowly rotate it keeping his or her eyes closed until he or she feels the laser pointer is shining on the target. The child then opens his or her eyes to see if he or she was correct.

Ways to modify: You can turn the stool more than one rotation.

Arrow Clues

Area of attention: Focused

Materials: Index cards with arrows and clues. One arrow and two clues per card.

Procedure: Briefly show the child the card as he or she is seated in front of you. He or she is to name the letter the arrow is pointing to but not the other letter. If the arrow is pointing up or to a shape, he or she does not say anything. Make as many cards as you can to keep the stimulus fresh.

$$B \rightarrow A = A$$

$$R \uparrow D = \text{Nothing}$$

$$T O \leftarrow = O$$

$$\square \leftarrow E = \text{Nothing}$$

Color and Shape 1

Area of attention: Focused

Materials: Paper with colored figures

Procedure: Put the paper with colored figures in front of the child. He or she is to start at the top left line and, as quickly as he or she can, go left-to-right without using his or her finger. He or she is to call out the color and direction of each arrow and the shape and color to which it is pointing. If the arrow is pointing down or up, he or she is to name the colors and shape of both figures on either side of the arrow.

Ways to modify: You can use a mask target right after you show him or her the two figures. You can increase the time you show him or her the figures.

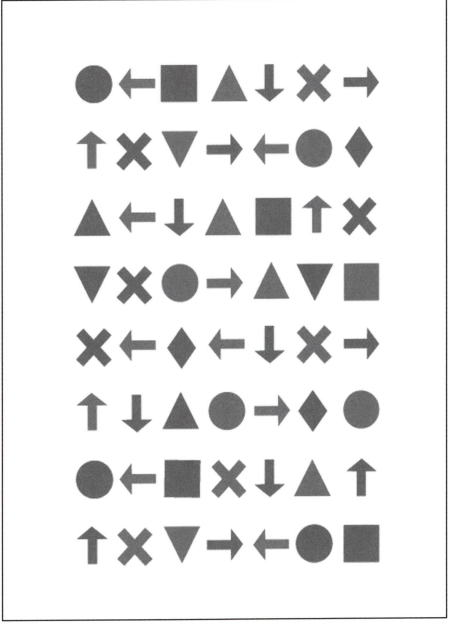

To see this image in color, please see page CA-4.

Color and Shape 2

Area of attention: Focused

Material: Target with colored letters around an "X"

Procedure: Tell the child to look at the "X." He or she is not to take his or her eyes from the "X." While he or she is looking at the "X," ask him or her questions, such as:

1. How many red letters are there?

2. Name the blue figures.

3. What is the figure at 2 o'clock?

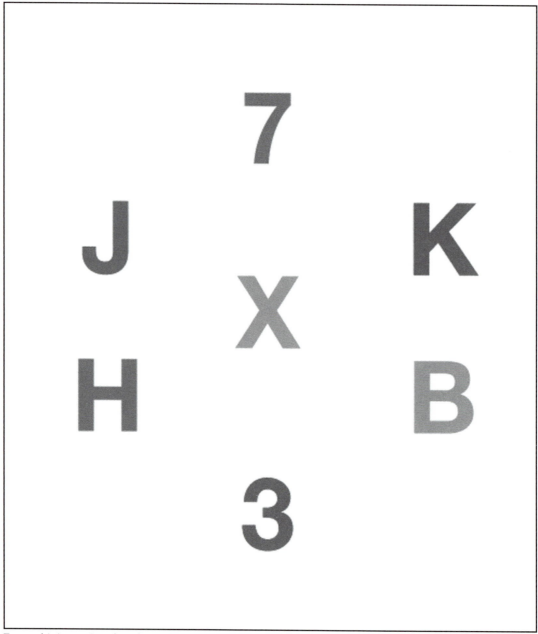

To see this image in color, please see page CA-4.

Divided Stimuli

Area of attention: Focused

Materials: Targets of stimuli and mask. Make more of these on index cards.

Procedure: Briefly (2 seconds) show the child the target with three figures and then the mask for 2 seconds. After you show the mask, ask him or her questions, such as:

1. "What was the direction of the tilted line in the left figure (toward or away from the opening)?"
2. "Was the line in the center figure tilted toward the opening?"

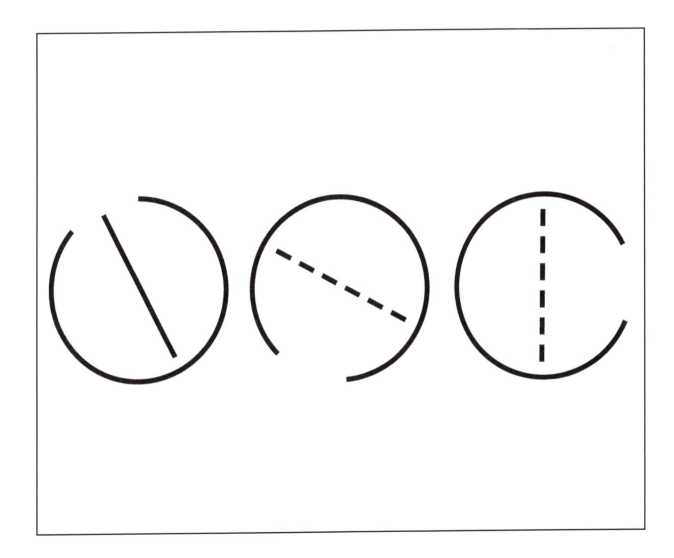

Magazine Picture and Hole

Area of attention: Focused

Materials: Page from a magazine, sheet of paper with a ½-inch hole in its center. Make sure the paper is much larger than the magazine picture.

Procedure: Have the child close his or her eyes as you put the paper over the magazine picture. Hold the paper so the hole is over the center of the picture. Slowly move the hole over the picture until he or she can tell you what the picture is. The key is to move the hole slowly and not let him or her see any of the picture except through the hole.

Ways to modify: You can use a larger hole or have two holes, each ½ inch.

Arrows

Area of attention: Focused

Materials: Index cards with arrows in groups of five—some with tails and some without tails

Procedure: Have the child sitting across the table from you. Show him or her one of the rows for about 2 seconds (longer, if necessary). When you take the card away, the child will raise his or her right hand if he or she sees three out of five with tails. He or she will raise his or her left hand if he or she sees three out of five without tails. If he or she sees no tails, he or she does not raise a hand.

Ways to modify: Add color to one of the arrows to catch his or her attention. If raising a hand is difficult for the patient to learn, he or she can tell you if three out of five had tails, etc., and not raise a hand.

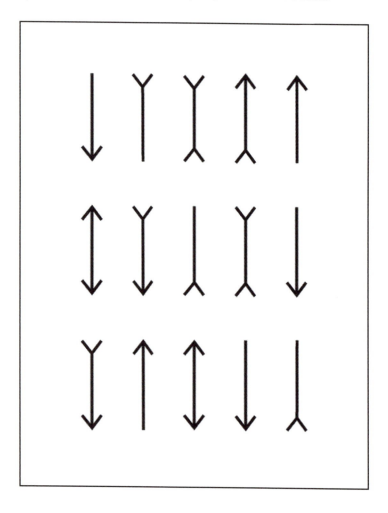

SUSTAINED ATTENTION

High Card One Back

Area of attention: Sustained

Materials: Two decks of cards

Procedure: Have the child seated across the table from you. Have a deck of cards face down in front of each of you. You each turn a card over (face up). You start this activity on the second card. If he or she turns over a card that is not as high as your card, he or she has to tell you what your previous card was. For example, you show a 10 and then a jack, and the jack is higher than his or her card. He or she has to say 10. If both cards are the same or if his or her card is higher than yours, then he or she says nothing, and the activity continues. It is only if your card is higher than his or her card that he or she has to tell you your previous card.

Find the Word

Area of attention: Sustained

Materials: Page from a book, an index card with five to seven words

Procedure: The child sits at a table and has a page from a book in front of him or her. You show him or her an index card with one to seven words on it that are on the page in front of him or her. The child has 5 to 10 seconds to memorize the words. Now, take the list of words away, and tell him or her to find the words on the page of print in front of him or her. The child cannot use his or her finger. If the child forgets some of the words, use another page, and do it again but without as many words for him or her to memorize.

Ways to modify: Make it selective by adding music as background noise.

Alphabetize

Area of attention: Sustained

Materials: A page from a book

Procedure: Start with the first sentence, and have the child put the words in alphabetical order. Once he or she has had done the first sentence, have him or her continue with the second sentence. For young patients, just use the first letter of the words to put in alphabetical order.

Ways to modify: You could make the activity selective by having him or her listen to a CD story while he or she is doing this.

Letter Flash

Area of attention: Sustained

Materials: Cards with single letters on them

Procedure: You show the child a card with a letter on it. He or she has to quickly name as many animals or objects that start with that letter. This really trains the executive function but, by doing this for 5 to 10 minutes, we can train the sustained system as well as the executive. Do not show him or her the next card until he or she can name at least five animals or objects. Keep track of his or her answers. He or she is not to use the same word twice.

N–Back

Area of attention: Sustained

Materials: Deck of cards

Procedure: N can vary from 2 to any number. The child turns over the top card of a deck of cards that is laying face down. If you designate N as 2, this means that when he or she turns over a face card, he or she has to remember and tell you the identity of the number card that was 2 before the face card. Mix the deck so that the first two cards he or she turns over are number cards, and then he or she proceeds through the deck of cards. For example, if he or she turned over 7, then 10, then a jack, he says that N is 7. For very young patients, you could even make N = 1, and he has to remember the last number card before the face card.

From Lane, K. A. (2012). *Visual Attention in Children: Theories and Activities*. Thorofare, NJ: SLACK Incorporated. © 2012 SLACK Incorporated.

Red/Green Pursuits

Area of attention: Sustained

Materials: Red/green glasses, p-d-p-q target

Procedure: The child sits across from you at a table. He or she has the red/green glasses on. You hold the card in front of the child, and he or she covers the left eye. You slowly move the card in a horizontal direction, and he or she starts on the top line and calls out the letters in correct sequence. (With the red/green glasses, he or she will only see every other letter.) Continue this after a few times by having him or her cover the other eye and do the same procedure. He or she will now see the letters not seen on the first try. After a few tries, have him or her do it with both eyes open. He or she should see all the letters. Some may look like they fade but he or she should see all of them. If he or she cannot see some of the letters, this means that the child is not using one of his or eyes and should have an eye examination.

The patient should not move his or her head or body, only his or her eyes. He or she is to correctly call the letters starting in the top row left side and proceed in a left-to-right sequence.

```
pdpqanxdpctdbpv
pklpddbppdpqdbbp
dpbyfgpdbqbbkhjc
rwhsmddbgjkepqdi
bpdrtbnmqzsbpqqd
ppqqhjuirdbmnitsn
jilpbbdqqfcgtsprqp
pfgdpcqqspdlmnop
tvqqddppbbrsbnqp
pbbqbgrddphqrstxv
```

To see this image in color, please see page CA-5.

The Wall

Area of attention: Sustained

Materials: A square piece of wood with holes cut into it. The holes should be in rows. The side facing the therapist has numbers under the holes to help the therapist remember the proper sequence. The patient's side does not have numbers.

Procedure: The therapist puts his or her finger through the holes in a sequence. Start with three and work up to seven. The child must remember the holes, and when the therapist tells him or her, he or she must put his or her fingers through the same holes in the same order. Have the patient use his or her left hand for this activity.

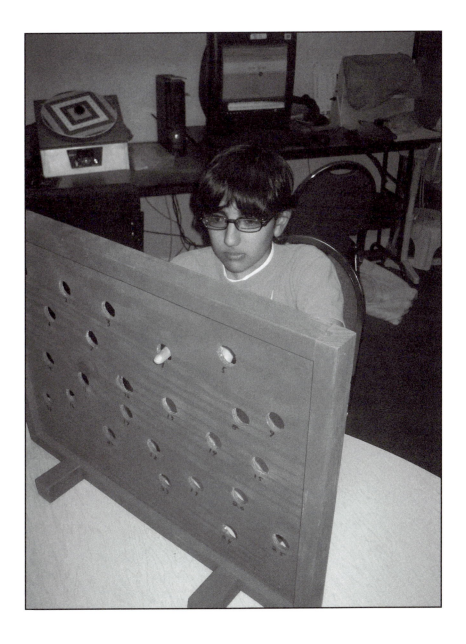

Shape Drawing

Area of attention: Sustained

Materials: Paper and pencil

Procedure: The child is to draw as many shapes as he or she can in a period of time. He or she cannot scribble. It must be a shape, and they must all be different. This is harder than it seems. Start with 3 minutes as a period of time, and then increase the time to 10 or 15 minutes.

Playing Cards and Sequence

Area of attention: Sustained

Materials: Playing cards, two decks

Procedure: Put 10 cards from one deck face up in a row. Have the child look them over for a period of time and turn them face down, keeping them in a row. The child takes the second deck of cards and starts to turn them over (face up). When he or she sees one of the cards that is in the sequence (face down) in front of him or her, he or she has to remember its location and turn it over. If the child is correct, the card is taken from the row and put back in the deck. If he or she picks the wrong card, the card goes back in sequence face down, and he or she continues. When he or she has correctly found all the cards, the activity is over.

Dominoes—Cards

Area of attention: Sustained

Materials: Dominoes, playing cards

Procedure: This is similar to "Playing Cards and Sequence," except the dominoes are used instead of one deck of cards. Show the child the dots on the dominoes and how they translate into numbers. For example, four dots are the same as the number 4. Because dominoes have two ends with numbers, it is the total number of dots on the domino that is the number used. For example, a domino with two dots on each half is the same as the number 4. Put 10 dominoes in a random order in front of the patient. Let him or her look it over for a period of time, and then turn the dominoes over. Now, take a deck of cards (face down), and have the child turn a card over. If its number is the same as one of the dominoes, he or she has to remember the location of that domino and turn it over. If he or she is wrong, the domino is turned back face down. If he or she is right, the domino is taken away. Face cards do not count and are not used, except an ace, which is the same as 1.

Disorganized Letters and Numbers

Area of attention: Sustained

Materials: Chart with random letters and numbers, metronome

Procedure: The child is to alternate between the letters and numbers. He or she cannot go in a sequence. At the beat of the metronome, he or she is to call out a letter, then a number, and continue in this fashion. The key is that he or she is not to repeat any. You will have to keep track. He or she is not to repeat the same letter or number twice.

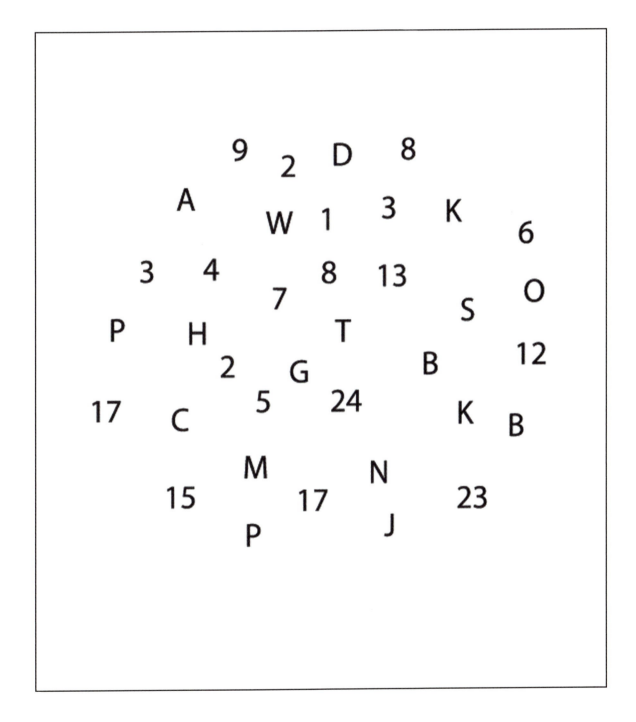

Make That Number

Area of attention: Sustained

Materials: Dominoes

Procedure: Have the child seated across the table from you. Tell the child that you want him or her to use his or her dominoes to add up to a certain number. The child can use any pattern and any domino he or she wants. The areas of the dominoes that touch must add up to the number you say. The key to this exercise is that you are going to limit the number of dominoes he or she can use. For example, "I want you to use only four dominoes and add up to the number 15." Remember, you add the number of dots from the ends that touch.

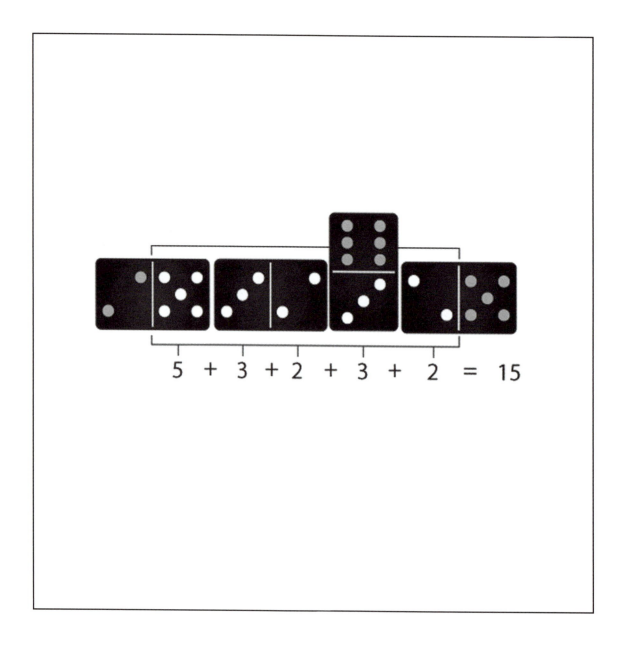

Ascending/Descending Letters and Numbers

Area of attention: Sustained

Materials: A sequence of letters and numbers, such as $C_2 K_1 M_4 P_3$

Procedure: Depending on what number is next to the letter, the child has to call out the correct letter in ascending order. You can also do descending. For example: in ascending order the letter C would be the second letter in the sequence and K would be the first letter per the example under materials.

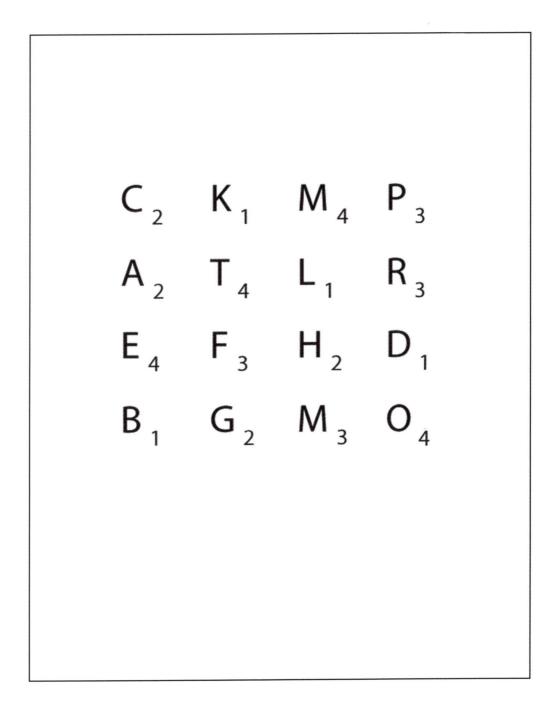

X Counting

Area of attention: Sustained

Materials: A sheet of paper with Xs in a row. Every few Xs, there is a + or a – sign, for example:

XXXX + XXX – XX + XXXX – XXXX = 5

You may have several rows of Xs to make it longer and more difficult. In fact, a whole page of these will make it more of a sustained test.

Procedure: Have the child start at the top row and count or subtract the Xs. You will have done this ahead of time and know the correct answer. Start with a single row and build up to a whole page.

Ways to modify: Have a CD player with a story at the same time he or she is counting.

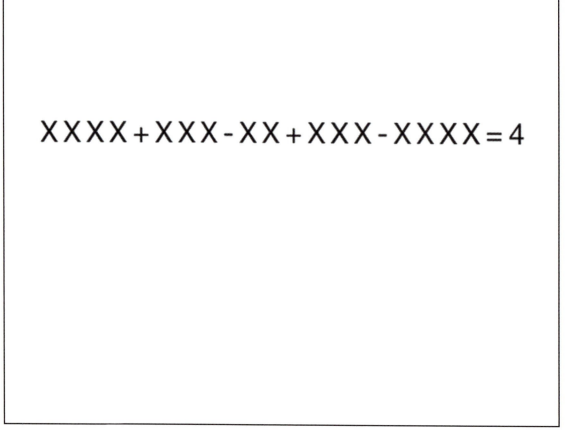

Target Card

Area of attention: Sustained

Materials: Two decks of playing cards

Procedure: You show the child several cards from your deck that will be his or her targets (for example, 2 of diamonds, 4 of clubs, king of spades) and then put them back into your deck. He or she is to remember the list and start to turn his or her cards over one at a time. When he or she sees one of the targets, he or she puts it face up and continues until he or she finds all of the target cards.

Estimate Time

Area of attention: Sustained

Materials: Stopwatch

Procedure: This is to teach the child to estimate time in seconds. Have him or her sit across from you, and you hold the stopwatch. Practice by showing 5 seconds and then 10 seconds. Now, tell him or her you want him or her to guess a certain amount of time. For example, "Raise your right hand, and hold it up for 15 seconds." When he or she drops his or her hand, show him or her the stopwatch to let him or her see how close he or she was to the correct time.

Withhold Response

Area of attention: Sustained

Materials: A page of print from a book

Procedure: The child must call out the letters of the words in a left-to-right sequence. Before he or she starts, tell him or her three letters that he or she must not name, for example, e, w, n. If he or she calls out any of these letters, the child has to start over. If three letters is too difficult, start with one letter.

Antisaccade

Area: Executive function

Materials: Two pen lights

Procedure: Stand in front of the child while holding two pen lights. The child is to stand by, fixating on your nose. Tell him or her that when you flash one of the pen lights once, he or she is to quickly move his or her eyes to the pen light and then back to your nose. If you flash one of the pen lights twice, he or she is to quickly move his or her eyes to the other pen light (the one not flashed) and then back to your nose.

SHIFTING ATTENTION

Near/Far Sequence

Area of attention: Shifting

Materials: Two targets with random letters and numbers in sequence. Both must have the same sequence. For example, both targets are: K   B   2   3   P   o   1   Q   C   T

Procedure: You hold one target about 6 feet from the child, and he or she holds the other target directly in front of him- or herself. At your command, he or she is to shift his or her eyes from his or her sheet to yours and call out the letters and numbers in the proper sequence. The child must alternate between his or hers and yours on every other figure. Time the child to see how quickly he or she can do this. Vary the targets at each session.

Cubes With Letters

Area of attention: Shifting

Materials: Purchase small cubes with letters or numbers on them.

Procedure: Dump the cubes on the table in front of the child. He or she is to point and move his or her eyes in the proper sequence from first letter in the alphabet to the last or the lowest number to the highest. Make a game of this, and see how fast he or she can do this exercise. Keep the child's score and see if he or she can beat it.

Delayed Saccades

Area of attention: Shifting

Materials: Index cards or white board with letters around an "X"

Procedure: Hold the card, or stand the child in front of the white board. Let the child look at it for about 3 to 5 seconds, and then cover the board or take the card away. The child must look at where the "X" was and not move his or her eyes until you tell him or her to move. Then, call out a letter, and he or she must make a quick movement to where that letter was located. When the child does this, he or she then moves his or her eyes back to where the "X" was located and waits for your instructions. It is a good idea to let the patient practice the eye movement a few times before you remove the card or cover the board.

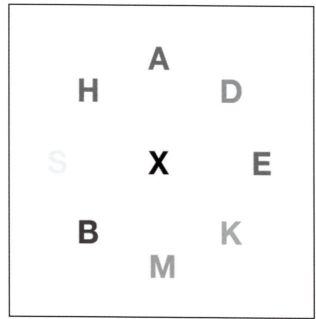

To see this image in color, please see page CA-5.

From Lane, K. A. (2012). *Visual Attention in Children: Theories and Activities.* Thorofare, NJ: SLACK Incorporated. © 2012 SLACK Incorporated.

Trail Making

Area of attention: Shifting

Materials: White board or chart in book, red/green glasses

Procedure: The child puts on the red/green glasses. He or she is to use his or her finger, and, as quickly as he or she can, connect the letters and numbers in the correct sequence. The sequence is first a number and then a letter, for example, 1-A, 2-B, 3-C, etc., until he or she finishes without losing his or her place. You can time the child and see how fast he or she can do this. Use a white board to vary the locations of the letters and numbers.

To see this image in color, please see page CA-6.

From Lane, K. A. (2012). *Visual Attention in Children: Theories and Activities.* Thorofare, NJ: SLACK Incorporated. © 2012 SLACK Incorporated.

Visual Motor Control Bat

Area of attention: Shifting

Materials: Visual motor control bat (a bat with colored sections), Marsden ball, balance trainer. (The example does not show colored sections. Put colored tape on bat. For example, blue on ends, then yellow, red, and white center.)

Procedure: Have the child hold the bat with both hands palm down as shown in the picture. You call out a color sequence, and he or she pushes the ball with the bat, hitting the ball with that colored portion of the bat you call out. While he or she is doing this, he or she is standing on the balance trainer. You call out a sequence, and he or she has to push the ball in the correct sequence, for example, red, blue, white, red, etc.

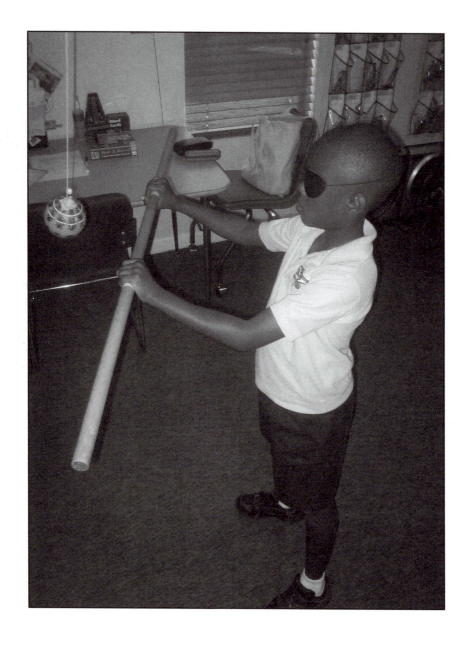

Alphabet Pencils

Area of attention: Shifting

Materials: Alphabet pencils (pencils with alphabet vertically on pencil)

Procedure: The child sits across a table from you. He or she is to use both of his or her eyes (binocular). Hold the pencils so they are about 1 foot apart. The patient is to start at the top of the left pencil and call out the top letter. He or she then quickly, without moving his or her head, moves his or her eyes to the right pencil and calls out the top letter. He continues to alternate between pencils, calling out all the letters from top to bottom. You can vary the positions of the pencils while he or she is doing this, for example, move the pencils 3 feet apart or slightly in front of the other pencil.

Ways to modify: Use a metronome, and the child must call out a letter at each beat. You can also do this one eye at the time before you go binocular. Remember that he or she cannot move his or her head or body, just his or her eyes.

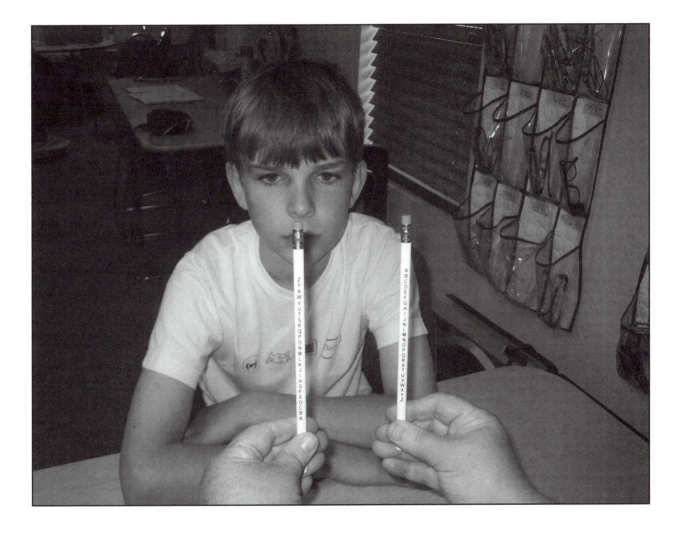

Occluder Numbers

Area of attention: Shifting

Materials: Index cards with a single number or letter. Make a way to partially occlude your card so only top of the letter or number is shown. Always occlude the bottom half, because the brain gets most of the information from the top half.

Procedure: Both you and the patient have cards with a single letter or number. Only your cards have the bottom half covered. The child's cards are in front of him or her and lying face up. You show one of your cards for a few (2) seconds, and he or she has to quickly find the same card in his or her stack of cards. The child's cards are not covered.

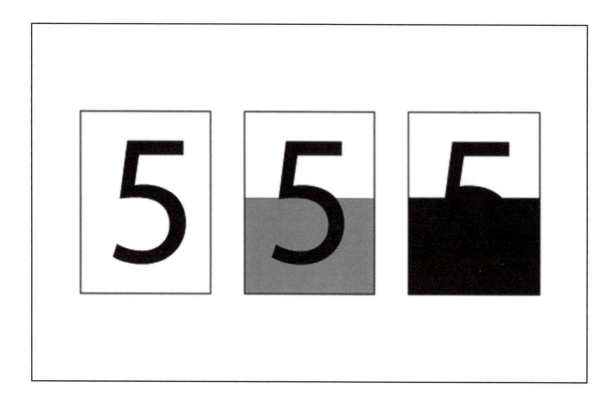

Color Atlas

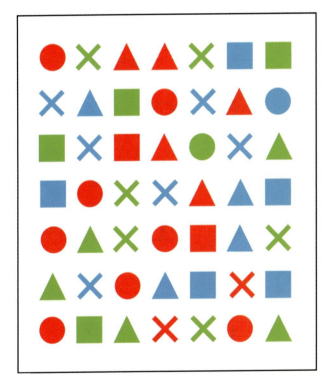

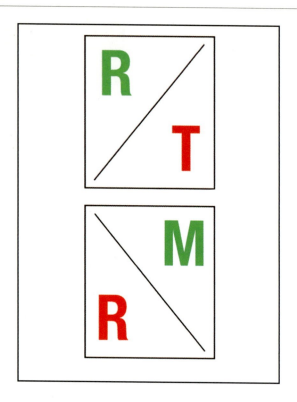

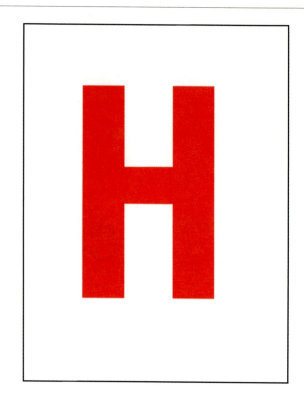

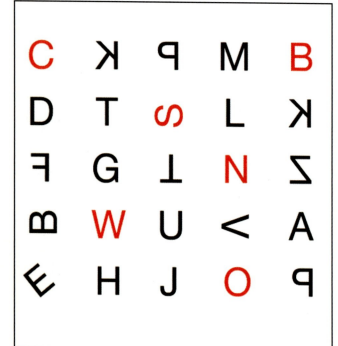

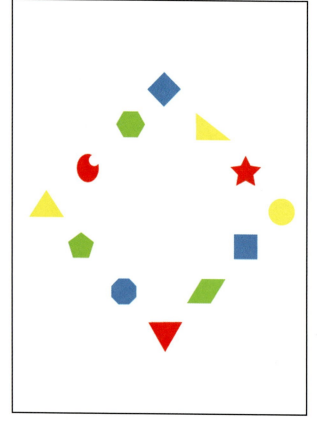

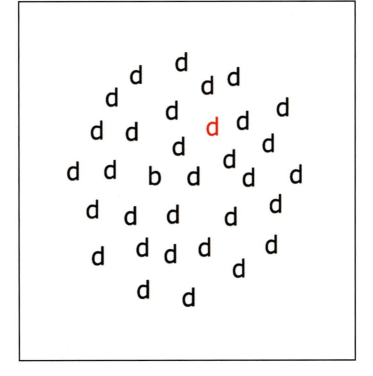

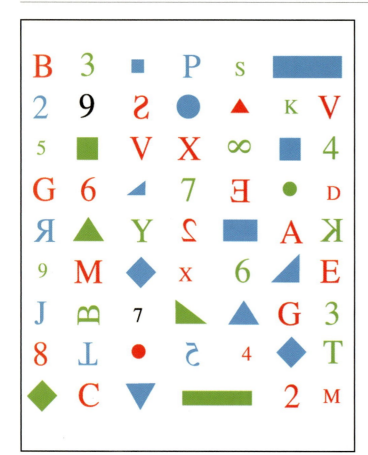

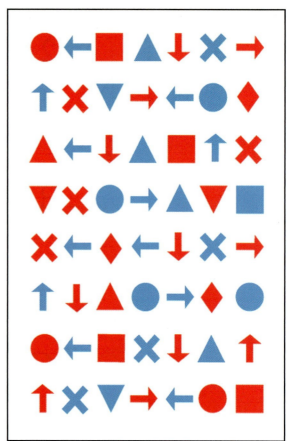

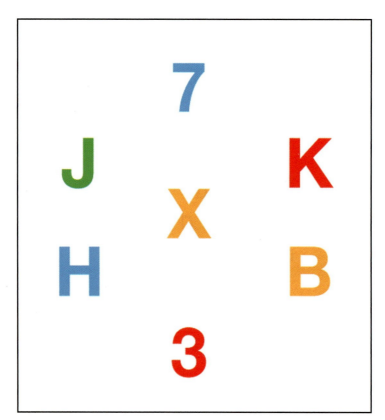

From Lane, K.A. (2012). *Visual Attention in Children: Theories and Activities.* Thorofare, NJ: SLACK Incorporated. © 2012 SLACK Incorporated.

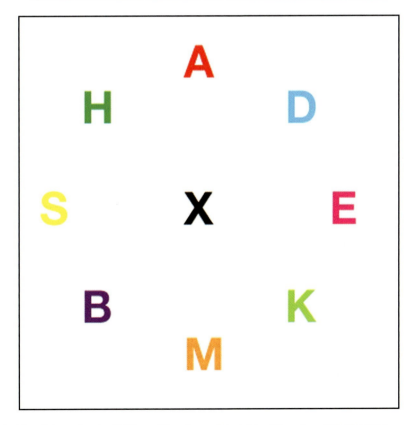

pdpqanxdpctdbpv
pklpddbppdpqdbbp
dpbyfgpdbqbbkhjc
rwhsmddbgjkepqdi
bpdrtbnmqzsbpqqd
ppqqhjuirdbmnitsn
jilpbbdqqfcgtsprqp
pfgdpcqqspdlmnop
tvqqddppbbrsbnqp
pbbqbgrddphqrstxv

A

H   D

S   X   E

B   K

M

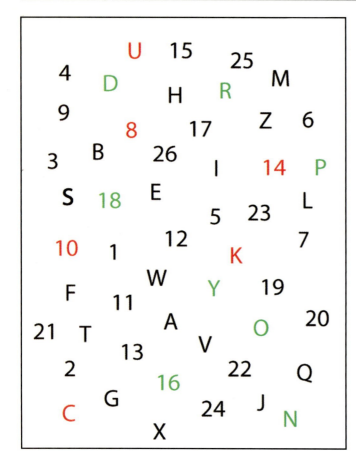

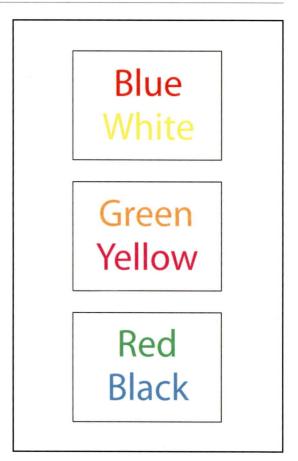

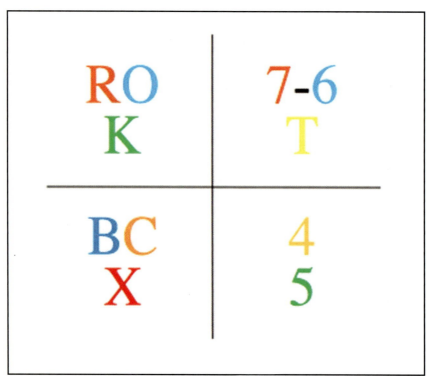

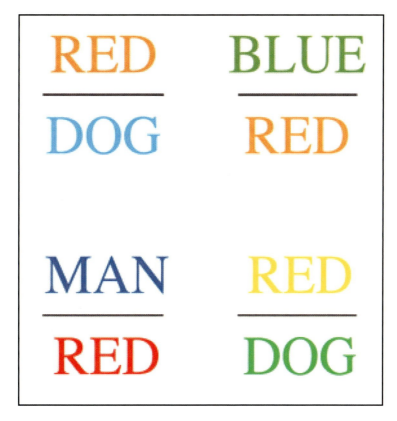

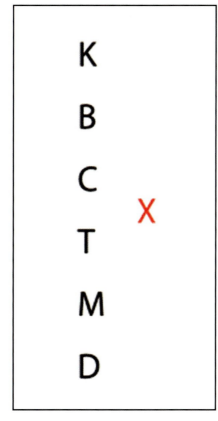

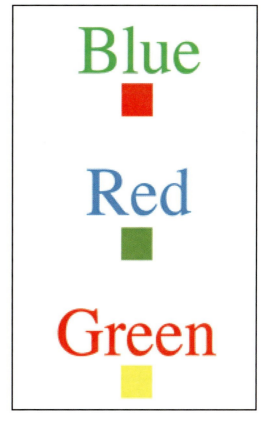

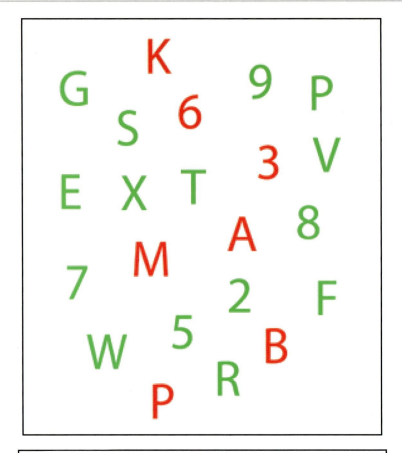

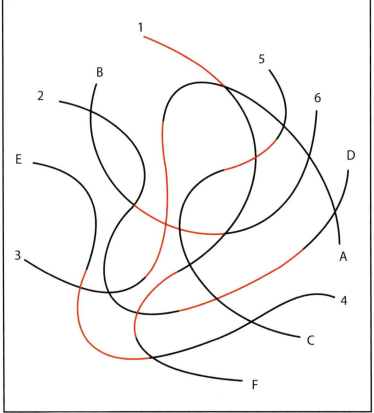

From Lane, K.A. (2012). *Visual Attention in Children: Theories and Activities.* Thorofare, NJ: SLACK Incorporated. © 2012 SLACK Incorporated.

Antisaccade

Area of attention: Shifting
Materials: White board, laser pointer, target with X in center:

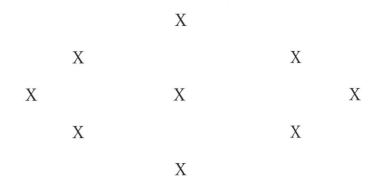

Procedure: The child looks at the center X. He or she is not to move his or her eyes off of the center X. You shine a laser pointer at one of the Xs in the periphery. The child, as quickly as he or she can without moving his or her head, shifts his or her eyes to the opposite X from the one the pointer is shining on. For example, you shine on the X at 2 o'clock he looks at 8 o'clock. The child then moves his or her eyes back to the center X and waits for your next directive.

Pen Light

Area of attention: Shifting
Materials: Pen light or laser pointer
Procedure: Have the child sitting or standing and looking straight ahead. You hold a pen light at different locations and blink it. If you blink it once, the child makes a quick eye movement to the light and then back straight ahead. He or she is not to move his or her head. If you blink it twice, the child does not move his or her eyes. You can vary the commands, for example, two blinks are movement, and for one blink, he or she does not move his or her eyes, etc.

Bell and Location

Area of attention: Shifting
Materials: Small bell
Procedure: Have the child close his or her eyes. Have the child sitting in a chair or standing about 6 feet in front of you. Hold a small bell or something that makes a soft noise at a location in front of or to the side of the child (not behind him or her). Keep it in his or her field of view so that when he or she opens his or her eyes, the child can make a quick eye movement to the location that he or she heard the sound. Wait a few seconds after you make the sound so you can move before he or she opens his or her eyes. The child is to keep his or her head straight and just move his or her eye to the location of the sound—not to where you are standing. Repeat this several times.

Brockstring

Area of attention: Shifting

Materials: Brockstring (a string or metal rod about 2 feet long with beads at various positions), metronome

Procedure: The child holds one end of the string at his or her nose and the other at arm's length in front of him or her. Place the beads at various positions but do not put the first one closer than 4 inches from his or her nose. At the beat of the metronome, he or she is to quickly shift his or her eyes from bead to bead, starting with the first bead. When he or she reaches the end of the string, he or she starts back toward his or her nose again. The child continues to move his or her eyes until you tell him or her to stop. You can vary this by having the child move his or her arm to different positions, such as slightly to the right or up.

Ways to modify: Show the child a sequence of the colored beads on paper such as R-B-W-B-R. He or she will move his or her eyes to that sequence when he or she hears the metronome.

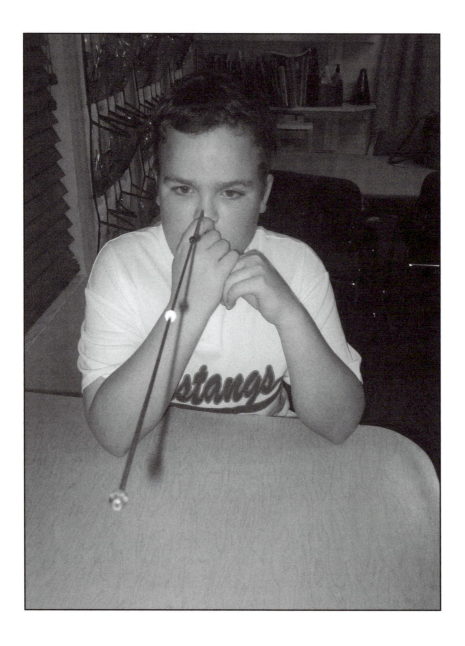

SELECTIVE ATTENTION

Domino Memory

Area of attention: Selective

Materials: CD player, dominoes

Procedure: Have all of the dominoes on the table in front of the child (face up). Pick out one to five dominoes and show them to the child. Have him or her close his or her eyes and mix them up with the rest of the dominoes. He or she is to listen to the CD player while he or she does this. Tell the child you are going to ask him or her questions about the CD story. After you mix the dominoes, have him or her open his or her eyes, and see how quickly he or she can find them. Put a time limit on this. For example, you have 30 seconds to find all five of the dominoes.

Spatial Memory

Area of attention: Selective

Materials: CD player, blank grids, target grid—make several target grids.

Procedure: The child has a blank grid sheet of paper in front of him or her at a table. You hold up one of the target grids for about 3 seconds, and then take it away. After you take it away, tell the child which feature you want him or her to remember and its location. The child is to point to his or her blank grids, where the feature was located on your target. For example, you show the child the target below and then tell him or her, "Point to where the X was located." The child points to his or her grid top right.

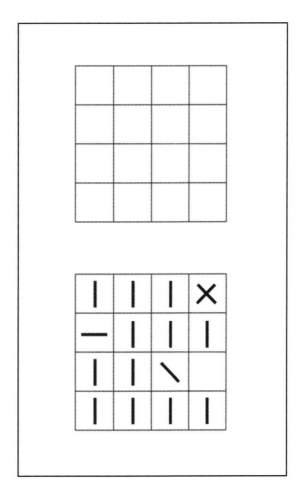

Stroop Words

Area of attention: Selective

Materials: Card with colored words

Procedure: Have the child seated in front of you. You hold up the colored words, and the child is to quickly name the color of the ink, not the name of the word. He or she must answer quickly or take the card away.

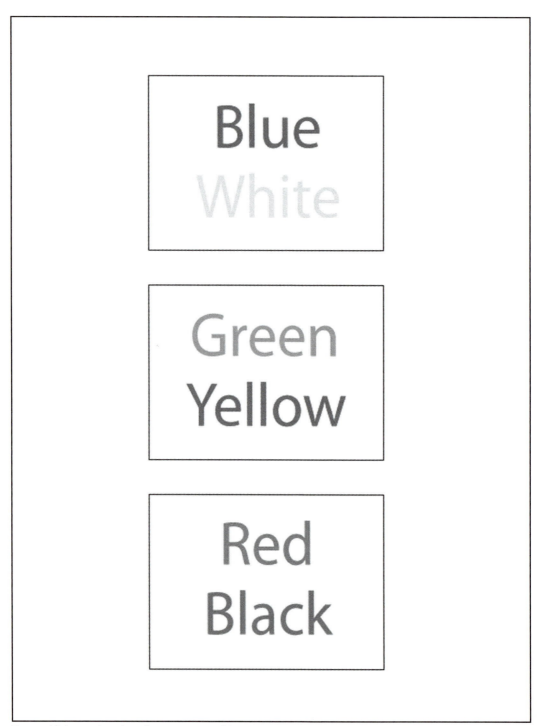

To see this image in color, please see page CA-6.

From Lane, K. A. (2012). *Visual Attention in Children: Theories and Activities*. Thorofare, NJ: SLACK Incorporated. © 2012 SLACK Incorporated.

Categorize

Area of attention: Selective

Materials: CD player, target cards—make several cards with some letters and numbers in red and blue like the ones below.

Procedure: Show the child the card with the four choices, while he or she is listening to the CD. Give him or her about 10 seconds to look at the card (more if the child needs it). After you take the card away, you are going to ask him or her categories, such as:

1. Name all the red letters.

2. Name the figures in the top right, etc.

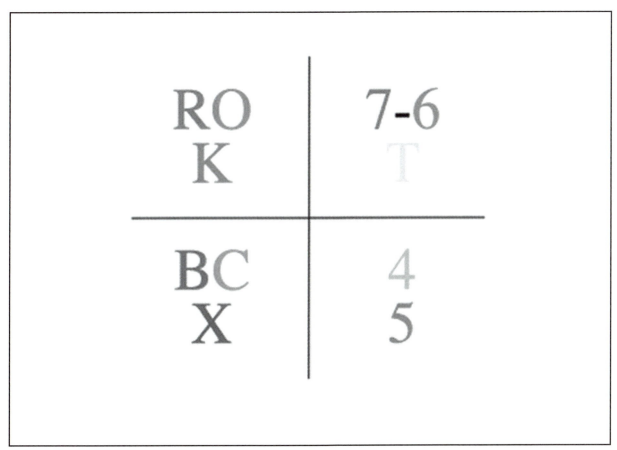

To see this image in color, please see page CA-6.

Mirror Drawings

Area of attention: Selective

Materials: Mirror, white paper with dots drawn on it in random order

Procedure: Start with the activity by only having two dots. Gradually build up to as many dots as you feel he or she can handle. Lay the paper on the table in front of the mirror. Cover the paper with another sheet of paper so the child can only see the paper by looking into the mirror. The child is to only look into the mirror and, with a pencil, connect the dots on the sheet of paper on the table. He or she is allowed to lift his or her pencil off the paper, but he or she should try to do it without lifting the pencil off the paper.

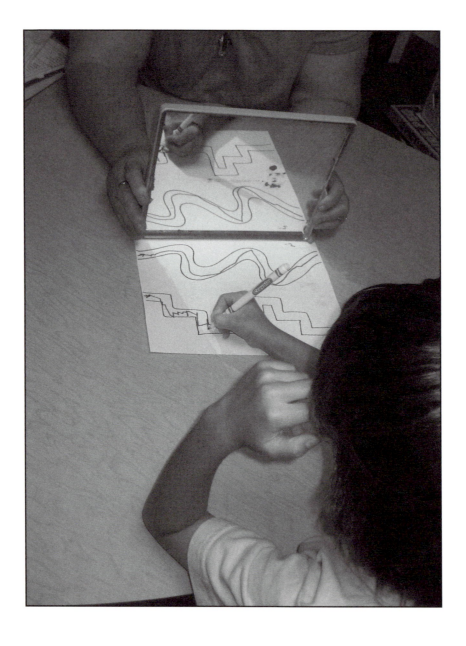

From Lane, K. A. (2012). *Visual Attention in Children: Theories and Activities*. Thorofare, NJ: SLACK Incorporated. © 2012 SLACK Incorporated.

Multiple Stimuli

Area of attention: Selective

Materials: Mask card, cards with a word above and one below the line like the ones below. The mask card is one of the other targets with a word below and above the line. You make the mask card.

Procedure: Have the child seated across the table. Briefly show the child a card (about 2 seconds), and then the mask for 2 seconds. Ask the child questions, such as:

1. What was the word above the line?

2. What was the color of the word below the line?

3. What were both words and their colors?

4. It is suggested that you cut this chart into four targets.

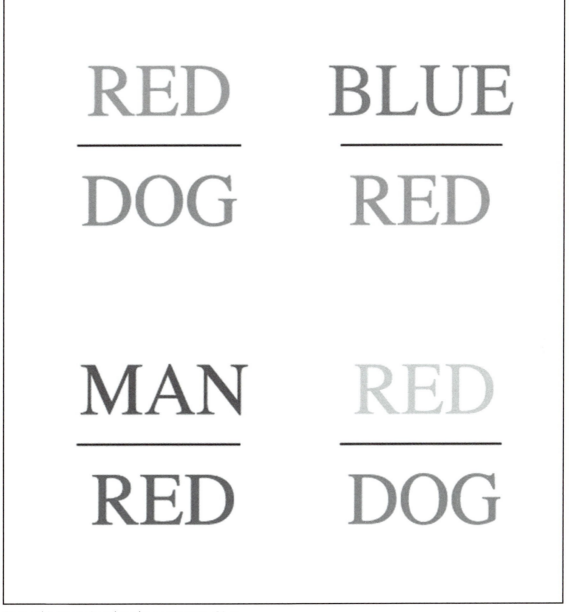

To see this image in color, please see page CA-7.

From Lane, K. A. (2012). *Visual Attention in Children: Theories and Activities*. Thorofare, NJ: SLACK Incorporated. © 2012 SLACK Incorporated.

Faces

Area of attention: Selective

Materials: A sheet of white paper with faces and numbers and letters.

Procedure: Hold the target in front of the patient for 3 seconds. Tell him or her you want him or her to remember as much of the target as he or she can. Then, ask the child questions, such as:

1.   Name as many letters as you can.

2.   Name the numbers.

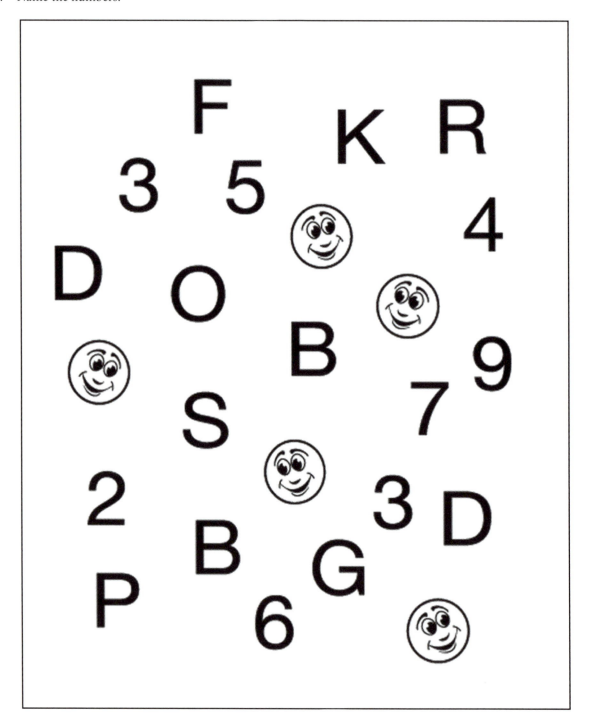

Line Tracing

Area of attention: Selective

Materials: White marker board or white paper.

Procedure: On the board or a piece of paper, draw the lines like you see in the example. The child is to start at the A, and, without using his or her finger and only his or her eyes, the child is to follow the line to the correct number. If the child cannot do this, let him or her use his or her finger in the air to follow the line. If the child still cannot do it, let him or her use his or her finger on the board or paper.

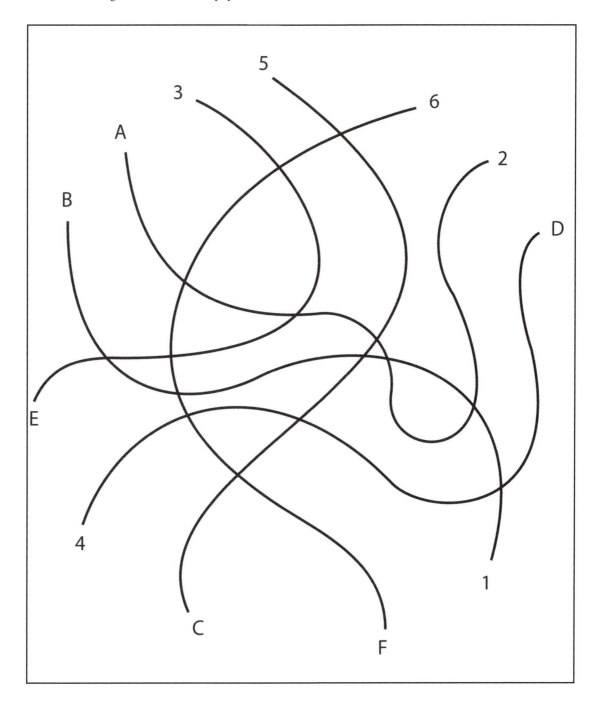

Global to Small

Area of attention: Selective

Materials: Global to small worksheets

Procedure: Hold the worksheet in front of the child and have him or her, as fast he or she can, do one of the following:

1. Name the word.

2. Name the small letters that make up the letters in the word.

3. Name the large letters and ignore the small letters.

4. Alternate between naming the small letters and naming the large letters.

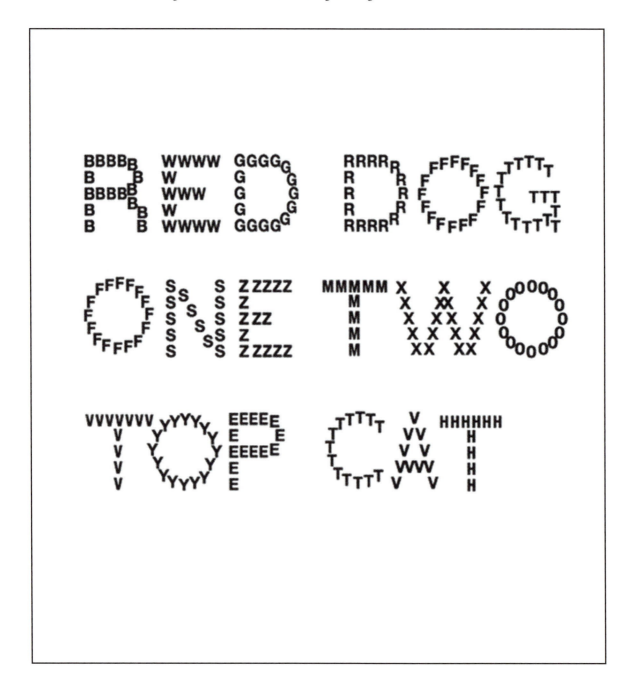

Vertical Letters

Area of attention: Selective

Materials: Index cards with letters in a vertical column and a red X at the side

Procedure: Show the child the card for a short period of time (about 2 seconds). He or she is to remember as many of the letters as he or she can. The card is designed so the red X attracts his or her attention first. The child must learn to ignore the X.

Ways to modify: Substitute the X with other distractors, such as colored words or a human face.

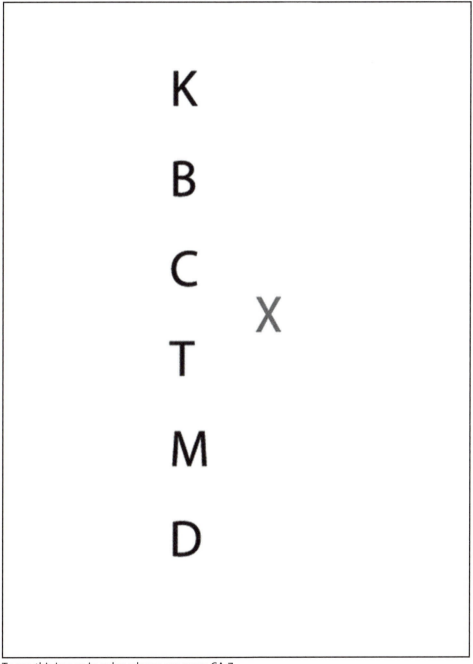

To see this image in color, please see page CA-7.

Delayed Stomp and Hit

Area of attention: Selective

Materials: Marsden ball, stopwatch, eye patch

Procedure: The child stands in front of the Marsden ball. At your command, he or she is to stomp his or her right foot and then push the ball with his or her right hand. Alternate between hands. The main point is that the child must stomp his or her foot and then push the ball. Start one eye at a time.

Vary this activity by having the patient postpone hitting the ball for a period of time after the foot stomp. Use the stopwatch, and show him or her 3 or 5 seconds and get him or her used to estimating time. Once the child has a good idea on time, tell him or her that, after his or her foot stomp, he or she must wait a period of time before he or she hits (pushes) the ball. Vary the time from a couple of seconds to 10 to 15 seconds.

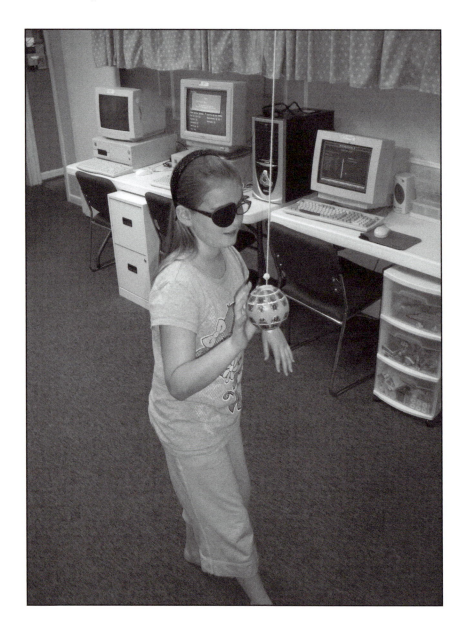

Trails

Area of attention: Selective

Materials: White board or white paper. Draw random letters and numbers.

Procedure: The child stands in front of the board or paper and must first point to the correct sequence and then connect the correct sequence. The sequence is 1-A, 2-B, 3-C, 4-D, 5-D, etc., alternating between numbers and letters.

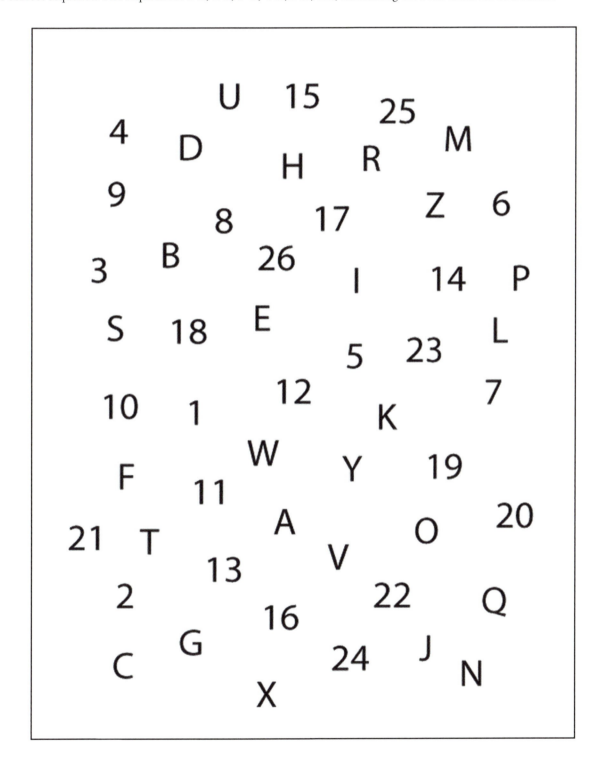

Variation of Stroop

Area of attention: Selective

Materials: A pen light. Make a target with a colored square and a colored word in a different color than the square.

Procedure: Flash on the target. The child is to tell you the name of the color of the square. You will probably have to speed the flash to about 1 second.

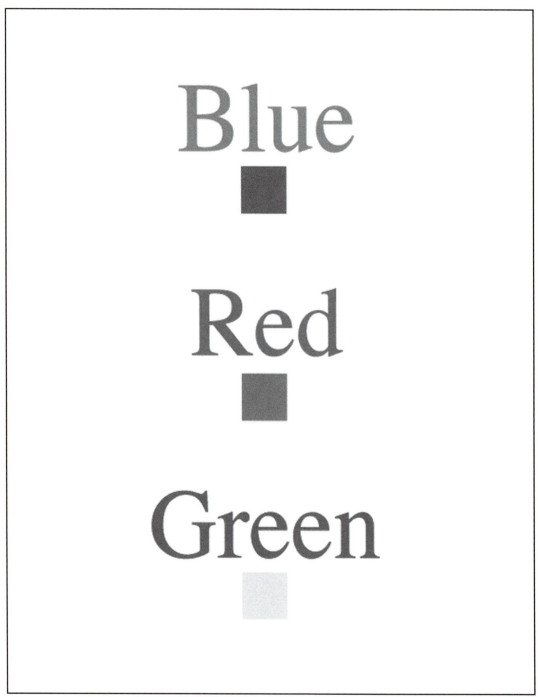

To see this image in color, please see page CA-7.

Word Counting

Area of attention: Selective

Materials: CD player with story, reading book

Procedure:

1. The child reads a paragraph out loud, and at the end, you ask him or her how many times the word "and" was in the paragraph. You can tell him or her this before he or she reads the paragraph. Make this more difficult by playing a CD player with another story.

2. After he or she reads the paragraph, ask the child to name the words that ended the sentences.

3. After the child reads the paragraph, ask him or her to remember as many of the verbs as he or she can.

Word List

Area of attention: Selective

Materials: CD player with story, word list with letter written after the words

Procedure: Have the CD player on. He or she is to read aloud the sequence of words. When he or she has completed the sequence, ask him or her to name as many of the letters as he or she can that followed the words. At first, he or she does not have to remember them in correct sequence, but, to make it more difficult, have him or her repeat the letters in sequence.

Boy - A, Dog - T, House - C, Car - X, Airplane - M, Cat - K, Girl - W

Ball - V, Ride - F, Bike - T, Work - C, Train - S, Seat - M, Shirt - Q

Bus - G, Talk - J, Stop - N, Hard - O, Bake - E, Pool - W, Party - T

Plant - R, Light - O, Chair - F, Bug - P, Ride - A, Pole - Y, Sofa - K

Blue - Y, Talk - E, Hard - S, Buy- Z, Soup - U, Fast - L, Draw - M

Hair - S, Arm - D, Neck - L, Eye - G, Drive - P, Art - U, Picture - F

Door- T, Rug - X, Knob - O, Seat - J, Run - A, Draw - L, Post - U

Soft - Z, Build - P, Work - B, Walk - J, Window - E, Eye - W, Red - H

Frame - R, Swim - D, Red - A, Huge - L, Call - J, Bath - Y, Easy - Y

Road - H, Face - J, Chip - S, Deer - J, Have - K, Good - P, Sense - E

Red/Green Trails

Area of Attention: Selective

Materials: Red/green glasses, white paper. You draw a pattern with some of them in red.

Procedure: The child wears the red/green lenses, which will make all of the red figures with the eye behind the red lens and the green figures with the eye behind the green lens fade. Before he or she puts the red/green glasses on, let him or her look at the chart for a few seconds. Then he or she is to put the glasses on and try to alternate between calling out a letter then a number in the correct sequence. For example, all letters in alphabetic order and the numbers in order. In this example, the letters would be E, F, G, K, etc., and the numbers would be 2, 3, 5, etc.

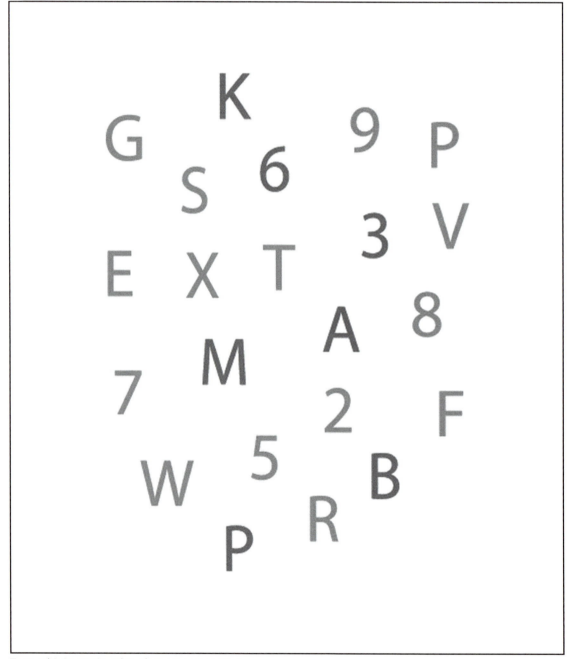

To see this image in color, please see page CA-8.

From Lane, K. A. (2012). *Visual Attention in Children: Theories and Activities.* Thorofare, NJ: SLACK Incorporated. © 2012 SLACK Incorporated.

Maze With Red/Green Lenses

Area of attention: Selective

Materials: Red/green glasses, white paper. You draw a maze as shown below but have parts of the lines in red and green, which will fade when he or she wears the red/green lenses.

Procedure: The child first looks at the maze. Then, he or she puts the red/green glasses on and tries to follow the lines to the correct location without using his or her finger.

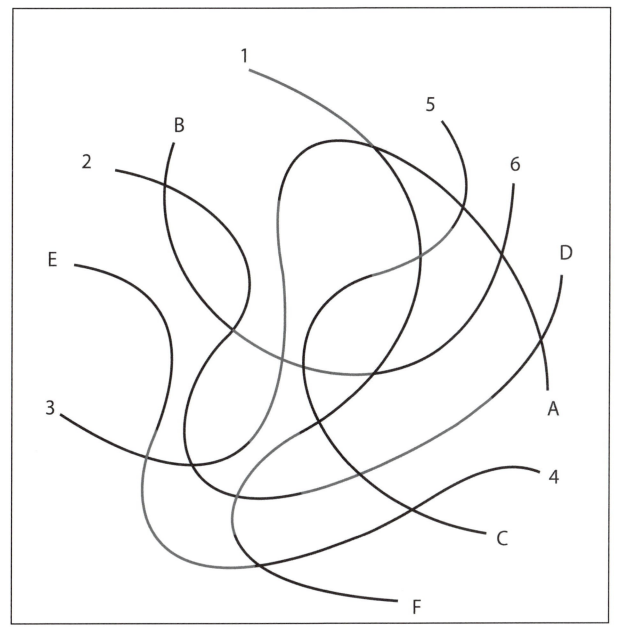

To see this image in color, please see page CA-8.

DIVIDED ATTENTION

Walking Rail Math

Area of attention: Divided

Materials: Walking rail, fixation chart with letters or numbers in rows. This can be on a white board or paper.

Procedure: Have the child walk in a heel-to-toe manner on the walking rail without shoes. He or she is to call out the letters on the chart in a left-to-right sequence as he or she walks on the walking rail. While he or she is doing this, you ask him or her a math problem, for example, "How much is 20 from 55?" He or she is to answer the question as he or she continues on the walking rail and calling out the letters on the chart.

Marsden Ball and Spelling

Area of attention: Divided

Materials: Metronome and Marsden ball

Procedure: The child does this with his or her "left" hand. He or she stands in front of the Marsden ball and pushes it with his or her left hand. At each beat of the metronome, he or she says a letter of a word you want him or her to spell. The child does not say the letter until he or she hears the metronome. If it is a young patient, show him or her the word you want him or her to spell. Hold it next to the Marsden ball. The key here is to use only his or her left hand and not to say the letter until the metronome beats. The child is not to stop pushing the Marsden ball.

Dominoes and Counting

Area of attention: Divided

Materials: Two sets of dominoes

Procedure: You lay all of the dominoes on the table in front of the child, and show him or her a pattern made from three to seven dominoes. The child must find the same dominoes and match the pattern, but he or she must do it while counting backward from 50. You will need to vary the number he or she counts backward from, depending on the age of the child.

Marsden Ball and Pen Light

Area of attention: Divided

Materials: Marsden ball and pen light

Procedure: The child stands in front of the Marsden ball and pushes it with his or her right hand. You stand in his or her peripheral vision and hold the pen light. If you flash it once, the child continues with his or her right hand. Two flashes means that the child changes hands and pushes it with his or her left hand. The child then continues with this hand until he or she sees two flashes. One flash means he or she just continues with the same hand.

Ways to modify: You can flash the light three or four times, and the patient must ignore this and continue with the same hand.

Number and Letter String

Area of Attention: Divided

Materials: A sequence of letters and numbers such as the following:

| A | 4 | T | 5 | O | 3 | C | 4 | K | 5 |

Procedure: Show the child the string of letters and numbers. Have him or her repeat the letters by saying the letter that follows it in alphabet and adding the numbers. For example, for the above, the child would say the following:

| B | 4 | U | 9 | P | 12 | D | 16 | L | 21 |

Ways to modify: Show a shorter string (about three to five) letters and numbers. He or she now has to look at this for 5 seconds and repeat the letters and add the numbers after you take it away.

Target Letter

Area of attention: Divided

Materials: Playing cards

Procedure: The child sits at a table with a deck of cards face down. He or she turns the first card over, and if it has the letter "e" in its spelling, he or she puts it face up in a new pile. If it does not have the letter "e" in its spelling, it goes in the new face down pile. Cards with letter "e" would be three, five, seven, eight, nine, ten, queen, and ace. If the child makes a mistake, he or she starts over. The goal is to get through the entire deck without making a mistake.

Walking Rail Counting

Area of attention: Divided

Materials: Walking rail, white light, red light

Procedure: The child is to walk in a heel-to-toe fashion, and you are to stand at the end of the walking rail. The child is to start counting by twos if you flash a white light. He or she continues until you flash a red light. Then, he or she counts backwards by twos until you flash a white light, and he or she counts by twos forward again.

Finger Touch

Area of attention: Divided

Materials: Target with letters in sequence, white board or index cards

Procedure: The child sits across the table from you with his or her left hand palm down on the table. You show him or her a card or white board with letters in rows. The child is to call out the letters in the proper left-to-right sequence. As he or she does this, you touch the fingers of his or her left hand in a sequence. Start with three and work up to seven. After the child has called out all of the letters in a row from the index card or board, he or she must show you the fingers you touched in the proper sequence. He or she must not stop calling out the letters as you touch his or her hand.

Adding 3

Area of attention: Divided

Materials: A sequence of numbers on the board or paper, metronome

Procedure: The child is to stand in front of a long sequence of numbers. At each beat of the metronome, he or she is to call out the numbers in sequence. The challenge is that from time to time, you are to call out a number, and, without losing his or her place or skipping a beat, he or she is to add 3 to the number you call out. Set the metronome at a slow beat to start.

Remember the Sequence

Area of attention: Divided

Materials: A list of words, a sequence of numbers

Procedure: Have the child seated in front of a list of words. Now show him or her a sequence of numbers. Start with three and work up to seven numbers. The child must remember the number sequence while he or she puts the words in alphabetical order and then tells you the number sequence. For example, you show him or her the sequence 5 7 6 3; then, take it away, and show him or her DOG BOY MOM. The child puts the words in alphabetical order (BOY DOG MOM) and then repeats the original number sequence.

Divided Attention

Area of attention: Divided
Materials: Target cards

K	*	2
W	*	3
M	*	4
L	*	1
O	*	7
C	*	8
D	*	4
R	*	3

Procedure: Hold the target in front of the child. He or she is to keep his or her eyes on the central dot, and as the child goes down the columns, he or she is to call out the letter on the left and number on the right without moving his or her eyes from the central dot. If holding a pencil at the dot helps to keep his or her attention, let the child do this. Watch his or her eyes. If the child moves his or her eyes, he or she starts over.

Read and Remember

Area of attention: Divided

Materials: Short stories

Method: The child is to read a short story to herself or himself for a 5-minute period. While he or she is reading the story, you ask simple questions such as:

"How old are you?"

"When is your birthday?"

"Where do you live?"

Continue to ask simple questions every 30 seconds. At the end of 5 minutes, ask him or her questions concerning the story just read. (This activity was adapted from Spelke, E. S., Hirst, W., & Neisser, U. [1976]. Skills of divided attention. *Cognition, 4,* 215-230.)

MOTOR AND RIGHT HEMISPHERE TRAINING

Domino Orientation

Area of attention: Motor and right hemisphere

Materials: Dominoes

Procedure: The child has his or her eyes closed. You put a sequence of dominoes in different orientations in front of him or her. Start with two and work from there. The child opens his or her eyes and looks at the dominoes for about 10 seconds. You then cover the dominoes, and he or she must find the same dominoes in his or her group of dominoes and put them in the correct sequence and orientation.

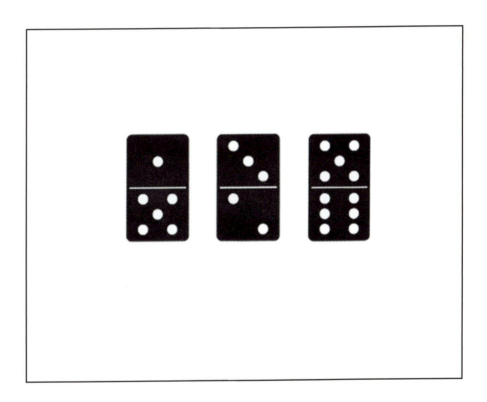

Hand Slap

Area of attention: Motor and right hemisphere

Materials: None

Procedure: This is a fun activity to start the therapy session. Have the patient hold out his or her left hand palm up, and lay it under your right hand palm down. Now, see if the child can quickly take his or her hand away and slap the top of your hand before you can pull it away. After a few attempts, reverse the procedure, and the child lays his or her hand (left) on the palm of your right hand, and see if you can slap the top of his or her hand.

One-Legged Balance

Area of attention: Motor and right hemisphere

Materials: Open box laying on its side

Procedure: Slowly roll the ball toward the child as he or she is balancing on one leg. The child is to try to kick the ball into the open box while keeping his or her balance.

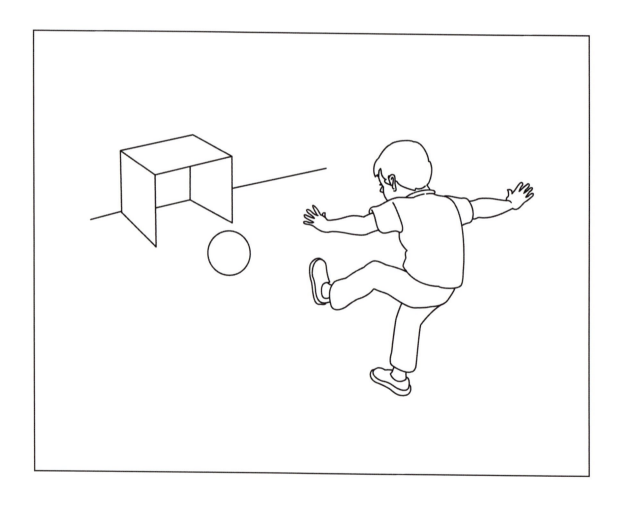

Train Right Hemisphere

Area of attention: Motor and right hemisphere

Materials: Right hemisphere glasses, kick ball, small ball or bean bag

Procedure:

1. Do as many activities as you can to stimulate the right hemisphere. All of the activities must be done with the child's left hand or left foot. This includes catching and kicking.

2. Have the child wear the right hemisphere glasses and do the same type of motor activities as you did in #1. With the glasses, he or she can use either hand or foot. Assign the right hemisphere glasses for home therapy, and have the child wear them for a couple of hours a day as he or she does normal activities.

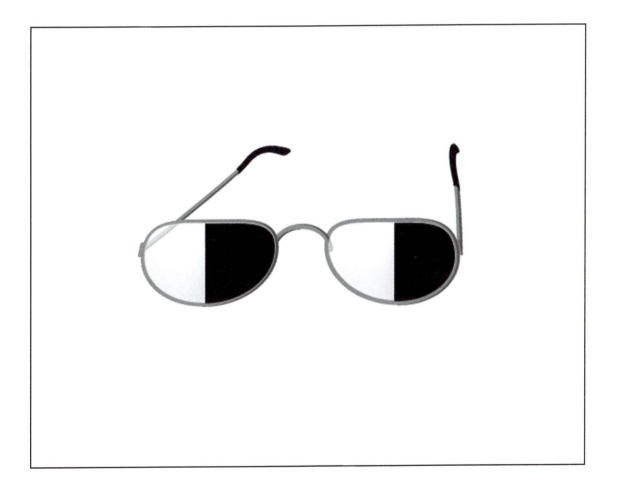

Mixed Font

Area of attention: Motor and right hemisphere

Materials: Have 10 lines of letters in mixed font, such as shown below.

Procedure: Put the mixed font in front of the child, and have him or her call out the letters in a left-to-right sequence. Record his or her time. The child is not allowed to use his or her finger.

Ways to modify: You can vary the size of the letters. For younger children, use larger letters.

a B m G K d L s O I

i t Y P e N K Z a r F

T p R b N m S l j o C

n F S r l k e M C H u

v g J w P t G L m F J

D l s M f w P z h A N r

M x T y Q V r p E b

H t Z L q F J g l t o A

R e G E S i M B W C

V H n U K l d l f w t

Tonic Neck Reflex

Area of attention: Motor and right hemisphere

Materials: Skateboard board

Procedure: Put the child in a prone extension posture on the skateboard board with his or her head, shoulders, and arms raised and legs held straight and hyperextended at the hip. See if the child can hold this position for 30 seconds while counting aloud to 30. The child's counting should help to keep him or her from holding his or her breath. "A normal child of age 6 and above can usually hold the position for 20 to 30 seconds" (Ayres, 1973).

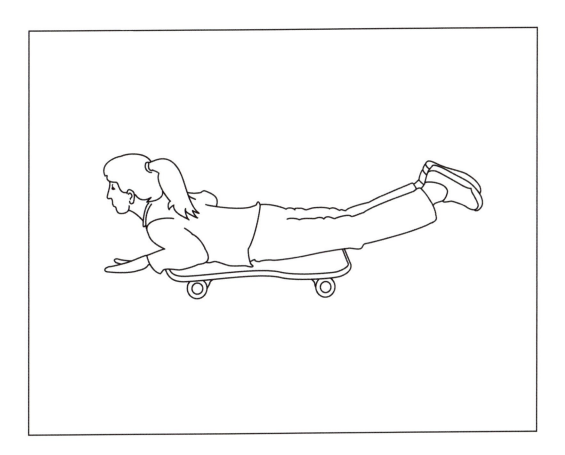

REFERENCES

Ayers, J. (1973). *Sensory integration and learning disorders.* Western Psychological Services.

Moro Reflex

Area of attention: Motor and right hemisphere
Materials: Straight chair, beanbag chair
Procedure:

1. Have the child sit on a beanbag or in a straight chair with pillows behind the back so he or she is inclined about 45 degrees.

2. Have the child open his or her arms and legs out in full extension, inhaling while moving the limbs out. As the limbs move out, the head moves backward. Hold for 5 seconds.

3. While exhaling, move the arms and legs simultaneously in toward each other in full flexion until the body is in a fetal position with arms and legs on the chest. As the limbs move inward, the head moves forward. Hold for 5 seconds.

4. Slowly have the child move the arms and legs back to the starting position in #1. Hold for 5 seconds. Repeat #3 with the opposite arm and opposite leg on top.

5. Repeat the sequence for three cycles, alternating which arm and leg are on top.

Tonic Labyrinthine Reflex

Area of attention: Motor and right hemisphere
Materials: None
Procedure: Have the child be on the floor on his or her stomach with his or her legs straight out behind, arms bent, in front of his or her face, with thumbs touching.

1. Have the child lift his or her arms, head, and upper body as high as possible, while fully relaxing the lower body. The child should feel tension in his or her lower back. Have the child hold his or her thumbs about an inch off the floor with his or her visual focus on the thumbs.

2. Keeping his or her left thumb still in front, have the child move the right thumb to the right as far as possible so that it straightens out at the end of the arc, while turning his or her head to follow the movement of the thumb with his or her eyes.

3. Have the child bring his or her right arm and head back to the starting position so that his or her two thumbs are again touching.

4. Repeat the same procedure to the left. Each side should take about 30 seconds out and back.

5. Slowly have the child lower his or her thumbs, head, and upper body to a relaxed position and hold for 5 to 10 seconds.

6. Repeat for three cycles.

White Marsden Ball

Area of attention: Motor and right hemisphere

Materials: White Marsden ball, red/green glasses

Procedure: This exercise trains the M pathway, which is critical for visual attention. Have the child wear the red/green glasses and stand in front of the Marsden ball. The child is to alternate pushing the ball with his or her hands. See how long he or she can do this.

Ways to modify: Have the child stomp his or her left foot and alternate hands each time he or she pushes the ball.

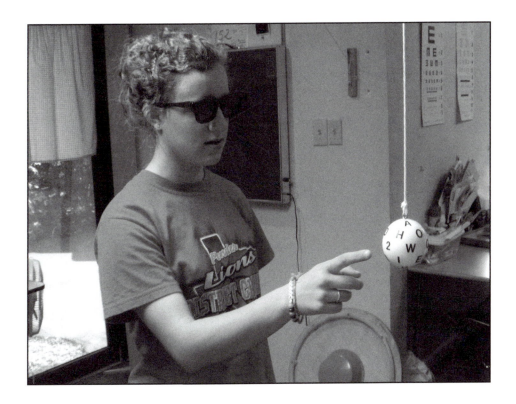

From Lane, K. A. (2012). *Visual Attention in Children: Theories and Activities*. Thorofare, NJ: SLACK Incorporated. © 2012 SLACK Incorporated.

Balance Trainer

Area of attention: Motor and right hemisphere

Materials: Balance trainer, Wayne saccadic fixator

Procedure: Have the child stand on the balance trainer. The child should balance on the trainer and touch the lights in the correct order. See how fast he or she can do this, and record his or her time.

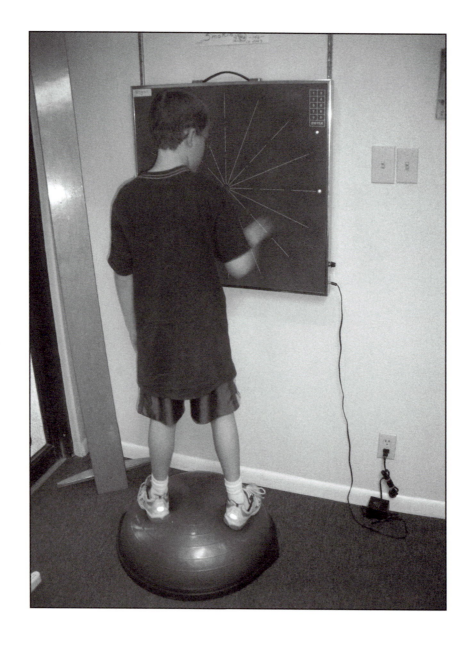

Stereopsis Training

Area of attention: Motor and right hemisphere

Materials: Random Dot E test (Bernell, Mishawaka, IN), balance trainer

Procedure: The child balances on the balance trainer with the polarized glasses. You start at about 3 feet in front of the child, and have him or her tell you if the E looks like it is in 3D. As the child is balancing, slowly move the target in a circular pattern, and have the child tell you if he or she can still see the 3D E. Do this for a few minutes; then, do it in a horizontal left-to-right pattern, and see if he still sees the 3D E.

Ways to modify: You can try to test the child by holding up the card in an upside-down position. This makes the E appear to go into the card instead of 3D. Ask him or her what is different.

Domino Patterns

Area of attention: Motor and right hemisphere

Materials: Dominoes

Procedure: Make a pattern with some of your dominoes and have the child make the same pattern with his or her dominoes. You can also ask the child to make a pattern that is upside down from your pattern.

Ways to modify: Put a time limit on this, and tell the child that he or she only has a certain amount of time to complete the pattern.

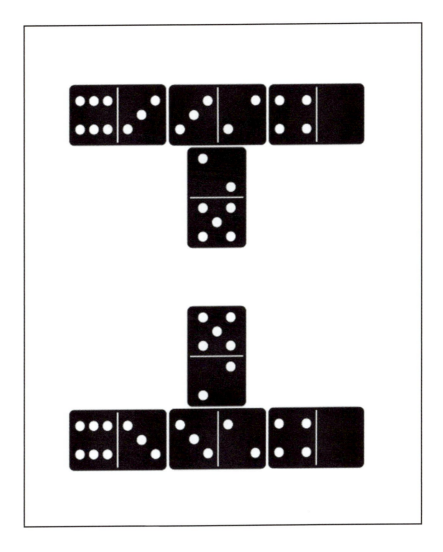

Peripheral Chart

Area of attention: Right hemisphere

Materials: Peripheral chart below.

Procedure: Hold the chart in front of the child at about 14 inches. He or she is to focus on the center X and not move his or her eyes from the X. While he or she is doing this, you point to one of the letters with a pencil and ask him or her what it is. He or she is not to move his or her eyes.

Ways to modify: Give the child a sequence of letters. He or she is to point to them without moving his or her eyes, or have him or her spell a word by pointing.

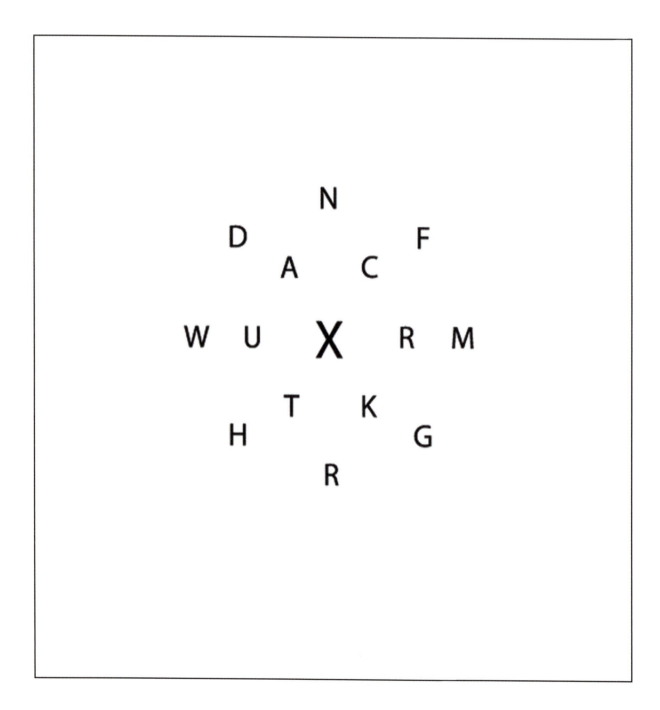

Peripheral Dots

Area of attention: Motor and right hemisphere

Materials: White board, seven dots per row in four rows about 12 inches apart

Procedure: The child is on his or her knees in front of the white board. He or she uses the left hand and draws a straight line through each of the dots, starting from the left dot in each row. He or she can go left to right or right to left. If the board cannot be moved, the child can stand to do this. If he or she misses a dot, the child starts over.

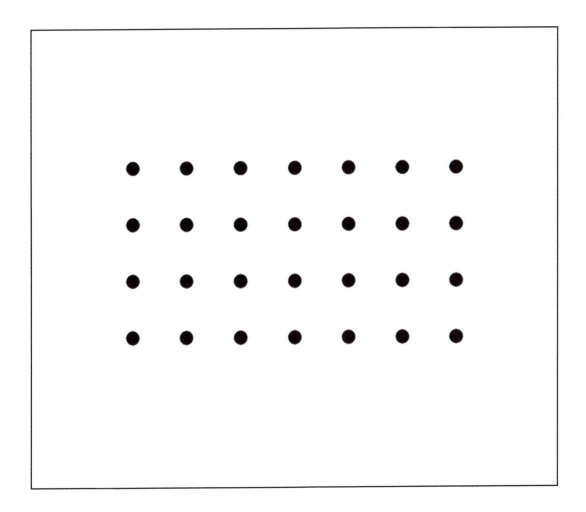

HOME TRAINING

End-of-Day Activity

Area of attention: Home therapy

Materials: This can vary.

Procedure: At the end of the therapy session, show the child what you want him or her to remember and show you at the next session. This can be a number sequence or a domino pattern or anything else. When he or she comes in for the next session, the child will show you what he or she was to remember. It is okay if he or she takes notes. This would be a good way to get him or her used to making lists or taking notes to help him or her remember.

Remember the Day

Area of attention: Home activity to get the child to pay attention to things in his or her environment

Materials: None

Procedure: Have the parent make a note of several (10) things that the child should have noticed during the day, such as the color of the car, his or her friend's dog, or what his or her best friend was wearing. At the end of the day, the parent asks the child the 10 questions to see how much he or she remembered.

Right Hemisphere

Area of attention: Home training to stimulate his or her right hemisphere

Materials: Right hemisphere glasses

Procedure: Put the right hemisphere glasses on the child, and have him or her wear them for 1 hour a day, but not on the same day he or she wears central occluder glasses. You may want to start with 15 minutes and build up to 1 hour. Keep the child in the house because part of the vision is blocked. He or she is to do his or her normal routine.

Central Occluders

Area of attention: Home therapy to train peripheral vision

Materials: Glasses with center area occluded

Procedure: Have the child wear the glasses at home for 30 minutes a day. These glasses block his or her central vision and force him or her to be aware of his or her peripheral vision. You may want to start with 15 minutes and work up to 1 hour. If the child is young, have the parents ask him or her questions, such as what he or she notices in his or her peripheral vision. Keep the child in the house because his or her central vision is blocked.

Peripheral Training

Area of attention: Home training to make him or her aware of his or her peripheral vision

Materials: None

Procedure: When the child's takes the child into a store or for a walk, he or she is to ask him or her to tell the parent what he or she sees in his or her peripheral vision. The child is not to turn his or her head and must keep looking straight ahead. For example, when in the grocery store and he or she is walking down an aisle, the parent should ask him or her what he or she sees in the peripheral vision.

Resources

Guided reader
Taylor Associates
1.800.READPLUS

DEM Saccadic Fixation Test
Bernell Corp.
www.bernell.com

Eye tracking and perceptual workbooks
Dr. Kenneth Lane, OD, FCOVD
www.lanelearningcenter.com

Oculomotor equipment
Bernell, Inc.
www.bernell.com
- Brockstrings
- Marsden ball
- DEM saccadic fixation test
- Eye port
- Peg board rotators
- Eye patches
- Alphabet pencils
- Fixation charts
- Red/green glasses
- Wayne saccadic fixator

Optometric Extension Program (OEP) also has oculomotor training equipment.
1-800-424-8070

College of Optometrists in Vision in Vision Development (COVD)
www.covd.org
A good source for a list of developmental optometrists in your area.

Workshops by Dr. Kenneth A. Lane, OD, FCOVD
E-mail: bookspublishing@slackinc.com

Lane, K. A. *Visual Attention in Children: Theories and Activities* (pp. 207-208).
© 2012 SLACK Incorporated.

Glossary

accommodation: The bending of the lens in the eye to focus the image clearly on the fovea. Many children have accommodation (focusing) problems. The symptoms include blurred print, headaches, and eye strain. Accommodation is improved in vision therapy by the use of lenses to stimulate and relax focusing.

acuity (visual): A measurement of what the average person can see and identify at a certain distance. For example, 20/20 means that you see at 20 feet what the average person sees at 20 feet; 20/100 means that you see at 20 feet what the average person sees at 100 feet. Therefore, 20/20 vision is only average vision. There is no perfect vision.

ambient vision: Refers to our peripheral vision, which we use at night, and consists mainly of rods while our daytime vision consists mainly of cones.

amblyopia: This means that the child is not corrected to 20/20 vision with glasses. Amblyopia is usually caused by one eye drifting either "in" or "out" (strabismus) or if one eye is extremely farsighted or has a lot of astigmatism compared to the other eye. This is corrected with patching the stronger eye and forcing the weak eye to be used. Patching is usually very effective up to 10 years of age.

binasal occlusion: This is covering the nasal part of a child's lenses in his or her glasses to make him or her use peripheral vision.

binding: Attention is needed to select a subset of items to receive perceptual processing. The binding problem means that only the features within the attentional area will be combined to reconstruct the object. Attention acts like the glue that combines the features to form the object.

binocularity: This is the ability to use both eyes together to focus light on each eye's fovea. Binocular problems include strabismus and convergence problems.

bottom-up processing: These processes refer to the perceptual, motor, or externally generated or cued inputs that require a response. They may also be subconscious and do not pertain to higher cognitive functions.

conjunctions: Two or more features such as color and orientation.

convergence: This is the turning of both eyes in toward the nose.

convergence insufficiency (CI): This is a condition in which the child's eyes tend to drift "out" when he or she looks at an object up close. Normal binocular vision has the eyes drifting out slightly when you look at a distant object. With convergence insufficiency, they drift out further at the near point than at the far point.

cortical mantle: The enveloping cover or layer.

209

Lane, K. A. *Visual Attention in Children: Theories and Activities* (pp. 209-212).

crowding: A condition in which features (such as letters) compete for recognition. For example, if there are too many letters close together, the brain does not have enough feature detectors to identify an individual letter quickly. The other letter competes for identification.

denervation supersensitivity: Areas of the brain that are partially denervated by the lesion become hypersensitive to the remaining input.

diaschsis: Refers to the re-establishment of unimpaired neurological systems.

divided attention: The ability to respond simultaneously to multiple tasks or multiple task demands.

dorsal stream: This is the magnocellular pathway from the lateral geniculate nucleus to the parietal lobe.

dyslexia: A severe reading disability. To qualify for a diagnosis of dyslexia, the child must be at least 2 years below grade level and is probably in the lower 4% of the population in reading.

executive function: A part of working memory. It forms an interface between long-term memory and short-term memory. Executive functions refer to cognitive abilities involved in the initiation, planning, sequencing, organization, and regulation of behavior. They constitute a superordinate system that mediates self-initiated behavior and governs the efficiency and appropriateness of task performance.

fixation: The process of directing the eye toward the object we want to see and identify. The image of the object will be centered on the fovea. In reading, the fixation is a pause as we process information.

focused attention: This is the ability to respond discretely to specific visual, auditory, or tactile stimuli.

fovea: A tiny pit, about 1 degree wide (1.5 mm), in the center of the macula (6 mm in diameter) of slim, elongated cones. It is the area of cleanest vision, because here the layers of the retina are spread apart, permitting light to fall directly on the cones.

ideomotor: Aroused by an idea or thought and is involuntary.

joint attention: Refers to a child sharing an activity or experience with another person, usually the mother, rather than just playing with a toy. The child and the mother play with the toys together.

lazy eye: *See* amblyopia.

learning disability: When it refers to reading, it has the same symptoms as but is not as severe as dyslexia. Usually, these children are in the lower 20% of the school population.

macula: An oval area in the retina 3 to 5 mm in diameter, usually located temporal to the posterior pole of the eye and slightly below the optic disk. It is characterized by the presence of yellow pigment diffusely permeating the inner layers. It contains the fovea in the center and provides the best photopic visual acuity.

magnocellular (M) pathway: A visual pathway from the optic nerve to the lateral geniculate nucleus and then to the parietal lobe. It deals a lot with motion perception, depth perception, and our peripheral vision.

Marsden ball: This is a small ball about 3 inches in diameter that is usually hung from the ceiling. It is used in oculomotor activities such as pursuit movements.

neglect: A visuospatial attention disorder leading to impaired perception of and diminished responses to stimuli presented in one side of space, more commonly the left side.

one degree of print: Approximately four letter positions on a normal page of print.

orthography: Deals with spelling patterns of words.

parietal lobe: The area of the brain that responds when we fixate or track an object of interest. It is responsible for directing visual attention and is involved with saccadic and pursuit eye movements. It is also involved with tasks that require hand-eye coordination for manipulation in reachable space. The parietal lobe is also the brain area where the magnocellular pathway terminates.

parvocellular (P) pathway: Is one of the two visual pathways from the optic nerve along with the magnocellular pathway. The P pathway deals with detailed analysis and object identification. The M pathway directs attention to the object to be identified by the P pathway.

pop-out: This type of target is so different from the others that it automatically catches your attention, such as a white square in the middle of all black squares.

pursuit eye movement: Eye movement following a moving object. This was the second eye movement after saccadics that developed in our evolution.

Rett syndrome: These symptoms include the onset of the following after the period of normal development: 1) deceleration of head growth between ages 5 and 48 months; 2) loss of previously acquired purposeful hand skills between ages 5 and 30 months with subsequent development of stereotyped hand movement (e.g., hand wringing or hand washing); 3) loss of social engagement early in the course; 4) appearance of poorly coordinated gait or trunk movements; and 5) severe expressive and receptive language development with severe psychomotor retardation.

saccadic eye movement: Rapid eye movement to a stationary object. It was the first eye movement to develop in our evolution.

selective attention: This is the ability to maintain a behavioral or cognitive set in the face of distracting a competing stimuli.

semantics: Deals with the interpretation of the meaning of words.

sequelae: A condition following and the result of previous disease.

shifting attention: Refers to the capacity for mental flexibility that allows us to shift our focus of attention. In this book, it also refers to the ability to move our eyes as we shift attention between objects.

strabismus: This is a binocular problem caused by the eyes either drifting "in" (esotropia) or drifting "out" (exotropia). The most common strabismus in a 2- to 3-year-old child is esotropia due to an uncorrected farsighted correction.

substitution: Existing intact brain structures can assume functions previously held by the lesioned areas.

sustained attention: This refers to the ability to maintain a consistent behavioral response during continuous and repetitive activity.

TBI: Traumatic brain injury.

TIA: Transient ischemic attack.

top-down processing: These processes indicate higher brain centers, such as the frontal lobe, and play a part in determining that sensory information is selected for further processing.

transfer: Being able to do one activity that will directly improve another activity. For example, some people feel that some types of computer games help in academic skills; however, this is not usually the case.

ventral stream: This is the parvocellular pathway past the lateral geniculate nucleus projecting to the inferotemporal cortex. Used in object recognition.

vergence: A disjunctive rotation movement of the eyes, such that the points of reference on the globe move in opposite directions. Convergence means that the eyes move "in" toward each other. Divergence means that they move "out."

version: While vergence means the eyes move in opposite directions, version means they move in the same direction, such as both eyes looking to the left.

vigilance: This is sustained attention that is maintained over time.

visual field: An area of space that is being processed by areas of the retina. For example, right visual field is the nasal part of the left eye retina and the temporal of the right eye retina.

visual lobe: The useful field of view. This is the area surrounding the point of regard from within which information is processed with each fixation. This is usually larger than the 4-degree angle usually associated with the fovea.

visual spatial: Deals with the organization of visual space, such as poor visual spatial skills with children who have very poor visual motor abilities.

visual tracking: This is the same as saccadic fixations. Problems in this area cause a child to lose his or her place reading or make mistakes copying from the board or a text.

working memory: The set of processes that permits us to hold on to information until it is used or encoded or to keep stored information readily accessible. For example, working memory allows us to hold on to information long enough to write it down and to temporarily divert our attention to a new task.

Index

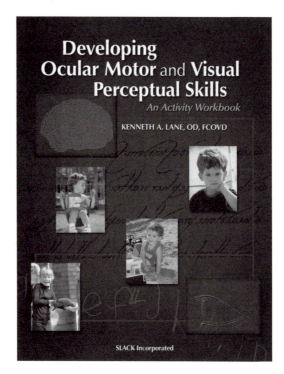

Attention Industry Partners!

Whether you are interested in buying multiple copies of a book, chapter reprints, or looking for something new and different — we are able to accommodate your needs.

MULTIPLE COPIES

At attractive discounts starting for purchases as low as 25 copies for a single title, SLACK Incorporated will be able to meet all of your needs.

CHAPTER REPRINTS

SLACK Incorporated is able to offer the chapters you want in a format that will lead to success. Bound with an attractive cover, use the chapters that are a fit specifically for your company. Available for quantities of 100 or more.

CUSTOMIZE

SLACK Incorporated is able to create a specialized custom version of any of our products specifically for your company.

Please contact the Marketing Communications Director for further details on multiple copy purchases, chapter reprints or custom printing at 1-800-257-8290 or 1-856-848-1000.

*Please note all conditions are subject to change.

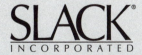